Hospital aesthetics

Disability, medicine, activism

Amanda Cachia

Manchester University Press

Publication of this book has been aided by a grant from the Millard Meiss Publication Fund of CAA.

Published by Manchester University Press
Oxford Road, Manchester, M13 9PL
www.manchesteruniversitypress.co.uk

British Library Cataloguing-in-Publication Data
A catalogue record for this book is available from the British Library

ISBN 978 1 5261 87864 hardback
ISBN 978 1 5261 87888 paperback

First published 2025

EU authorised representative for GPSR:
Easy Access System Europe, Mustamäe tee 50, 10621 Tallinn, Estonia
gpsr.requests@easproject.com

Cover image alt text: A small box, made from a wooden frame and glass panels, holds a small stack of books. The box rests on four bent and wobbly metallic table legs.

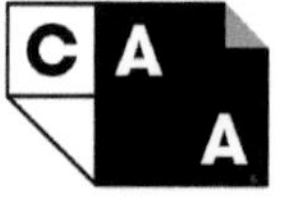

Advancing
Art&Design

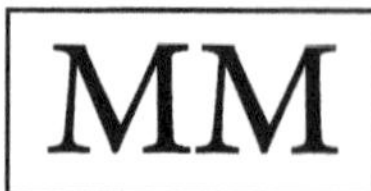

Typeset
by New Best-set Typesetters Ltd
Printed and bound by CPI Group
(UK) Ltd, Croydon, CR0 4YY

For Ryan and Finley

Contents

List of figures

Preface

When I was 11 or 12 years old, my naked body was put on display for the gaze of a white male doctor. He wanted to inspect it for its irregular shape and size. I was of medical interest to the industry because I was born with a rare form of dwarfism named brachyolmia. Conditions of my dwarfism include 4 foot 3 inch stature, faster bone degeneration than normal, spinal stenosis, and scoliosis. While I've never had to have any surgery as an outcome of my dwarfism, I have had to deal with the social and cultural stigma attached to having a body that is considered atypical, and startlingly noticeable to the public eye. As a consequence of having brachyolmia, I often have to negotiate the challenges of staring, occasional comments and questions, and living in a world that has been architecturally designed for the "average" 6-foot person. The doctor hadn't figured out my rare form of dwarfism yet; on that day I was asked to go behind a curtain and take off my clothes in his office. My parents were sitting at his desk, looking worried. I vividly recall standing behind the curtain after removing all the garments from my body, and feeling mortified. I didn't want to go out there, in front of my parents, and him. But he summoned me to come out. So I slowly walked out from behind the curtain. I remember the simultaneous sensation of my cheeks burning and the cold wooden floorboards gripping at my feet and legs. On this stage, exposed to the medical gaze. Apart from his stare, my parents looked at me. But I couldn't look at them. I could tell they felt bad, embarrassed for me. I can't remember what the doctor said then. But after a few minutes, I was asked to go back and get dressed.

I tell the reader this story because this experience, among many others, has shaped the person I am today. Feeling denied my privacy and stripped (no pun intended) of any dignity in the doctor's office, I told myself that I never wanted to be put in that position again. But it took me a long time to get there. For a while, I just didn't like my body. Societal images of bodies had a powerful impact on me. In this first story, the doctor's gaze on my naked body emanated from a position of medical privilege and authority. He felt he knew what was "normal," and was attempting to detect my so-called "abnormality." Back in that doctor's office, all those years ago, I was made to feel that my body was wrong, that it was limited. Finally, I am now able to identify personally as disabled. It took me a long time to reach that point, because I never thought I was disabled. While it is sometimes difficult to reach items on the top shelf in a grocery store or see a bank teller over a high counter, I saw these challenges as easy to overcome. I have come to see that I am disabled because I share characteristics with others who are disabled.

When I was a teenager, my mother took me to a children's hospital in Sydney to meet with a specialist in genetics and skeletal dysplasia. I still remember this white male doctor's name, but I choose to keep him anonymous. While my family and I understood that I had a bone growth disorder, up until this visit we didn't know what my diagnosis was. We learned from this doctor the official name of my condition, and that there were only a small handful of people in Australia who had it. To this day, I have never met anyone else with brachyolmia (I'm 45 years old). The part of the visit that was memorable was that as the doctor was examining my body (fully clothed this time, I'm relieved to say) and turning over my hands in each of his hands to inspect them, he made a comment, mostly to himself: "She's quite attractive." I could feel my mother bristle at this, as did I. He spoke about me as if I wasn't in the room, but it also felt invasive and creepy, even if I did have my clothes on! When the doctor left the room, my mother expressed her shock and indignation that the doctor would say such a thing about her daughter. I felt the same way. To this day, I struggle to unpack that moment. It was obviously wrong on so many levels that he said it. The objectification was two-pronged: apart from treating me like a medical specimen that he was clearly marveling at, he was also treating me like a sexual object. On top of this, the doctor made clear that he was almost surprised that I was attractive – disabled people and people of short stature are not considered attractive or desirable in society, so I was an anomaly in that sense too. It was disappointing that this doctor, in whom we placed such great respect and trust, would make such a thoughtless, flippant comment.

In 2018, I gave birth to my daughter Finley, who has the most common form of dwarfism, achondroplasia. I distinctly recall one visit to the doctor during my pregnancy, with my husband Ryan, who also has achondroplasia. During this visit I had to get a sonogram, and the doctor's office also delivered the results of my amniocentesis, a test where a small amount of amniotic fluid is collected from the area surrounding the baby in the gestational sac. The test measures all kinds of things, including protein levels, but it can also uncover birth defects. They informed me and my husband that Finley had inherited my husband's gene mutation, which is autosomal dominant, meaning that my husband has a 50 per cent chance of passing his achondroplasia down to his children. Finley was in luck; she had indeed inherited achondroplasia. However, the doctor saw this as a stroke of bad luck rather than good, and they asked if I still intended to keep the pregnancy based on this newly acquired knowledge. My husband and I went quiet in shock at the doctor's assumption that we wouldn't necessarily want the baby any more owing to her achondroplasia diagnosis, and eventually those feelings turned into indignation and anger. We never attempted to try and correct the doctor in their assumption. We simply said we would be keeping the baby.

In reality, and quite antithetical to the doctor's expectation, I had long fantasized about having a baby with achondroplasia, after having encountered so many gorgeous achondroplasia children at the Little People of America conventions. Finley was my dream come true, and I will never forget the little smile she flashed at me, my husband, and my mother (who was visiting from Australia at the time) that was captured on a sonogram, and later a print which I still have today in a frame by my bed. Indeed, Finley's cherub grin in the sonogram foretold what was to come: a bundle of energy, happiness, sunshine, and joy wrapped into one exquisite package. Even today, five years after Finley was born, I still shake my head in disbelief that the doctor would have had us do away with Finley forever. Their insensitive question came on the heels of a difficult two-year period of trying to have children, so their question was, for us, not just out of left field, but from an entirely different planet.

Many of my fellow disabled community members understand these stories intimately. They are not unusual. We could fill an entire library with stories of our encounters with the medical industrial complex. Some of my dwarf friends are academics who write on disability and bioethics, such as Joseph Stramondo, and in this book I draw on his thinking that works to undo the assumptions that the medical world makes – the same kind that guided the doctor who delivered the news of my daughter's achondroplasia. I'm very proud to be part of my community, and it is this pride that continues to be tested by the medical industrial complex. Since 2012, Little People of America has engaged in conversations regarding a new drug called vosoritide, developed by the US company BioMarin Pharmaceutical. The goal of the drug is to prevent medical complications associated with achondroplasia, which can include sleep apnea, hearing loss, and spinal problems, but one of the most immediate byproducts of taking the drug is that it can increase height. For many folks with achondroplasia, their short stature is not a disability that needs to be corrected, and Little People of America promotes dwarf pride and the fact that little people can live fulfilling lives. The drug therefore threatens an erasure of dwarf identity that many do not consider an illness or a defect. But there are also many families who support this intervention, who are not so familiar with dwarf pride, so the community remains divided. There are often heated debates and tensions at the conventions and online around the medical world's role in supposedly curing dwarfism.

This tension is what I seek to probe (this time pun intended) in this book. I've been captivated by the new generations of contemporary disabled artists who want to share their own stories of the medical industrial complex, using contemporary art as an expression of a medical critique and, by extension, a critique of the medical model of disability. What I'm learning is that these artists have political intentions, and this is why I have developed the term *hospital aesthetics*. This concept is distinct from the work of clinical arts workers in clinical settings, who instead focus on the well-being of patients through the therapeutic benefits of art. What I see in the artwork in this book, then, is the same spirit of defiance and pride in one's body that I observe in my own nascent experiences with the medical world as a child and as a teenager, in my experience as a geriatric pregnant woman in 2018, and through Little People of America. This work speaks to a desire to express agency, empowerment, and a loud(er) voice over the clamor of convoluted medical language and impersonal bedside manner. But it is also more complicated than this. This is what I will uncover in the upcoming chapters, and why I wanted to write this book.

Acknowledgments

I would like to acknowledge that the land in which this book was written has served as a site of Indigenous peoples, specifically the Atakapa-Ishak, Tāp Pīlam Coahuiltecan, the Sana band of the Tonkawa tribe, and Karankawa nations.

This book was written during the first year of my tenure-track position as Assistant Professor of Arts Leadership in the Kathrine G. McGovern College of the Arts at the University of Houston. During the longer writing jags of this book, I was quite ill with various colds and flus. The irony of this is not lost on me, given that I have written a book about disability, health, and illness. My convalescence put me into the shoes of many of the artists whom I write about in this book. Through illness comes periods of great creativity and reflection. During my periods of recovery, I was able to think and write, which was a gift. So I am grateful for illness, for giving me time and allowing me to explore the creativity that has presented itself through the many artists in this book. I want to thank these artists for their time and generosity, including Dominic Quagliozzi, Robert Andy Coombs, Bhavna Mehta, Lauryn Youden, Sharona Franklin, and Carolyn Lazard, as well as Black Womxn Flourish. I also interviewed a number of groups at earlier periods before this book was fully conceptualized, including the Sickness Affinity Group, Power Makes Us Sick, and the Feminist Health Care Research Group.

I would like to acknowledge the Creative Capital/Andy Warhol Foundation Arts Writers Grant, which has critically supported me with the development of this book thanks to a $50,000 stipend. Beyond the financial benefits this prestigious grant has afforded me, it is an honor to be recognized by a body that is dedicated to the highest rigors of research, writing, and scholarship supported by like-minded professionals in the field of contemporary art. I am also grateful to the University of Houston Division of

Research for providing a grant to support the production of this book, and to the College Art Association Millard Meiss Publication Fund.

The faculty and students in the Masters in Arts Leadership program at the University of Houston have provided much nourishment and support, particularly my partner-in-crime, Fleurette Fernando, and Dean Andrew Davis. Fellow art historians Natilee Harren and Sandra Zalman have been reliable mentors, colleagues, and friends. Other colleagues in the Kathrine G. McGovern College of the Arts also deserve thanks, including Megan Topham, Keliy Anderson-Staley, Roberto Tejada, Rex Koontz, Evan Leslie, Melissa Noble, Katherine Veneman, former Director of the School of Art, Beckham Dossett, and new Director of the School of Art, Beth Merfish. I also appreciate the support of Woods Nash, Assistant Professor of Bioethics and Medical Humanities in Behavioral and Social Sciences in the Tilman J. Fertitta Family College of Medicine at the University of Houston.

Thank you to my editor, Emma Brennan at Manchester University Press, and editorial assistant Christian Lea. I also wish to thank my anonymous peer reviewers for insightful and incredibly helpful feedback. The book has more dimension thanks to your thoughtful comments and suggestions. There were many others who assisted in the development of this book along the way, including Cara Jordan, James Cui who assisted with line editing, Beth Lee-De Amici for indexing, and Kaylee Alexander for citation editing and compiling the bibliography. I am also grateful to Madison Zalopany for writing the image descriptions, and James Toftness for assisting with image compilation and permissions. I especially want to thank all the individuals and organizations who granted permission to use images for this book. Images are the critical backbone of the book and truly give readers insight into the work of the artists.

Portions of this book have been previously published elsewhere: sections of the Introduction were published in "Here's Looking at You: Disability Art at the Turn of the 21st Century" in the *For Dear Life: Art, Medicine, Disability* catalogue published by the Museum of Contemporary Art San Diego, curated by Jill Dawsey and Isabel Casso; sections from Chapter 2 were previously published in "Crafting Disability: Re-envisioning Indian Textile Traditions," *Journal of Modern Craft* 17, no. 2 (2024), "The (Narrative) Prosthesis Re-fitted: Finding New Support for Embodied and Imagined Differences in Contemporary Art," *Journal of Literary and Cultural Disability Studies* 9, no. 3 (2015), and *Contemporary Art and Disability Studies*, edited by Alice Wexler and John Derby (Routledge, 2019); and lastly sections from Chapter 4 were previously published in "Networks of Care: Collectivity as Dialogic Creative Access," in *Curating Access: Disability Art Activism and Creative Accommodation*, edited by Amanda Cachia (Routledge, 2022) and "Constructing Elastic Worlds: From Avant-Garde Exhibition Design to Crip Comfort," *Journal of Curatorial Studies* 13, no. 2 (2024). I thank the publishers for generously giving permission to reprint these sections in this book.

This book was written very quickly on the heels of my first book, *The Agency of Access: Contemporary Disability Art and Institutional Critique* (Temple University Press, 2024). This book fell into my lap because it was already written in my mind. I only take this to mean that the work is all there, in front of us, and it demands to be recorded, discussed, and theorized, now more urgently than ever.

My family, as always, continue to sustain me outside of my writing time. But my husband Ryan has been particularly supportive, making sacrifices to accommodate my career goals and my dreams. I am fortunate to have someone in my life who wants everything for me. I dedicate this book to him, and to my daughter Finley.

Introduction

Riva Lehrer's nuanced approach to portraiture is exemplified in the drawing *Zoom Portraits: Alice Wong* (see Figure I.1), which offers a captivating likeness of disability activist Alice Wong. Here, Wong gazes at us intently, perhaps confrontationally, as if returning the gaze to which disabled people are always subjected in an ableist world, particularly in medical contexts. Wong's act of staring back at us is what may strike us first – her dark eyes bright and sharp – but then we notice Wong's breathing apparatus, which covers part of her face, as well as the ventilator tube itself, front and center.[1] Underneath the tube, Wong's lips are partially visible and painted with bright red lipstick. As Wong has said, "every breath from my ventilator is a ferocious feline roar of defiance and joy."[2] The framing device and backdrop of Lehrer's portrait is also important, because the artist has recreated her engagement with Wong as she sits for the portrait on Zoom. The knowledge that the portrait was mediated through this technology situates the sitting during the COVID-19 pandemic, which disproportionately impacted disabled people, including Wong. However, unlike in most paintings in the history of portraiture, the Zoom frame positions the sitter in relationship to an interlocutor on the other side – first the artist and then the viewer. The power in this is that a disabled artist is gazing at a disabled sitter from the outset, and they share an understanding of how meaningful this exchange is. They also share an immense understanding of the struggles disabled people face with the medical industry, as both Lehrer and Wong have spent extensive time in hospital, undertaking surgeries and enduring interventions to help them survive.[3] Typically, the power of the gaze rests with the nondisabled medical practitioner or with the viewer, and the disabled body is placed under scrutiny. Here, Lehrer gives her impressions of Wong, which come from a fierce place of care, comfort, and allyship. While Lehrer gives us insight into her personal perspective on

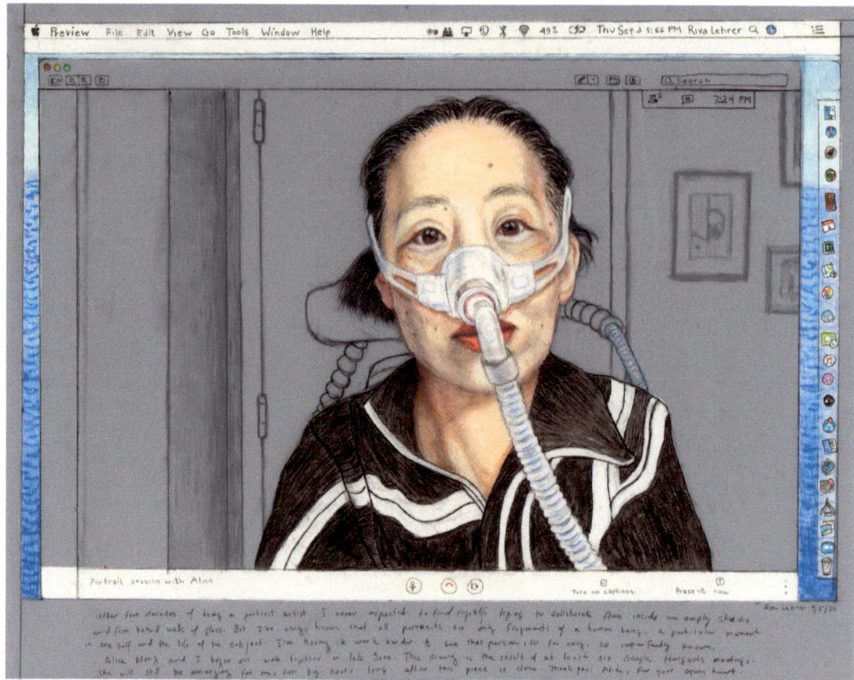

I.1 Riva Lehrer, *Zoom Portraits: Alice Wong*, 2020. Graphite and colored pencil on paper, 25.25 × 31.25in. (65 × 79.5cm). Courtesy of the artist.

Image description I.1: A color pencil drawing of disabled activist, Alice Wong, framed in a floating Zoom window. Alice is a thin Chinese American woman. She faces us directly with a stoic expression wearing a respirator over her nose and ruby red lipstick on her lips. Alice's portrait is carefully and naturalistically rendered in color, however, the details of her home have been roughly sketched in graphite. Below the Zoom box is handwritten text scribbled in tiny and neat lettering.

Wong, she equally offers an unflinching portrait of a disabled person who is reclaiming her body and her breath, where even the lipstick contributes to a new hospital aesthetics.

Hospital Aesthetics: Disability, Medicine, Activism argues that contemporary disabled artists are offering a new hospital aesthetics, taking health and care into their own hands and body-minds. Hospital aesthetics is defined as artwork that explores the ever-subjective experience of being sick and disabled, set apart from and outside of a clinical and therapeutic setting, and in opposition to the medical model of disability. This hospital aesthetics is not interested in art therapy's clinical concern with the well-being of hospital patients, but rather it wants to challenge the oppressive master narratives in the medical model of disability, a philosophy in which disability is bad and must be fixed or corrected. In doing the work of hospital aesthetics, contemporary disabled artists are contributing to a type of disability activism that can improve both mainstream bioethics and ableist museum and gallery culture. This is because the work of contemporary disabled artists extends the imperative of decolonizing the gallery into the act of decolonizing the hospital; the artists I examine work against the medical industrial complex's tendency to treat disabled bodies as specimens, and eventually as archives. Instead, their hospital aesthetics shows a different side to disabled bodies that attempts to undo the social and cultural impacts the hospital has had on its disabled patients, both historically and in the contemporary moment.

The visual culture of medicine generally undermines and controls disabled bodies at large, ultimately resulting in unfavorable outcomes for the physical and psychological care of disabled bodies. It is imperative, then, that disabled artists seek to establish a hospital aesthetics in which to rescript these medical images of disability, both past and present, which was particularly true in the age of the COVID-19 pandemic. While the term *hospital aesthetics* evokes its etymological neighbor *hospitable* – to be kind or cordial to strangers and guests, a practice demonstrated in contemporary disabled artist communities, where health and care are necessarily interdependent – the term also does much more than this. In doing the work of hospital aesthetics, both as process and product, contemporary disabled artists unleash a form of radical activism to empower themselves and the disabled and sick population to consider illness on their own terms, revealing the inadequacies of the medical industrial complex. The binary of hospitable versus inhospitable within the medical industrial complex has additional resonance as it relates to the art gallery, a space that has historically privileged audiences based on class, race, education levels, and more. Hospital aesthetics can help to challenge and transform both the hospital and the art gallery into more welcoming sites, where the two venues can share critical dialogue and resources regarding the treatment of disabled bodies. In the following five chapters, I will examine the work of nine contemporary disabled artists and four care collectives from the United States, Canada, and Europe who use a range of mediums including drawing, sculpture, installation, painting, performance, video, and socially engaged art practice to illustrate hospital aesthetics. I use the term *contemporary disabled artist* to refer to an artist who explores themes connected to disability, often drawing on personal experience. In this way, the reader will understand that the work is not conflated completely with the artist's authorship, which is multifaceted.

Around 2020, as I was completing my first book, I began to notice that many new disabled artists were drawing on their personal experiences in hospitals, with doctor's visits or long-term illness as inspiration for their art practices. I was drawn to thinking and writing about these artists because they are part of a new and younger generation of disabled artists who are quite forthright and unafraid to present their assertions about the complicated relationships between the medical industrial complex, capitalism, the state, and their bodies. Like many of their artist peers, they frequently turn to social media platforms, particularly Instagram, to share their experiences in hospitals, with medications and other prosthetic supports, both human-made and natural, and with pain. While their interdependent experiences in institutional and at-home care settings are diverse, emotional, and political, the through line is a robust activism which I argue is powerfully shaping generative conversations around disability and its relationship to toxic environments – and ultimately all our lives while we lived through the "inhospitable" coronavirus moment. While in the 1980s and 1990s artists like Jo Spence, Hannah Wilke, Mike Parr, Félix González-Torres, and Bob Flanagan were lone figures in the field of capturing illness in their art practices, today artists are charting their experiences in noticeably greater numbers. I find that the reasons this topic has increased in popularity and criticality in the last few years are twofold: first, disabled artists are much less inhibited than they were just a decade ago and now feel more inclined to make bold statements about their encounters with the medical industrial complex; second, the world went through the COVID-19 pandemic, and suddenly almost everyone understood the complications, challenges, and nuances of being inconvenienced, ill, sick, and temporarily or permanently disabled.

This book was also shaped by an exhibition that I curated at the University Art Gallery at San Diego State University in fall 2022. I realized that the theme of that exhibition, *Script/Rescript*, has become so ubiquitous that it needed to become the impetus for something larger: it made most sense to develop the premise of the exhibition into a monograph. A detailed study could trace what I recognized as a prominent new aesthetic in contemporary art practice that has now become an integral and important contribution to art history at large – what I call a hospital aesthetics, or the aesthetics of the hospital.

Initially, I had planned to title this book "Hospitable Aesthetics," but after a suggestion from an editor, I realized it would be more provocative to call the book "Hospital Aesthetics" instead. I hope that the pathos and tension this title captures will give the book and its attendant arguments a critical edge. "Hospitable Aesthetics" seems too kind, warm, and fuzzy. Disabled artists don't want to be warm and fuzzy, or "hospitable." They want to be contrarian. Given the very loaded history of associations that hospitals have for disabled people, and the medical model, I want the words *hospital* and *aesthetics* to butt heads, and I want to make complex an aesthetics of the hospital that extends beyond pleasing interiors.

The study of the intersections between contemporary disability, medicine, and the visual culture of the hospital has been limited, but there are a few significant texts that this book will acknowledge and draw from. Lisa Cartwright's seminal book *Screening the Body: Tracing Medicine's Visual*

Culture (1995) is an especially important touchstone for this book. It is foundational for positing that the visual culture of medicine seeks to objectify and control bodies, negatively impacting how disabled bodies are cared for both physically and psychologically. It is imperative, then, that artists seek to establish a hospital aesthetics in which to rescript these medical images of disability, both past and present. Petra Kuppers's *The Scar of Visibility: Medical Performances and Contemporary Art* (2007) looks at the trope of the scar as a generative place for transforming the limitations of medical imagery in contemporary art praxis. While I, like Kuppers, show how contemporary disabled artists transform medical imagery into images that become empowering for self-narratives of illness, in my book the locus of the investigation is the hospital in the COVID-19 era, and how the word *hospital* manifests in both the hospital itself and the art gallery. I also turn to other contemporary studies of the disabled body entwined with the philosophy and ethics of care; even though these books do not reference visual culture, their thinking is still important for their contributions to how disabled philosophical frameworks press up against the medical model of disability. This book aims to develop critical relationships between contemporary disability art, hospitable aesthetics, the medical industrial complex, visual culture, and disability justice and activism, and to expand the conventions of display in museums and hospitals alike.

I want to re-emphasize that the hospital aesthetics in this book is very much political, and not tied to studies on how the interior design of the hospital room can inhibit or enhance patient well-being. I have already noted how this hospital aesthetics is separate from the work of art therapists too, but this does not in any way diminish the work of interior designers, art therapists, and other clinical workers who work in hospital environments with patients' well-being in their minds as their primary duty of care. In fact, several powerful art collectives are working closely with hospitals to change the nature of the artwork that is hung in hospital rooms so that it is inherently challenging rather than soothing. Naturally I find this a more interesting approach because it moves a little closer toward provoking critical thought rather than merely dispelling anxiety. For example, the UK-based art collective Hospital Rooms commissions world-famous artists to create site-specific installations for hospitals that specialize in treating patients with mental health challenges, anxiety, and depression. The Arts & Medicine program of Cleveland Clinic also strives to curate museum-quality art experiences for hospital visitors, patients, and staff. Many hospitals now also have Art in Medicine programs, which aim to promote healing across the full plethora of art forms, including the visual arts, music, and performance. The mission of the Center for Performing Arts Medicine (CPAM) at Houston Methodist Hospital is to translate the collaborative potential of arts and medicine to the holistic healthcare environment. The center engages in specialized healthcare and wellness education for performing and visual artists, alongside research that seeks to harness the broadest potential of the arts in therapy, rehabilitation, and human performance.

The reader should also understand that I do appreciate the benefits of images that contain sandy beaches with palm trees and crisp, sun-filled ocean air which hang on the walls of medical settings. Since I turned 40 years old, I have been getting mammograms at the University of California San Diego Women's Breast Health Imaging Clinic. These annual screenings spark numerous weeks of spiraling anxiety prior to my appointment; it hasn't helped that I've had several false alarms and a biopsy that ended up revealing a harmless cyst. Those same beaches and palm trees that are strategically hung in the waiting room and X-ray room are undoubtedly soothing. Still, it seems as if there is a disconnect across these worlds, and perhaps an irony too. While there are art therapists and music therapists employed by the hospitals, indicating that hospitals are aware that patients' well-being is paramount, a lingering conservatism toward disabled bodies persists. This is because, ultimately, the training that young doctors get is still centered on fixing, even if they now have more exposure to the art world than ever before as a means to be more empathetic. Nonetheless, the world by and large has come to acknowledge and recognize the doctor's poor bedside manner. The worlds of the hospital and the art gallery have come together to address this issue (signaling that, indeed, a relationship does already exist – albeit not necessarily a politically conscious one – across these sites).

The Director of Education at the Blanton Museum of Art at the University of Texas in Austin, Ray Williams, has established robust partnerships with medical educators and clinicians, beginning during his time as an educator at the Harvard Art Museum. Williams argues that medical students benefit from class time spent in museums using artwork to build empathetic communication, teamwork, and cultural competency. In a 2023 book he edited with Ruth Slavin and Corinne Zimmermann entitled *Activating the Art Museum: Designing Experiences for the Health Professions*, the authors offer descriptions of their teaching practices to support a more humanistic approach in healthcare for the benefit of medical workers and their patients.[4] The W. T. and Louise J. Moran Chair of Learning and Interpretation, Caroline Goeser, and Jenn Beradino, the Senior Manager of Object-Based Learning at the Museum of Fine Arts, Houston, also engage extensively with local medical students to fulfill the same objectives that Ray Williams advocates for. In a conversation I had with Goeser, she stated that her team looks to fill the gaps in medical students' education, asking how they can find room for more empathy and care in their attitudes and treatment toward their patients.[5] As meaningful and effective as all these interventions are, there is still a missing piece that provides a critical space for the disabled patient. In the next section, I will explore both the praxis and theory that ground this book's approach, examining the work of other influential scholars and artists, all of whom are equally invested in exploring this critical space.

Disability art's history of critiquing medicine

One of the first major focuses of contemporary disabled artists was the imperative to critique the medical model of disability. While it is true that several contemporary artists such as Félix González-Torres and Bob Flanagan made work about their own forms of health and illness throughout the 1980s and 1990s, these artists were the exception to the rule. But their work was still part of the mainstream, while the work of contemporary disabled artists was sidelined. Also, to my knowledge González-Torres and Flanagan never identified as disabled, nor did they use the language of disability to engage with their work, either in private or public settings (i.e. the studio and the art gallery). While in the following five chapters I pay tribute and draw a connection to artists from earlier decades, who provide an important foundation and precedent for the work we see gaining momentum today, in this section I would like to center the work of the artists who were most on the margins. Yet if it wasn't for the work of Flanagan and company, we would not be witnessing the turn to hospital aesthetics that contemporary disabled artists are deeply engaged with in the current moment.

Before providing a brief history of disability art's critique of medicine, I'd like to take the reader on an equally brief journey through the historical treatment of disability in medicine at large. The response to disability in medical contexts has long been the "curative imperative," as coined by Joseph Stramondo. During the eighteenth and nineteenth centuries, the curative imperative was much more sinister, as the hospital wasn't necessarily the first place where treatment was sought for disabled people. Instead, people with both physical and cognitive disabilities would be sent to psychiatric institutions, colloquially known as "insane" or "lunatic" asylums. Unfortunately, electric shock therapy and experiments were also practiced on disabled patients in these institutions, without the necessity of a prognosis that warranted such intervention. The study of eugenics also greatly influenced doctors in this period. Eugenics, the biosocial movement embraced by the Nazi Party, advocates the use of practices aimed at improving the genetic composition of a population, usually focusing on the medical manipulation of human populations. The movement was influenced by physiognomy, a classification process that emerged in the nineteenth century and purported to assess a person's character or personality from his or her outward appearance, especially the face. Disabled people (and other minority subject positions) were particularly marginalized by this process because they were considered disposable members of the population. Physiognomy was used by the police in criminal profiling. It was not uncommon for doctors to practice forced sterilizations on disabled women, whom they deemed unfit to reproduce, or to perform lobotomies, removing sections of a disabled person's brain to reduce so-called "mania."[6] Over time, these forced surgical practices were questioned and replaced with medication as the main form of treatment in the 1950s and 1960s. While this problematic historical response to disability by the medical industrial complex impacted a broad range of disabled people, including those with neurodivergence, the genealogy of the contemporary disability art response to the medical model that I trace here focuses on physical disability. Thus, the reader will note that I do not tackle the vast literature on art and mental illness. This means that there is still much work to be done to write all the multiple histories of a truly diverse disability art history.

Some of the earliest and most influential disability studies scholars who have detailed the various medical injustices wrought on disabled bodies include Rosemarie Garland-Thomson, Lennard Davis, Tobin Siebers, Susan Schweik, Beth Linker, and Catherine Kudlick. Linker and Kudlick agree that a history of medicine that incorporates a disability perspective and, conversely, a history of disability that incorporates a medical historian's perspective could prompt a productive dialogue that closes the divide (and thus the tensions and misunderstandings) between the two subfields. In a brilliant positioning paper by Kudlick, she examines *why* there has been a distance between the two subfields in the first place, and states that "the crux of the difference lies in politics."[7] The subfields have been incompatible because there are different political realities between each "opposing intellectual past."[8] While disability studies is concerned with a politics of empowerment for disabled people, the medical field wants to correct disabilities, with little regard for the agency of disabled individuals. Despite conceding that breaking down the divide between the history of medicine and the history of disability would be useful, Kudlick ultimately maintains that the divide should not be completely erased just yet. More time is required to appreciate the nuances within both sets of histories, and to thoughtfully "reframe our primary questions and concerns."[9] It is clear, then, that disabled artists have much material to draw on within this complex history of disability as it intersects with medicine. Based on Kudlick's assertions, it is up to the historian of disability to put pressure on – and thus question – the intentions of medicine's approach toward disabled embodiment, and this is certainly how the earliest contributors to the visual art discourse of disability and medicine have proceeded.

Riva Lehrer and other disabled artists of her generation in the 1980s and 1990s benefitted from a greater degree of awareness around disability justice, practicing during the years when the academic field of disability studies was taking root. She and others have deployed the medical model of disability as a vehicle for articulating a politics of resistance. The medical model of disability encompasses how disability is conventionally and persistently perceived in mainstream society – that is, as something inherently wrong that needs to be fixed. The social model of disability flips the script on the medical model and instead suggests that it is society that disables the individual. We can trace these strategies and the beginnings of a critical disability arts movement to 1995, when a significant convening on disability arts and humanities, the This/Ability conference, was held at the University of Michigan in Ann Arbor, Michigan. Organized by scholars Susan Crutchfield, Marcy Epstein, and Joanne Leonard, the event heralded a moment in which disabled artists could not stay silent any longer. The conference established a forum in which disabled artists could network and find a mutually supportive space for organizing. Attending the conference were disability studies scholars David T. Mitchell and Sharon L. Snyder, who have been critical figures in providing scholarly and creative forums for the disabled community, including artists. In their documentary, *Vital Signs: Crip Culture Talks Back* (1995), the scholars shine a light on disabled activists and artists as they record three days of the conference. Well-known advocates such as Eli Clare, Kenny Fries, Cheryl Mae Wade, Simi Linton, and Mary Duffy are interviewed amidst footage of performances, conversations, and debates.[10]

Figure I.2 shows a still from a performance by prominent disability studies scholar Carrie Sandahl, who was a graduate student at the time, and is now a major figure in the field that has become known as crip theory (originally coined by Robert McRuer).[11] Sandahl stood in the middle of the gallery wearing a white medical jacket covered in red graffiti, protesting how her body had been manipulated and probed by doctors. Sandahl explains that the piece was an acknowledgment of her feeling "that people with disabilities are always situated within a medical discourse. That's why I got the lab jacket and why it's written in red to signify blood. And the fascination that people seem to have with a medical discourse of your body – as if it's always been written on your body whether you're wearing it or not."[12] I consider Sandahl's work to be a seminal piece in disability performance art, and one of the first overt critiques of the medical industrial complex.

In the first exhibition I curated for Pro Arts Gallery in Oakland, California in 2011, entitled *Medusa's Mirror: Fears, Spells and other Transfixed Positions*, I included three works on paper by disabled artist, scholar, and activist Sunaura Taylor (see Figure I.3). In these three works, entitled *Fig 121–124* (2010), Taylor appropriated images from a medical textbook, displaying four photographs in a grid of a young boy who is being fitted for a prosthesis consisting of two legs. While today a prosthesis itself is not considered to be a harmful or unwanted intervention on a disabled person with either congenital or acquired limb differences, during the earlier years of prosthetic technology many prosthetics were ill-fitting. In one of Taylor's images, the boy is slouched to one side as his body rests precariously

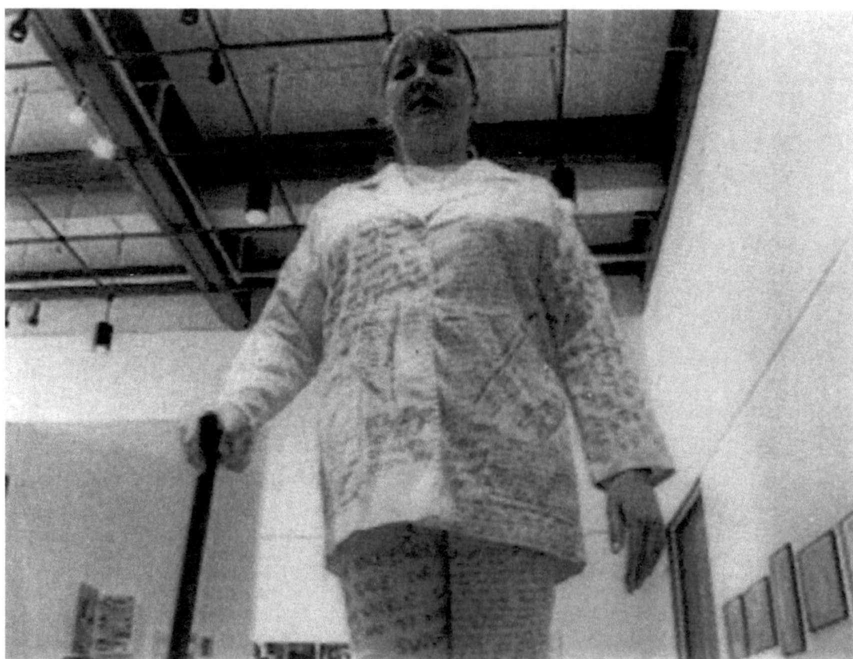

I.2 Carrie Sandahl performance, 1995, "This/Ability: An Interdisciplinary Conference on Disability and the Arts," University of Michigan, Ann Arbor, Michigan. Courtesy of David T. Mitchell.

Image description I.2: A grainy black and white photo of a white person seen from below. They stand, looming over the camera looking down at us with a blank expression. They wear a white lab coat and pants that have illegible text scribbled all over the garments. Their right hand holds onto a black cane.

on the two mechanical legs. In another, he is using crutches which are not the right size for his frame. Prosthetics were not always necessarily an effective means for assisting an individual with moving through life's everyday activities. This was especially true with children, who are more often able to adapt to their environment than adults. Children may have been forced to wear uncomfortable or even painful prosthetic devices for the sake of appearing "normal," even if the practical applications did more harm than good. In Taylor's piece, the artist interrupts the images with paint to change their meaning into something more political. Taylor says, "By whiting-out the individuals in the medical images I am removing disability from the gaze of medicine and pathology, while simultaneously giving back privacy to the individuals in the images."[13]

The images struck a chord for me because they reminded me of the pain, trauma, and shame I felt in my body under the gaze of a doctor when I was a child (as described in the Preface). The experience was

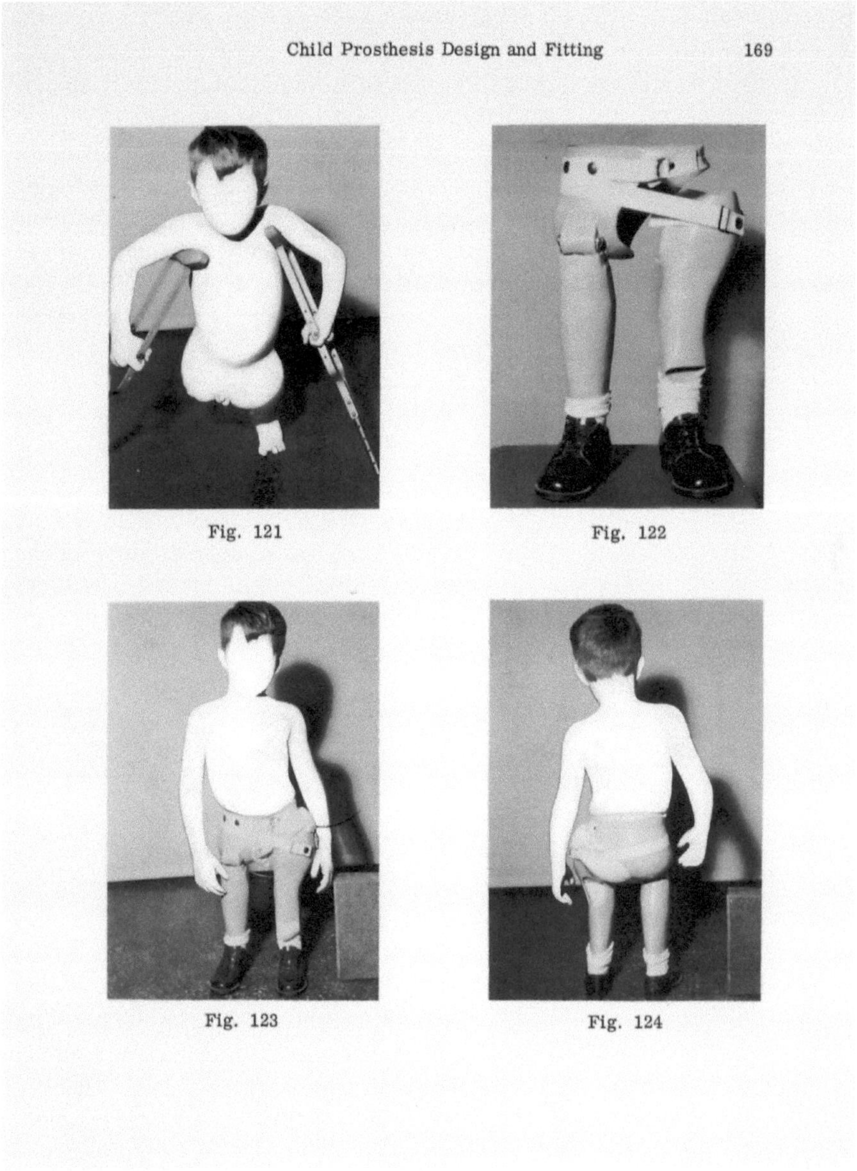

Child Prosthesis Design and Fitting 169

Fig. 121

Fig. 122

Fig. 123

Fig. 124

I.3 Sunaura Taylor, *Figure 121–124*, 2010. Oil paint on digital print on paper. 4 × 6 ft (48 × 72 in.) (122 × 183 cm). Courtesy of the artist.

Image description I.3: Four black and white photos in an even grid formation, two rows with two photos each. Each image features a White disabled child with their face erased. The child is an amputee with an assymetrical body often associated with scoliosis. The images feature the child shirtless and using crutches or prosthetic legs. Each image is numbered as if from a medical textbook.

intensely relatable. Further, I recall through various visits with specialists at a children's hospital in Sydney when I was a young teenager that solutions to my dwarfism were presented to my parents, including injections to add a few inches of growth to my height or, more drastically, reconstructive surgery to insert lengthening rods into my legs which would allow them to lengthen over time. This type of surgery involves breaking the femur and/or tibia, making for a long and arduous recovery process. I remember recoiling in horror at these "solutions" or "cures" for my dwarfism, even at that young age. Taylor's images reminded me of how the medical world had tried to normalize me, like the young boy in the medical textbook. Taylor's painterly solution to reclaiming and so thwarting the medical gaze felt empowering, agential, and as though a wrong was somehow being righted.

Taylor's work has influenced me to this day, where in the hazy aftermath of COVID-19 a larger assemblage of artists are immersed in an aesthetics of the hospital than ever before. On May 28, 2020, Taylor wrote an article entitled "What Would Health Security Look Like?," published in the *Boston Review*.[14] She begins the paper by stating what is now understood as the obvious: "If there is one thing this [coronavirus] pandemic is making abundantly clear it is that our individual health is interconnected – to each other, to our political and economic systems, to the broader ecology, and the other species we share the planet with."[15] Shortly after this powerful opening line, she writes about how the pandemic, as portrayed through the media, provided us with various visualizations that prove how leaky and porous our bodies truly are in response to our immediate environments. Never have we been more aware of how the fluid that emanates from our bodies on a daily basis can easily and unpleasantly be shared with those around us, giving birth to what became the ubiquitous 6-foot rule of social distancing. Taylor discusses the popular illustrations and graphics depicting the cough droplets, sneezes, and breath which float within a 6-foot radius of our mouths, so that any other person who comes into contact within this zone will plough unceremoniously through the murk, unbeknownst to them.

The visual culture of the pandemic as disseminated through the media is an important backdrop for the artwork discussed in this book. While the artists analyzed here do not talk of potentially deadly coronavirus droplets affecting the globe on a mass scale, they do nonetheless illustrate toxic residue left behind after their encounters with health challenges. They meticulously and creatively document artifacts from their medicalized rituals, giving viewers an opportunity to look at them as material forms in their own right – indeed, aesthetic forms, devoid of needy bodies or anxious minds. Viewers might imagine how their own bodies would engage with these props and tools of the medical industry in their own lives. One senses that the artists' engagements with the tool kits that sustain their bodies through their creative practice are a meditation of sorts, where they embrace their own individualized crip-ecologies and interdependent networks of care that are a necessary part of their lives. Disabled artists have, in fact, taken the pandemic moment of 2020–21 as an opportunity to speak of how the world is starting to walk in their shoes, so to speak, learning to cope with barriers and other disruptions and challenges to their daily lives and their environments – physically, mentally, financially, socially, medically – that disabled folks always already experienced well before the pandemic came along. It is as if the pandemic has highlighted the challenges of disabled folks.[16] As chronically ill artist Ezra Benus states, "Suddenly, people are realizing that better hygiene and access to remote work and learning are societal obligations. Until something like the coronavirus affected the general population, these things were presented to disabled people as impossibilities."[17]

During a conversation I had with Benus, I asked him if he felt that the changes caused by the pandemic could serve the needs of disabled people. Now that the world was forced to, for example, work from home during quarantine and communicate virtually through internet platforms such as Zoom, perhaps employers, businesses, and other capitalist institutions would give the green light to these conditions full time for those who need them for health reasons. Benus said that while it would be nice to think that the able-bodied world could recognize the benefits of some of these new post-coronavirus conditions, he wasn't overly optimistic that employers would grant these measures permanently to chronically ill, disabled, and immunocompromised folks. It will therefore be interesting to see how temporary pandemonium over a world health crisis may have contradictory, chronic, and generative applications for marginalized artists.

All of these ideas help to illuminate the genesis of hospital aesthetics and the ongoing legacy of disability art's history of critiquing medicine.

American novelist, editor, and journalist Dodie Bellamy's interestingly titled book, *When the Sick Rule the World*, shows how disability art and culture are drawing from, and refuting, practices of medicine.[18] Bellamy's book, full of witty stories that oscillate between the sick, social, and individual body, has been the topic of a number of group-curated exhibitions in Europe and North America in the past few years that include the work of disabled artists and their explorations of illness and care. One iteration of a *When the Sick Rule the World* exhibition was hosted by Gebert Stiftung für Kultur in Switzerland in 2019, curated by Fanny Hauser and Viktor Neumann. Another relevant exhibition of note is *Sick Time, Sleepy Time, Crip Time: Against Capitalism's Temporal Bullying* by disabled curator Taraneh Fazeli and held at Redbull Arts Detroit in Michigan. A nonfiction book that has gained attention for its reflections on personal illness is the novel *Sanatorium* by British disabled artist and author Abi Palmer.[19] The author shares her experiences of healing in the thermal baths of a famous rehabilitation facility in Budapest. Palmer's book depicts some respite, as her body is healing in an environment that is the antithesis of toxic. These kinds of books have proliferated over the past few years. Overall, contemporary artwork which delves into these topics is emerging at astonishing speed, alongside groups of artists who have formed collectives under this umbrella. Apart from the artists who are the subject of this book, a sampling of others include Park McArthur, Constantina Zavitsanos, Annie Sprinkle, Emily Barker, Johanna Hedva, and the We Are Canaries collective in New York. The We Are Canaries collective developed to provide a more self-empowering network of support among artists and cultural workers when confronting an ableist medical system consumed with concepts of productivity and rivalry as opposed to concepts of collective care and self-care. Within this circle of allies, artists share stories of fragility, sickness, crisis, and exhaustion. I discuss the work of collectives in Chapter 4.

The most important point I want to elaborate in this section is that there is a bridge and a comparison between my term *hospital aesthetics* and the contributions that contemporary disabled artists make toward institutional critique within an art world discourse. In my monograph, *The Agency of Access: Contemporary Disability Art and Institutional Critique* (2024), I argued that contemporary disabled artists experiment with the materials and forms of access to critique the institutions that have for too long excluded their work, while asserting their agency, voice, and insistence on disability justice. Institutional critique as an art genre stemmed from the conceptual art movement of the 1960s. It was the art practice of critiquing the institution, debunking the myth of a supposedly neutral gallery space. Artists who worked within this genre challenged mimetic representation, iconography, and artists' production. Some of the mechanisms of the art museum and gallery that institutional critique focused on for its subject matter included funding, curation, acquisitions, leadership, power, and knowledge. In this second monograph, the artists are still doing the work of institutional critique, although in this instance they critique the medical industrial complex as well as the ableist values of the museum. As I mentioned at the start of this section, while a cultural critique of the medical model has been articulated by disability studies scholars and artists since the 1990s, very little scholarship has been produced that engages with this same critique while also fully immersed in art history, theory, and criticism.

As a trained art historian, I intend not only to continue to show how contemporary disabled artists are part of the canon of art history, and that their powerful artworks contribute to a unique disability art history, but also that the version of institutional critique that I have termed hospital aesthetics continues to reveal the pain, anger, and vulnerability of disabled artists today, and perhaps even more so than in my first monograph. While access aesthetics is certainly motivated by frustration and anger, hospital aesthetics reveals raw emotion that is stark, confrontational, and bold. Hospital aesthetics is thus a powerful form of institutional critique that artists with disabilities wield, and warrants a book-length study, much like my analyses of the access aesthetics which has stimulated disabled artists and their practices for the past decade. In this book, I'm suggesting that hospital aesthetics may have an even longer temporal arc than access aesthetics. This is because the momentum we are witnessing today in work by contemporary disabled artists was always already present in work by earlier disabled artists such as Riva Lehrer, Carrie Sandahl, and others during the 1980s and 1990s. This is cause for deep admiration, respect, and gratitude to disability art elders who have paved the way for all of us, because they have enabled us to make art about disability and the medical model, and thus to make change.

Hospital aesthetics theory

In this book, I argue that hospital aesthetics is an extension of the theorizing of radical health already developed by other scholars in other disciplines: philosophy and bioethics, communication, ethnic studies, critical race studies, art therapy, women's, gender, and sexuality studies, trans studies, and English and Latino/a studies. In academic disability studies, the medical model is used to explain how disability is conventionally and persistently perceived in mainstream society as inherently wrong, in contrast with the social model of disability, which points to the disabling effects of society. In the social model of disability, the hospital, ironically, is ableist, as well as the breeding ground for the medical model of disability. Through a longer lens, the artists in this book also inadvertently rescript the medical model of disability by showing that disabled people do not need to be fixed, while reminding us of the power of the social model, which posits that it is society that needs to be corrected in its poor attitude toward disabled people. However, they also move past the social model and come into a new space – a care model, which is more about turning toward each other for support and offering a more personal and nonabrasive touch, the antithesis to the majority of experiences that these artists cite as they encounter hospitals firsthand. In each chapter of the book, I explore what this care model looks like through the work of several artists, particularly in Chapter 4 through the care collectives. It is here that I need to center the work of feminist care scholarship as integral to my analyses in all of the chapters. In the field of disability studies, multiple theorizations of concepts of care have been generated by feminist activist scholars, particularly by Eva Feder Kittay in her groundbreaking work on "ethics of care," where she suggests that care work is often cast as "feminine."[20] Other noteworthy scholars who have developed extensive writing and theories on the intersections of feminism, disability, and care include Kristina Gupta, Christine Kelly, and Akemi Nishida with her book *Just Care: Messy Entanglements of Disability, Dependency, and Desire* (2022). Nishida is particularly notable for coining the term "bed activism." I weave their work into the upcoming chapters.

I also center the scholarship of queer women of color in feminist theory across numerous chapters in the book, and I reference their work alongside the artists I discuss. For example, in her lauded book *Care Work: Dreaming Disability Justice*, Leah Lakshmi Piepzna-Samarasinha, who identifies as a queer disabled nonbinary femme writer, educator, and disability/transformative justice worker, discusses creative collective access. She begins her first chapter, entitled "Care Webs: Experiments in Creating Collective Access," by asking the following question: "What does it mean to shift our ideas of access and care (whether it is disability, childcare, economic access, or many more) from an individual chore, an unfortunate cost of having an unfortunate body, to a collective responsibility that's maybe even deeply joyful?"[21] The writer takes us on a journey, where she asserts that disabled people need to find care and support of their own accord so that they are afforded autonomy and dignity throughout the process from beginning to end. Too often, disabled folks are neglected, ignored, and told that their care and access needs are a burden to society, the economy, the state, and even to family members and friends. This has resulted in numerous situations where public healthcare is denied, disrupted, or policed according to a very rigid, ableist mentality held by the mainstream public and the medical system. These kinds of negative encounters, ranging from one-on-one conversations with doctors to lengthy negotiations with health insurers and pharmaceutical companies, wreak traumatic effects on those who want or need these services. Unfortunately, although not surprisingly, care has also been afforded (or not) to disabled people based on race, class, gender, and location. Piepzna-Samarasinha also cites a long history of disabled people who have been abused under the auspices of so-called care, including being locked up in mental asylums, where they were robbed of their civil rights and were subject to abuse by those in power.[22] Given this long, problematic history, disabled people remain fearful, suspicious, and mistrustful of the medical system. Prior to the feminist health art collectives emerging in this current moment, which are the subject of Chapter 4, disability activists were energized and motivated to collectively organize for other important purposes; in particular, the disability rights liberation movements that emerged in the 1960s and 1970s demanded independent living and deinstitutionalization. It is against this historical backdrop that we can consider how Piepzna-Samarasinha's thinking provides an important theoretical and philosophical context to the work discussed in this book.

In 2023, English and Mexican American scholar Julie Avril Minich published a groundbreaking book entitled *Radical Health: Unwellness, Care, and Latinx Expressive Culture*, which not only gave me an opportunity to frame my own research against another scholar's important insights in a related topic, but also fueled my realization that artists are indeed creating work that can "offer a powerful intervention in contemporary US health politics."[23] Focusing on the work of contemporary disabled artists practicing across a range of artistic disciplines, Minich shows how these artists envision health as a communal responsibility through a disability justice approach. She also rejects the stereotypes and assumptions that poor health in Latinx populations – such as obesity, diabetes, addiction, and high-risk pregnancies – is a result of irresponsible lifestyle choices by the racialized poor. Minich acknowledges her own positionality as a white crip woman and how she came to the topic and politics of her book through lived experience. Minich's book shows how numerous minority groups (particularly Latinx communities) continue to be dismissed by the care industrial complex, particularly when health concerns are wrongly assumed to be caused by – and the fault of – the patient/complainant. Racism and discrimination continue to be regular fixtures in healthcare.

Similarly, queer Black disabled scholar Sami Schalk's important book *Black Disability Politics* (2023) provides a foundation for understanding the intersections between Blackness and disability.[24] Her core argument is that not all disability activism looks and functions in the same way, and that within Black activist communities, "disability" shows up in specific ways, such as police violence, medical neglect, or lack of access to resources. Sometimes disability activism is harder to recognize in Black communities because the language of disability is not necessarily used, but Schalk powerfully argues that disability activism is nonetheless being practiced. Like Minich, Schalk offers evidence of medical racism and medical neglect in the health industry, and she draws on the archives of both the Black Panther Party and the National Black Women's Health Project, where she identifies that public health initiatives must also be grounded in the experience and expertise of marginalized peoples. The National Black Women's Health Project represents another powerful women's collective, equivalent to those discussed in Chapter 4, where women are taking health and care into their own hands. I perceive Schalk's work to be parallel to the work I seek to accomplish in this book, as we both reflect on the injustices in the medical industrial complex and how disability justice seeks to redress these issues through community collaboration. Schalk's work is also most helpful to my work because she shows how disability activism within Black disability politics centers on medical racism and medical trauma for Black disabled communities, in contrast to white disability politics which she argues is more conventionally focused on topics like disability pride and inclusion. One of the major topics of concern among many of the artists discussed in this book is intersectional medical racism, and Schalk's work helps me to show not only the centrality of hospital aesthetics in the output of contemporary disabled artists, but that hospital aesthetics embeds queer of color critique politics too. Carolyn Lazard, Panteha Abareshi, Bhavna

Mehta, and the Black Womxn Flourish collective are some of these artists/groups.

While James Kyung-Jin Lee's *Pedagogies of Woundedness: Illness, Memoir, and the Ends of the Model Minority* (2021) is not queer women of color theory, his work is powerful because he examines another bias built into the medical industrial complex.[25] He shows how the Asian American population are a "model minority" in that they are expected to be exemplars of good behavior and a good life. This means that young Asian Americans have pursued well-respected and high-paying careers, such as medicine. What happens when someone from a model minority is a physician, and the physician is on the other side, that is, the side that most of us are critiquing? Lee argues that Asian Americans' roles as providers of care and as medical authorities comes with its own segregations and discrimination, and that, critically, Asian American investment in a medical career path comes as a knee-jerk reaction to the historical perception that Asian American bodies are diseased. I appreciate Lee's work because he shows how it is not easy on the other side of the fence, as it were, for racialized groups either, and that minorities experience this entrenched bias in different forms and shapes.

Joseph Stramondo's writing at the intersection of philosophy and bioethics has helped to reframe bioethics by centering the lived experiences of disability as a crucial source of moral knowledge that should guide clinical practice, biomedical research, and health policy. He has published scholarship on topics ranging from informed consent procedures to reproductive ethics to pandemic triage protocols to assistive neurotechnology. I apply Stramondo's work to the analyses in this book by suggesting that artists are also centering their lived experiences both inside and outside the hospital as a source of knowledge to guide clinical practice and correct biased assumptions about the disabled and sick body. I'm especially drawn to Stramondo's article "A Critique of the Curative Imperative," where the scholar brilliantly points out that while it is true that disabled people will most certainly not eschew certain medical interventions that will save their lives – surgery, chemotherapy, or radiation – the vast majority of medical interventions are not directly aimed at saving lives.[26] The interventions that do not fall under this remit, Stramondo states, are motivated by the "curative imperative."[27] This is a term he has coined that aligns with the critique of the medical model of disability, wherein the medical industrial complex aims to fix, heal, or cure. Stramondo ultimately argues that the curative imperative should be replaced "with a more nuanced view of when and why disability ought to be cured [and that this] would go a long way toward improving the health care disabled people receive."[28] While Stramondo's term *curative* no doubt is the adjectival form of *cure*, it also suggests the act of curating, which resonates in the field of art where I am positioned as both an art historian and curator. Stramondo's term inadvertently shows how curating is an act that has problematic applications in the medical world as it intersects with disabled bodies, but it also points to how curating and disability have never exactly been easy bedfellows in the art world either. In the next section, I will discuss how curators have started to address these issues through museum and gallery exhibitions, where the curative imperative is dissected.

The writing of artist, art therapist, and disability art advocate Chun-Shan (Sandie) Yi is also particularly important for this book. In both Yi's generative theory and praxis, she acknowledges the inherent tension that exists between art therapy and disabled people. Yi has a unique and important role to play as a professional who operates in both nonclinical and clinical settings. On the one hand, she has trained within ableist clinical frameworks and has been exposed to interventionist therapies for the so-called common good, but on the other hand, she makes artwork about the oppression she herself has experienced from the medical industry. She truly understands the bias around disability on the clinical side from her own personal lived experience as a disabled woman of color, and she is able to reflect on that bias in a powerful way.

In her essay entitled "Res(crip)ting Art Therapy: Disability Culture as a Social Justice Intervention" (which coincidentally echoes the title of my *Script/Rescript* exhibition), Yi discusses the tension that derives from stigma toward disabled individuals, where art therapy can actually be oppressive instead of healing.[29] This is because therapeutic practices, inclusive of art therapy, "overlook social justice for disabled people."[30] Yi further notes that art therapy typically has an interventionist "impulse," but that this assumption may not always be the most culturally appropriate or responsible.[31] Art therapy operates according to a deficit model of disabled people, in line with the medical model itself, where both frameworks assume something is missing and must therefore be fixed. Yi instead argues for a working definition of disability culture that can expand art therapy. She insists that art therapists need to take a more reflexive approach, and to consider how their own positions in an ableist world might intersect or conflict with their patient's. Furthermore, art therapists need to incorporate disabled people's stories and self-narratives, instead of following the impulse to erase and to correct. Yi concludes that "if art therapists want to embrace a social justice framework informed by a radical social model of care, they will need to become equal partners with the disability culture community and fellow activists, shedding the clinical role of the expert."[32] Yi therefore calls out art therapists for being unknowingly complicit with ableist frameworks akin to their medical practitioner peers in the hospital and clinical health setting. If the overarching imperative is to intervene – whether through surgery or therapy – then this can still bring an oppressive approach to bear on disabled body-minds. This book shows how the powerful expressions of sick, immunocompromised, and disabled artists share their stories as a measure of disability social justice, as an empowering voice and an equalizer with the medical industrial complex, where dialogues about disability are indeed rescripted. It is my hope that this book will build on Yi's excellent scholarship, and that both our work will provide a critical tool for art therapists as they learn how to navigate the needs of their disabled patients.

While I have discussed how these theoretical discourses frame the politics and the art explored in this book, I would be remiss if I didn't acknowledge the philosophy of aesthetics itself, and my decision to use *aesthetics* as an interlocutor in my new critical term, *hospital aesthetics*. Aesthetics is a set of principles that is concerned with the appreciation of beauty in art. The German philosopher Alexander Baumgarten introduced the term in the eighteenth century, and while Baumgarten originally meant aesthetics to apply to the entire realm of sensory experience, over time the term narrowed in its application to a discussion of beauty, and thus the implied function of the visual sense alone, in fine art. I point out this unfortunate theoretical development in the application of aesthetics in my book, *The Agency of Access: Contemporary Disability Art and Institutional Critique*. I suggest that contemporary disability art helps to open up Baumgarten's original definitions of aesthetics again, given the great interest contemporary disability art has in translation, movement, sound, and tactility. Contemporary disability art is sensorial because the disabled body opens channels of the senses that are generative and help to expand sensorial definitions. While my earlier argument is certainly still relevant to this book, the critical concept of hospital aesthetics aims to take us even further. To elaborate on this, I appropriately turn to a construction of aesthetics that is grounded in disability studies, rather than conventional art historical approaches.

I'm indebted to the work of Tobin Siebers, particularly his groundbreaking book *Disability Aesthetics*, published in 2010. Siebers paired the words *disability* and *aesthetics*, and my own term, *hospital aesthetics*, echoes his theoretical move. By pairing my words in the same manner that Siebers did more than ten years ago, I aim to bring a new ontology to aesthetics, as well as to build on Siebers's construction. In *Disability Aesthetics*, Siebers argued that trends in contemporary art brought a much-needed corporeal emotional response to art objects, expanding the definition of aesthetics. He claimed that the disabled body had a large role to play in this, which is much in line with my own previous argument. He states that "disability aesthetics refuses to recognize the representation of the healthy body – and its definition of harmony, integrity, and beauty – as the sole determination of the aesthetic."[33] The disabled body, then, in all its manifestations can be an aesthetic. Thrillingly and by default, it is also clear that the *unhealthy* body is an aesthetic too. And as with Siebers, pairing *aesthetics* with the word *disability* or with the word *hospital* is a contrarian move. As I noted earlier, the two terms rub up against one another. It's exciting. Just as Siebers makes a convincing case for how disability does work to unpack aesthetics, in turn, disability aesthetics does work to unpack the hospital. *Hospital aesthetics* takes into account conventional literal aesthetics of the hospital – scrubs; cold, hard surfaces; hospital beds; medical assistive devices; masks (the *exterior*, if you will) – and shows how the politics of the disabled body can both indulge and plunder these material and epistemological (*interior*) associations. The surfaces and innards of the hospital are necessarily appropriated, used up, and reconstituted by disabled artists who critique the *inhospitable* role it has played and continues to play in disabled people's lives, just as aesthetics itself has been epistemologically rehabilitated by disability. The work by the artists in this book powerfully illustrates how *hospital aesthetics* expands *disability aesthetics*, ultimately demonstrating that the philosophy of aesthetics is porous and has a remarkable capacity to evolve.

Health, hospitality, and healing in the museum

In this section, I further consider how the museum and the hospital might come together: how young medical students are being trained by educators at art museums to take a more humanistic and empathetic approach to patients. Since the COVID-19 pandemic shook the world, the art world has understandably taken a greater interest in health and, by extension, notions of hospitality and healing. This is not least because museums and galleries had to determine a way for visitors to still engage with their programs virtually as their buildings were forced to shut down. When I first started thinking about this book and some of the outcomes I hoped to achieve, I fantasized about approaching Houston-based hospitals (such as Houston Methodist's Center for Performing Arts Medicine) to host some of the artists in this book for short-term residencies. I began to look eagerly for funding opportunities so this could be realized. I wanted to pair the artists, who all have different disabilities, illnesses, and/or immunocompromised conditions, with the various units in the hospital so that they could share their experiences with others through their contemporary art praxis. My goal for these residencies was to offer a new kind of so-called therapeutic experience in the hospital environment, not only for the artists themselves, but also for the patients. Wrapped up in these therapeutic experiences was art-making using unconventional mediums, live performances and events that bring gallery-like programming into the hospital, exhibitions that can take place in hospital rooms and galleries simultaneously, and a shared critique of the hospital experience that may come into tension with traditional art therapies and medical staff. The idea was that artists bring hospitable aesthetics as both a process and a product into the hospital and gallery environment to generate revitalized notions of hospitality, but also to challenge the medical industrial complex itself, which is often at odds with disability studies communities and scholarship. But then I realized that this goal was unrealistic, because the hospital wasn't ready for the types of challenges and critiques I wanted to roll into the hospital, which after all, I was told, is a space for healing, and not a space for agitation. It seemed the only option for me was to continue to use the gallery as a site for critique and display of the hospital, instead of the hospital itself. This realization came as a disappointment, but not as a surprise.

In Irina Aristarkhova's book *Arrested Welcome: Hospitality in Contemporary Art*, I was struck by how the word *welcome*, as it connects to hospitality – and by extension, hospitals – is arrested. Aristarkhova wants us "to be mindful of positionality and inherent inequalities that bear on a claim to welcome."[34] As some of the writings I've discussed above have illustrated, it is important for us to recognize that hospitality is finite, and a line is often drawn regarding who is welcome and under what circumstances. Aristarkhova's discussion of hospitality also leans toward a critique of accommodation, a word that always already resonates with my previous scholarship: I have long stated that the art museum must be more accommodating – and so hospitable – toward disabled artists and audiences. In my edited volume *Curating Access: Disability Art Activism and Creative Accommodation*, forty authors from around the world individually and collectively share case studies for how accommodation can be creatively instigated in the art museum and in the artist's studio. There are also disability studies scholars and artists who contest the word accommodation, noting that disability is not a condition that should be accommodated for, as this indicates an intervention of fixing. This critique is similar to that made by Sandie Yi on art therapy, and to disability studies' entire critique of the medical model of disability. It is important to distinguish that the type of accommodation I am interested in – and this is indeed why I use the phrase *hospital aesthetics* instead of *hospitable aesthetics* – is inextricably tied up with a political outlook. My account of accommodation, in the edited volume and in all the other professional work I do as both a curator and a consultant, is very much rooted in a desire for action and transformation. My previous scholarship and activism then connect to the topic of this book by virtue of its political nature. For this reason, I am an ally of the artists who develop a radical aesthetics of the hospital.

The Finnish contemporary arts organization Frame organized a comprehensive series of programs and publications entitled *Rehearsing Hospitalities*, taking place from 2019 to 2023, which critically examined artistic practices "that are hospitable towards an array of knowledges and ways of knowing; [and] that challenge dominant, singular, and linear forms of knowing."[35] The many texts that have been published under the rubric of this series make clear that hospitality is a complex matter, and has many associations with hierarchies and power dynamics, particularly those originating from capitalism, colonialism, and patriarchy. Yvonne Billimore states:

> More often than not, the rhetoric of host/guest is used as a tool not to include but to divide and reinforce social hierarchies and norms, such as those of gender, class, race, ability and so on. Inscribed in hospitality is hostility. Those who do not follow the house rules or inconvenience its running order are treated as hostile threats and are not welcome. They are not afforded security, safety or care.[36]

These remarks ring especially true in relation to all the artists discussed in this book, and to my own encounters with the medical industry in both personal and professional contexts. Anything that threatens stability and the imperative to cure and to care as defined by the hospital and the state needs to be eliminated, or certainly to stay on the margins. Many philosophers have traced this larger problematic history of how bodies have been subject to questionable medical perceptions and approaches since the eighteenth century, such as Michel Foucault through his concept of the medical gaze, and Francis Galton and eugenics, which has a particularly sinister application to disabled bodies through distinctive periods of history and warfare. Jacques Derrida's seminar series, *Hospitality*, also wrestles with the notion of responsibility to the foreigner, and when we welcome them and when we turn them away.[37] The idea of the foreigner – or the hospital patient or the contemporary disabled artist, as the case may be – can reveal much about friendship, citizenship, migration, assimilation, xenophobia, and ableism. Ultimately, we can conclude that hospitality is finite, and this is especially true within the hospital. Yet we can equally regard hospitality as something capacious, with possibility.

While the gallery similarly cannot offer these unconditional qualities of hospitality owing to its colonialist origins and its ongoing attempts at reparation, the gallery nonetheless is a space that will display work by artists that challenge and critique the institution and the state. From late 2023 to early 2024, the Migros Museum für Gegenwartskunst in Zurich, Switzerland, hosted an interesting exhibition curated by Dr. Michael Birchall entitled *Interdependencies: Perspectives on Care and Resilience*. This exhibition investigated all the themes and ideas that have been prevalent since the pandemic began in 2020. It focused on three models of care – self-care, political care, and collective care – all of which are imbricated and sewn into the work of the artists in this book (some of whom also participated in the Zurich exhibition). One of the participating artists in the Zurich show was British-Kenyan artist Grace Ndiritu, whose recent solo exhibitions have been received with great acclaim by critics and curators around the world. In 2023, Ndiritu had a mid-career survey exhibition at SMAK in Ghent, Belgium, entitled *Healing the Museum*, which presented "spirituality as the impetus for an alternative museology during a time defined by ecological crisis and global conflict."[38] Ndiritu's work is steeped in shamanic studies and suggests that these non-Western methodologies should be radically applied to European institutions. Within Ndiritu's spiritual museology, art moves beyond representation, and instead aims to include and repair.[39] She lays the groundwork for redemption by inviting museums to play host to concepts they have long ignored or excluded. Ndiritu's work is therefore incisive for showing how one host can meet another host head-on in a meaningful exchange and encounter. In other words, museums have reciprocated and hosted Ndiritu's shamanistic hospitality as a welcoming gesture, instead of acting as conventional sites of refusal based on tired colonialist ideologies. Ndiritu's work also demonstrates how the museum's doors are indeed open to rethinking the way it operates, rendering it a hospitable venue for hospital aesthetics now and in the future.

In 2024, Senior Curator Jill Dawsey and former Assistant Curator Isabel Casso curated a comprehensive exhibition for the Museum of Contemporary Art San Diego entitled *For Dear Life: Art, Medicine, and Disability*. It was an ambitious historical and thematic survey covering the period 1965 to the COVID-19 era, and staged work with artists who had/have mental and chronic illness alongside sensory and mobility impairments, and those with HIV/AIDS, cancer, cystic fibrosis, substance abuse disorders, diabetes, and a range of other maladies. The curators wanted to emphasize finding common ground among all these experiences of exclusion, and they were careful not to essentialize similarities among the various forms of illness and impairment. Like me and Birchall, Dawsey has recognized the great visibility of this topic in the current moment, and also acknowledges that all this work was preceded by artists from the 1960s and 1970s who used the body as an artistic medium, including Suzanne Lacy, Lynn Hershman Leeson, and Emory Douglas. Dawsey's interest in curating this exhibition stemmed from her own personal experience of having multiple sclerosis. This connection affirms an observation I made in my 2014 article in *OnCurating*, "Disability, Curating, and the Educational Turn: The Contemporary Condition of Access in the Museum," where I claimed that curators at museums typically take interest in disability arts when they have a personal investment and lived experience with this mode of being.[40] In the article, I suggested that it is typically museum educators who show leadership in thinking through issues of disability for audiences, and I questioned why curators are not collaborating with educators to present and display disability-informed objects, exhibition design, and crip curation. While I think this situation is slowly changing thanks to the recognition that the whole world was "cripped" in the context of the pandemic, there is still a long way to go for museums to host these topics without fear of getting it wrong, or hesitation in consulting disabled communities.

Like the art museum, the field of contemporary art history has also focused more attention on the health humanities. Art historian Suzanne

Hudson is currently working on a new book project entitled *Better for the Making: Art, Therapy, Process*, a study of the therapeutic origins of art-making in American modernism. Like Ray Williams and his work at the Blanton Museum of Art, art historian Siobhan Conaty is interested in how art history produces transferable skills for medicine and the health sciences. Conaty has even used Frida Kahlo as a case study for how applying art history methods can improve nursing education and clinical practice. She also has written papers on the imaging of illness in breast cancer, the connection of work by Käthe Kollwitz to empathy and medical education, and more. Conaty also teaches these topics in the classroom. A precursor to a syllabus on this topic was a class taught by Katherine Sherwood at the University of California, Berkeley, entitled *Art, Medicine, and Disability*, which covered both historical and contemporary work where artists responded to illness, healing, and disability. The first time I ever attended a class on disability arts, it was Katherine's at UC Berkeley in 2012. Megan Voeller is another art historian who has written on the critical intersections of art and health. And in 2020, the Whitechapel Art Gallery released an issue in its Documents of Contemporary Art series titled *Health* that showcases a series of writings by scholars, artists, and art historians reflecting on how the vulnerability of our bodies reveal structural biases in society.

Like Birchall and Dawsey, I have been keen to investigate the rapid proliferation of visual and scholarly frameworks around care that have emerged since the pandemic. I have already mentioned my exhibition *Script/Rescript*, which I curated in fall 2022 and was held at the University Art Gallery at San Diego State University. In spring 2022, I also curated *Crip Ecologies*, which included the work of ten artists who illustrate our complex relationships with medical systems and procedures and are informed by aesthetics of pain and care. This work shines a light on how both our built and natural environments shed toxic matter that disproportionately affects the lives of vulnerable disabled people. The artists, therefore, were advocating for a "crip-ecology" that calls for a greater degree of interdependence and reliance on one another, and a greater sense of responsibility and care toward our landscape. In fall 2023, I curated *Resistance and Respiration* for Contemporary Calgary in Canada. That exhibition included fifteen artists, and I turned to the scholarship of Jean-Thomas Tremblay as inspiration, in his 2022 book, *Breathing Aesthetics*. I considered how breathing as it relates to disabled bodies might stereotypically be associated with "spasmic bodies," with sharp inhales, gasps, gurgling, coughs, and labored muscle contraction, or breathing aided by technological apparatuses. Breathing is particularly fraught in the context of Black bodies and police violence, as well as the physical struggle that became commonplace in the pandemic era. In the context of this exhibition, I was interested in how breathing could offer other physical, metaphorical, and epistemological opportunities to recast the disabled body within a range of respiratory variations. The title of Tremblay's book, *Breathing Aesthetics*, echoes the title of my own book of course, and this is also indicative of how both of our projects (and I'm sure others in the humanities) are attempting to define the output we are witnessing in the current moment. The cumulative focus of all three of my recent exhibitions reinforces the importance of this topic, and also highlights my critical desire to name this artistic activity and action: hospital aesthetics.

Chapter overview

In each of the book's five chapters, I examine two to three artists in detail, while many other artists are briefly mentioned to give more context and thickness to the chapter themes. I have chosen to focus more deeply on some artists and their portfolios than others; it is important that I use specific case studies to demonstrate the persuasiveness of the arguments within each theme and the overarching argument of the book. The supporting artists are nonetheless vitally important, as they illustrate the critical mass of contemporary disabled artists working on these topics, and that the work of the two featured artists in each chapter is not happening in a vacuum or in a silo. Many artists have been compelled to make work about these themes. The reader also needs to be aware that I am examining primarily Anglophone literature. There are many histories that have not come to light or that are not accessible to me because of linguistic barriers.

In each chapter, I provide historical, social, and cultural contexts for each artist and their work, drawing from disability studies, feminism, queer studies, trans studies, and the health humanities at large. The artwork starts in a mode of self-reflection in Chapter 1, moving into showing a greater awareness of objects that can attach and detach from bodies to heal and help with health, mobility, and supposed harmony in Chapter 2. In the center of the book, Chapter 3, we reach a climax (pun intended) where artists are exploring the sexual and sensorial nature of their bodies, defying medical paradigms that otherwise consider disabled bodies to be asexual. As Chapter 3 concludes with the work of Sins Invalid, a collective of performance-based disabled artists, Chapter 4 takes up the mantle of collectives more deeply, exploring the work of feminist-based health collectives in Europe and the USA, and how caring for one another elevates solidarity and support – an affront to the anonymous and clinical nature of the medical industry. The final chapter of the book motions toward solution, albeit alternative solutions through alternative medicine. While alternative medicine, set apart from the state, comes with its share of stigma and taboo owing to its unverified nature, these alternatives show not only a comforting way forward, but also reveal a sense of humor, lightheartedness, and even joy, despite all the challenges. It is these objects that convey another quality and dimension of hospital aesthetics. All the work the reader will witness is proactive, provocative, and telling regarding our bodies and ourselves.

In more detail, in Chapter 1, the contemporary disabled artists that I examine chart the course of their illness in private and quiet modalities such as a pain scale on Instagram and a series of "get well" flowers on a bedside table by Carolyn Lazard, or hospital drawings, sculptures, and performances by Dominic Quagliozzi. I argue that the contemporary artists in this chapter use everyday materials in poetic and transgressive forms to empower sick bodies, and critique the medical system through their own journalistic observations and experiences with the hospital. As viewers of this work, we learn to see get well flowers, a pain scale, or a hospital gown from a completely different perspective, and consider that perhaps these rituals or benign barometers for gleaning degrees of wellness or unwellness deserve further examination for what they convey. In this chapter, I argue that artists perform their illness and their disability as a means by which to empower their bodies in medical settings and procedures, much like artists who came before them, particularly Bob Flanagan, but also others who boldly documented their treatments such as Hannah Wilke and Jo Spence. In Quagliozzi's performances, he directly riffs on Bob Flanagan as an ode to their shared condition of cystic fibrosis. Earlier artist Félix González-Torres used a mattress and pillows with the indents of sleeping heads and candy piles that diminished over time to symbolize the wasting body afflicted by AIDS. The contemporary artists in this chapter follow suit, using everyday materials in expressive and challenging ways to fuel a dialogue on so-called defective, sick, and diseased bodies.

In Chapter 2, I examine how medical objects such as prostheses, wheelchairs, canes, and X-rays can become personalized in revised forms; these forms are laced with thoughtful and warm engagements with bodies, in contrast to the ways these items are typically issued in the sterile environment of the doctor's office. Berlin-based artist Jesse Darling uses braces to make his props comical, surreal, and bizarre. Bhavna Mehta turns to X-rays as a canvas for her textile and embroidery-based practice, using needle and threads to create intricate patterns directly on the X-ray. I examine these artists by gesturing toward Katherine Sherwood's paintings as a backdrop and historical precedent. This includes her X-rays of her brain after a stroke and her appropriations of canonical nudes such as *Sleeping Venus* by seventeenth- and eighteenth-century white male artists, equipping these nude figures with canes and braces woven across their limbs. This chapter builds on the argument made in Chapter 1, showing how impersonal medical tools become personalized and imbued with the stories, memories, and archives of the disabled user. Here, a more fervent and literal script/rescript is taking place.

Chapter 3 builds on the energy from the first two chapters to present the most overt and boldest expression of hospital aesthetics. I analyze the work of several artists who explore sexuality and sensuality using the hospital as an interface for encountering sex that would otherwise be taboo. They work to debunk the assumptions that disabled people do not and cannot have intercourse, revealing the medical system's inability to see disabled people as whole people. The artists I examine here include Panteha Abareshi, Robert Andy Coombs, and the performance collective Sins Invalid. Panteha Abareshi performs mostly nude, wrapped in white bandages as she straddles and drapes her body across and through walkers, crutches, and other supportive devices. This signals a revised relationship to prosthetic medical devices that seems more sexually empowered and provocative than asexual or mechanical. The artists in this chapter use the mediums of photography and performance to explore eroticism, fetish, intimacy, and intensity. I argue that their work is contributing to a new form of hospital aesthetics that is a far cry from the docile and monotonous veneer of the hospital. Instead, these artists strip the hospital of its unrealistic views of sex and disability by being disruptive, playful, and uncompromising in both their sexual desires and a larger desire to overturn stereotypes.

Chapter 4 examines what happens when disabled people work collaboratively to refute the medical system. Building on the discussion of the collective work of Sins Invalid from Chapter 3, I argue that disabled, chronically ill, and immunocompromised women artists are formally gathering together to support one another, mentally, physically, and culturally, as a more collaborative form of hospital aesthetics that is tied to "dialogic aesthetics." This was a term originally developed by art historian Grant Kester. My concept builds on Kester's ideas through a disability justice lens: hospital aesthetics in this context is specifically a dialogue on disability and radical health. The feminist collectives I examine include the Feminist Health Care Research Group (FHCRG), the Sickness Affinity Group (SAG), Power Makes Us Sick (PMS), and Black Womxn Flourish.

In Chapter 5, I focus once again, as I did in Chapter 1, on a quieter form of hospital aesthetics, but now I show how contemporary disabled artists are finding solutions for the application and ingestion of medicine in comical and empowering ways. I examine how contemporary disabled artists lean into alternative medicine and therapies for self-medication, pain management, and more. Such therapies might include massage, acupuncture, t'ai chi, and medical marijuana. While alternative medicine can also be defined as integrative or complementary medicine in line with more mainstream treatments for ailing health, in this case, I argue that disabled artists are truly using alternative medicines as a political means to refute mainstream attitudes to correcting disabled bodies and body-minds. The artists I examine in this chapter include Lauryn Youden, Carmen Papalia, Maryam Jafri, and Sharona Franklin.

In the conclusion, I summarize the key findings of the book. The work of the contemporary disabled artists discussed contributes to a new visual language and culture of hospital aesthetics that documents, questions, and critiques medical industrial systems of care within a capitalist regime. Their practices are firmly ensconced within contemporary scholarship and rhetoric around the importance of collective care, interdependency, and how disabled life can contribute to new understandings of access. This new generation of contemporary disabled artists fold their disabled identities seamlessly into their art practice, where the struggle between the medical model and the social model of disability provides a conceptual framework alongside age-old philosophical iterations on the ethics of care. As the artists navigate the politics of visibility and standards of productivity, perhaps in the wake of the COVID-19 pandemic, when the entire world was seemingly "cripped," society will place less emphasis on the ideal of a self-reliant individual and instead realize we are all in fact interdependent and reliant on care of each other.

Notes

1 For more on disability and staring, see Rosemarie Garland-Thomson, *Staring: How We Look* (Oxford: Oxford University Press, 2009).
2 Alice Wong, "Alice Wong on Hospitalization, Crowdfunding Medical Care, and Finding Love in Community," *Teen Vogue*, February 14, 2023, www.teenvogue.com/story/alice-wong-hospitalization-crowdfunding-community [accessed December 5, 2024].
3 For more information, see Riva Lehrer, *Golem Girl* (New York: Penguin Random House, 2020); and Alice Wong, *Year of the Tiger: An Activist's Life* (New York: Vintage, 2022).
4 Ruth Slavin, Ray Williams, and Corinne Zimmermann, eds, *Activating the Art Museum: Designing Experiences for the Health Professions* (New York: Rowman & Littlefield, 2023).
5 Caroline Goeser, interview with the author on Teams, March 5, 2024.
6 Perri Meldon, "Disability History: Early and Shifting Attitudes of Treatment," National Park Service, www.nps.gov/articles/disabilityhistoryearlytreatment.htm [accessed December 9, 2023].
7 Catherine Kudlick, "Comment: On the Borderland of Medical and Disability History," *Bulletin of the History of Medicine* 87, no. 4 (Winter 2013): 540–59. https://doi.org/10.1353/bhm.2013.0086
8 Kudlick, "Comment."
9 Kudlick, "Comment."
10 David T. Mitchell and Sharon L. Snyder, dirs., *Vital Signs: Crip Culture Talks Back* (Brooklyn, NY: Icarus Films, 1995), video, 48 minutes.
11 Sandahl is now a professor and head of the Program on Disability Art, Culture, and Humanities at the University of Illinois Chicago.
12 David T. Mitchell and Sharon L. Snyder, "Talking About Talking Back: Afterthoughts on the Making of the Disability Documentary *Vital Signs: Crip Culture Talks Back*," *Michigan Quarterly Review* 37, no. 2 (Spring 1998), http://hdl.handle.net/2027/spo.act2080.0037.216 [accessed December 5, 2024].
13 Sunaura Taylor, "Statement," Wynn Newhouse Awards, www.wnewhouseawards.com/sunaurataylor2.html [accessed December 9, 2023].
14 Sunaura Taylor, "What Would Health Security Look Like?," *Boston Review*, May 28, 2020, www.bostonreview.net/articles/sunaura-taylor-title-forthcoming [accessed December 5, 2024].

15 Taylor, "Health Security."
16 Joseph Grigely, "Cripping the World," email to his SAIC students, shared by Corbett O'Toole with permission, Facebook post, April 24, 2020.
17 Ezra Benus quoted in Zachary Small, "For Chronically Ill Artists, Coronavirus is the Worst-Case Scenario," *ARTnews*, March 13, 2020, www.artnews.com/art-news/artists/coronavirus-artists-chronic- illnesses-resources-1202681100 [accessed December 5, 2024].
18 Dodie Bellamy, *When the Sick Rule the World* (Cambridge, MA: MIT Press, 2015).
19 Abi Palmer, *Sanatorium* (London: Penned in the Margins, 2020).
20 Eva Feder Kittay, *Love's Labor: Essays on Women, Equality, and Dependency* (New York: Routledge, 1999).
21 Leah Lakshmi Piepzna-Samarasinha, *Care Work: Dreaming Disability Justice* (Vancouver: Arsenal Pulp Press, 2018), chap. 1, Kindle.
22 Piepzna-Samarasinha, *Care Work*, chap. 1.
23 Julie Avril Minich, "Introduction: Radical Health/Radical Unwellness," in *Radical Health: Unwellness, Care, and Latinx Expressive Culture* (Durham, NC: Duke University Press, 2023), 1–23.
24 Sami Schalk, *Black Disability Politics* (Durham, NC: Duke University Press, 2022).
25 James Kyung-Jin Lee, *Pedagogies of Woundedness: Illness, Memoir, and the Ends of the Model Minority* (Philadelphia, PA: Temple University Press, 2021).
26 Joseph A. Stramondo, "A Critique of the Curative Imperative," *Surgery* 171, no. 4 (2020): 1121–22, www.surgjournal.com/article/S0039-6060(21)00966-1/abstract [accessed December 27, 2024].
27 Stramondo, "Curative Imperative," 1121–22.
28 Stramondo, "Curative Imperative," 1121–22.
29 Chun-Shan (Sandie) Yi, "Res(crip)ting Art Therapy: Disability Culture as a Social Justice Intervention," in *Art Therapy for Social Justice: Radical Intersections*, ed. Savneet K. Talwar (New York: Routledge, 2019), 161–77.
30 Yi, "Res(crip)ting Art Therapy," 161–77.
31 Yi, "Res(crip)ting Art Therapy," 161–77.
32 Yi, "Res(crip)ting Art Therapy," 161–77.
33 Tobin Siebers, *Disability Aesthetics* (Ann Arbor, MI: University of Michigan Press, 2010), 3.
34 Irina Aristarkhova, *Arrested Welcome: Hospitality in Contemporary Art* (Minneapolis, MN: University of Minnesota Press, 2020).
35 Yvonne Billimore, "Introduction: Matter(s) of Security," in *Rehearsing Hospitalities Companion 3*, ed. Yvonne Billimore and Jussi Koitela (Berlin: Archive Books, 2022), 13–29.
36 Billimore, "Introduction: Matter(s) of Security," 13–29.
37 Jacques Derrida, *Hospitality*, Vol. 1, trans. E. S. Burt, ed. Pascale-Anne Brault and Peggy Kamuf (Chicago, IL: University of Chicago Press, 2023).
38 Ella Slater, "Grace Ndiritu Heals the Museum," *Frieze*, April 24, 2023, www.frieze.com/article/grace-ndiritu-heals-museum-review-2023 [accessed December 5, 2024].
39 Slater, "Grace Ndiritu."
40 For more information, see Amanda Cachia, "Disability, Curating, and the Educational Turn: The Contemporary Condition of Access in the Museum," *OnCurating* 24 (December 2014), www.on-curating.org/issue-24-reader/disability-curating-and-the-educational-turn-the-contemporary-condition-of-access-in-the-museum.html [accessed December 5, 2024].

1

Charting immunocompromised bodies

A transformer may not be the first image one associates with a body affected by cystic fibrosis (CF), but contemporary disabled artist Dominic Quagliozzi compellingly makes this connection for us. Quagliozzi makes work that is informed by his lived experience with CF and as a recipient of a double lung transplant. While CF's effects on the body are often uncontrollable to the person inhabiting it, in Quagliozzi's Untitled (Transformers) series developed in 2022 (see Figure 1.1), he not only loosely documents the changes in his body through these abstract hybrid paintings/sculptures, but also provides himself with talismans through which to channel change that is self-empowering, and indeed which he is more able to control.

In the series, fabrics made from blue and green hospital gowns with a familiar medical motif are stretched over support frames in place of canvas and hung on the wall. On the left and right sides of the frames are wood-block arms, also wrapped with the same hospital gown fabric, that fold at various points on hinges. They are pliable and flexible under the fingers of audiences, who are invited to play with the transformers to render them into potentially unending new shapes and forms. Much like the original transformers (Hasbro's 1980s children's toys), these "bodies" can be transformed to imitate the gestures, folds, joints, and creases of human bodies. Perhaps, in this titling act, Quagliozzi lightens the gravity of his medical condition. That viewers can engage with the work may be a commentary on our complicity in his condition. On a symbolic level, transformers also showcases how a body with CF shifts and transforms over time as organs lose strength and typical operation. Having spent a great deal of time in hospital settings, Quagliozzi has also embraced the materials of the hospital, from the hospital gowns that feature in his transformers to the tissue paper used on examination tables, with which he renders beautiful graphic illustrations such as rainbows that float and flutter under small magnetic pins attached to the wall. In using the quotidian

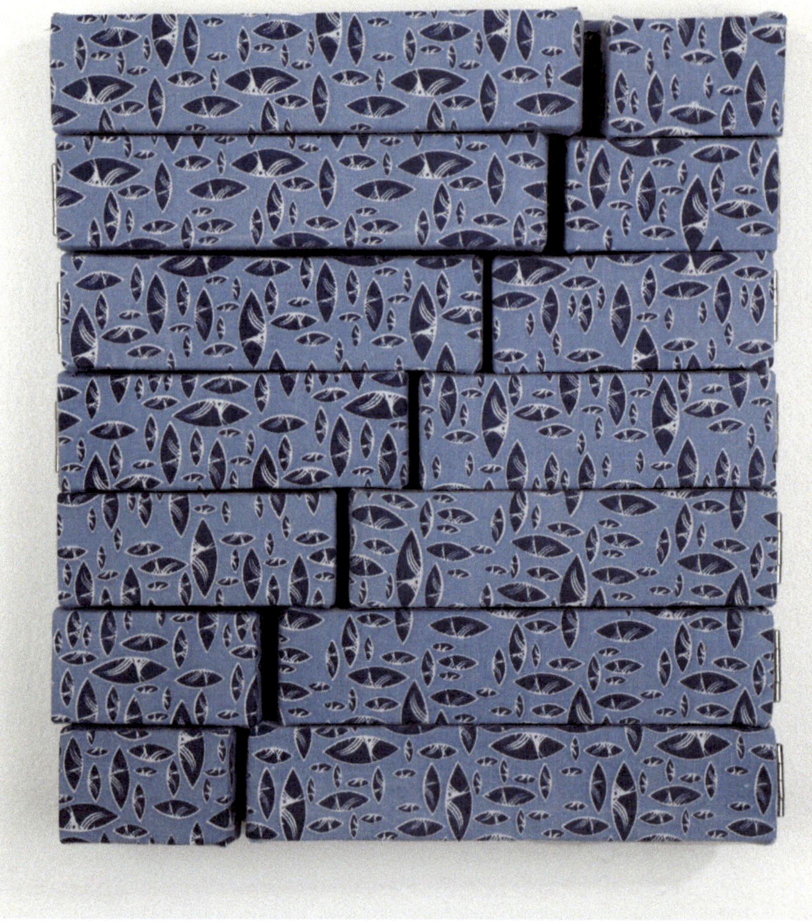

1.1 Dominic Quagliozzi, *Transformer (Blue Cyclops)*, 2022. Hospital gown, hinges on wood, 11.5 × 10.5 in. (29 × 27 cm) (closed). Courtesy of the artist.

Image description 1.1: A photograph of a blue sculpture which resembles a vertically oriented rectangular canvas that is composed of horizontal slats. These slats are covered in blue recycled hospital gown fabric and staggered in size, strategically creating a diagonal from the top right to the bottom left of the composition.

materials of the hospital gown, which Quagliozzi admits are sometimes stolen, or taken with permission when deemed out of commission by a hospital, he aims to make the familiar unfamiliar. Once decontextualized as works of art on a wall, these materials become humorous, heartwarming, and emptied of the vacant anonymity of rows of rooms full of hospital bodies lined up and down long hallways. Indeed, the hospital gown has been reconstituted into a hospital aesthetics.

This chapter explores how contemporary disabled artists have been "charting" their immunocompromised and disabled bodies. I adopt the verb "charting" in the chapter title from medical terminology, where hospital patients each have a chart of their ailments and diagnoses maintained by doctors. In the context of this work, it is the artists that are charting their own bodies instead of medical personnel. I will first study in detail Quagliozzi's work, which deconstructs his lived experience with chronic illness and disability through various media, including drawing, painting, photography, and performance. Using medical materials, he references new constructions of the body through both its presence and absence. By repurposing and recoding these materials into art, he explores the emotional and psychological moments of vulnerability, anxiety, fragility, and resilience experienced during hospital stays and while managing illness. I argue that Quagliozzi's work extends the imperative of decolonizing the gallery into the act of decolonizing the hospital; Quagliozzi opposes the tendency for the medical industrial complex to treat disabled bodies as specimens and, eventually, archives. Instead, his hospital aesthetics shows a different side to disabled bodies, aiming to undo the social and cultural impacts the hospital has had on its disabled patients, both historically and in the contemporary moment. In the second half of the chapter, I explore works by Carolyn Lazard, including a pain scale and a series of "get well" flowers on a bedside table. I argue that both of these contemporary artists use everyday materials in poetic and transgressive forms to empower sick bodies, and critique the medical system through their own observations and experiences with the hospital. As viewers of this work, we learn to see get well flowers, a pain scale, or a hospital gown in a different light, and to consider that perhaps these rituals or benign barometers for gleaning degrees of wellness or unwellness deserve further examination for what they convey.

The chapter also wrestles with an important politic that I addressed in the Introduction: that the way disabled and sick bodies are treated in the hospital varies based on gender, race, and class. Racism is disabling, gender is disabling, and so on, regardless of impairment itself. On a material level, this means that racist and sexist actions can be the cause of an acquired disability. A Black person's health can get worse owing to grave misdiagnosis by the white medical apparatus or a medical practitioner who dismisses a Black person's request for access to care. This is one of my main motivations in writing this book. It is not only about the disabled artist's desire to share their unsatisfactory experiences of the medical system and to find ways to restore their empowered identities as sick and disabled artists using hospital ephemera. This book also aims to share how rampant the intersecting acts of ableism, racism, and sexism are in the medical industry. The two artists this chapter focuses on exemplify these intersections. The first, Quagliozzi, is a disabled artist with CF who matter-of-factly understands his privilege as a young, white, conventionally attractive man with access to financial resources that help him navigate the medical system. The second artist, Lazard, is a Black disabled artist who has written about medical challenges and the stigma of race entwined with disability for the past decade. As the reader peels through their stories in this chapter, many layers of complexity will emerge, showing how the intersection of these identities play out in the artists' lives and in their artworks. By understanding these dynamics, the reader will better understand the work itself. As these artists chart immunocompromised bodies through their artwork, they also chart the implications of race, gender, and privilege, either overtly or with more subtle acknowledgment. These intersections are bound up in hospital aesthetics, which demands a diversity of perspectives on disability.

I start the chapter by discussing three distinct bodies of work produced by Quagliozzi at different periods during the last decade. In the middle of the chapter, I pause to introduce some philosophical and historical background on the origins of the medical gaze, the importance of the illness memoir, and why this work matters in a disability context. Then in the second half of the chapter I discuss five sets of work produced by Carolyn Lazard, examining how their politics is necessarily charged with racial overtones and a call for disability justice at every turn.

The hospital as an art studio

Dominic Quagliozzi received his Master of Fine Art (MFA) in Studio Art and painting from California State University in Los Angeles, and has shown his work in multiple solo and group exhibitions across the USA, Canada, and Australia. I will discuss three works by the artist, including *The Hospital Show* (2013), *Hospital Suit* (2019), and *Untitled (Transformers)* (2022). Quagliozzi lives and works in Massachusetts. During a particularly long stay in hospital in 2013, he started to use the hospital as if it were an artist's studio. He frequently talks about his hospital room as a surrogate art studio, because for CF patients who grew up in the 1980s and 1990s like Quagliozzi did, there were no preventative or prophylactic measurements or treatments for CF at the time, as it was a relatively underresearched disease. So patients lived their life, and when they had lung infections they would end up in hospital for weeks for intravenous (IV) antibiotics and undergoing airway clearance. Cystic fibrosis is a disorder that damages the lungs, liver, kidneys, pancreas, and intestines. It typically affects the cells in the body that produce bodily fluids such as mucus, sweat, and digestive juices. The symptoms of CF include persistent cough, lung infections, and problems with breathing and digestion. It can also impact longevity. Quagliozzi would have chronic lung infections two to three times a year, and he would be in the hospital for two weeks at a time. So he spent a lot of time in the hospital, which is where he started making art. He particularly wanted to start painting so he could identify as somebody other than just a sick person. Nurses and doctors, family and friends would visit, and they would see the artwork he was creating, so eventually he started to build this identity as an artist. At that point, his two identities as an artist and a sick person became intertwined.

Quagliozzi treated one particular stint in hospital as if it was an artist's residency, and the culmination of his stay would be an exhibition in his hospital room. The first week of his stay involved making the actual work, which used gouache on watercolor paper. He wanted to explore themes of human emotions and functions that are acceptable within the hospital walls but that aren't necessarily acceptable outside them. In some of the images, Quagliozzi depicted a simplistic, pared-down abstract figure in black wash paint, performing different actions and in different embodied states related to spending time in the hospital. He made eight to ten quick portraits as a kind of impression. He mixed his colors with Purell hand sanitizer instead of water, as this was plentifully available in his room. Every time someone came into his room, they would have to pump out the Purell and use it as a precautionary measure to avoid cross-contamination. Quagliozzi thought it was appropriate to use Purell as his part-medium of choice, contributing to his version of hospital aesthetics. Further, as CF is a respiratory disease, professionals who enter the room must also wear an isolation gown, a mask, and gloves to ensure that CF patients are protected from airborne illness, viruses, or bacteria. The way the medical professionals were covered up to both protect themselves and to protect him gave Quagliozzi a fragmented visual experience of these individuals, which served to reinforce the typical feeling of detachment stemming from a medical personnel encounter. The artist says, "So, I was only seeing the people that were coming into my room from the nose up. I am dealing with fragmented bodies and faces, but they are doing intimate things to me. They are measuring my blood pressure, taking my temperature, touching me, helping me dress and undress."[1] These visceral experiences framed the artist's aesthetic choices as he developed his drawings, in which the abstraction represented his inability to form detailed embodied features of the doctors and nurses.

In one drawing, the figure has a rash. In another, the figure has a bruise from a blown IV site. In another, called *Blood*, the figure is lying down with a big red blob connected to his arm (see Figure 1.2). In others, the figure is peeing yellow (titled *Piss*), or the figure is holding two big black bricks or walls, and he looks as though he is pushing them out. This is meant to symbolize a struggle with stress and anxiety. The artist was deploying this simple yet powerful iconography to project heavy concepts of mental and physical anguish, trauma, and bodily sensations.

For Quagliozzi, the process of working through those feelings in the artwork gave him agency over the fact that he was being listed for a transplant. The materiality of his body was being taken to another level.

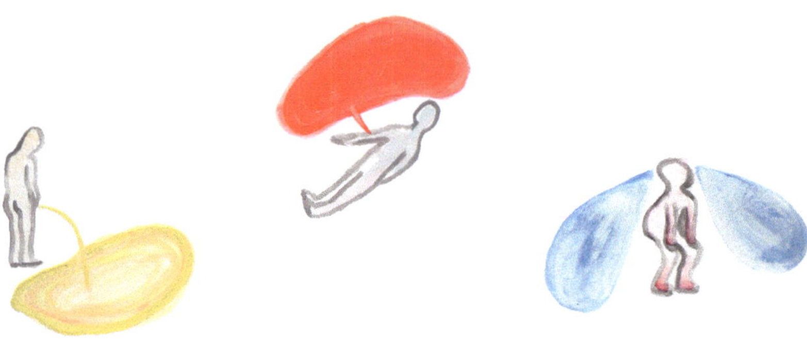

1.2 Dominic Quagliozzi, (left to right) *Piss*, *Blood*, and *Cry*, all 2013. Gouache on paper, 15 × 11 in. (38 × 28 cm). Courtesy of the artist.

Image description 1.2: A gouache painting of 3 gray figures with no facial features. Each figure is straight-sized, hairless, and has two arms and legs. The figure on the left stands with their back towards us as a stream of yellow arches outward from where their genitals might be and pools around their feet. The central figure lies on their back with their right arm extending toward an oblong splotch of red. The figure on the right has their hands resting on their bent knees. Two enormous droplets of blue fall from either side of their head.

By this, Quagliozzi means that before the lung transplant he was treated for infections with IVs. This was something he was used to and that he could handle in a matter-of-fact way. But the notion of the looming lung transplant was different; this was about taking parts of his body out and putting parts of somebody else's body inside of him. It was an entirely new existential situation that he was trying to figure out how to cope with.

After the first week of creating the works on paper, Quagliozzi made a press release announcing the opening of his show in his hospital room. He treated the press release like a work of art in and of itself, like a print (and somebody purchased it during the opening of the show). It used the hospital letterhead and included all the details of the opening (Figure 1.3).

He used the press release in the same way a gallery would to publicize an exhibition. However, instead of including an artist biography, which is part of the conventional template of an exhibition press release, he included his entire medical history. And in place of a dated list of all the exhibitions his work had been shown in, he provided details of all his hospital stays, his medical procedures, the diseases he had had, and the types of insurance he owned. So while the artist was reclaiming his identity as a sick person

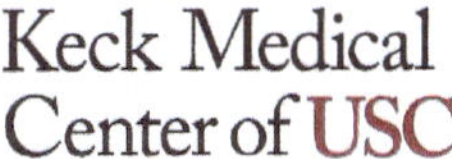
Keck Medical Center of USC

Keck Hospital of USC
USC Norris Cancer Hospital

The Hospital Show
Dominic Quagliozzi

April 10- 13, 2013
Opening Reception: Wednesday April 10, 7-9 PM.
By Appointment: April 11-13, call (323-442-8871)

KECK Hospital of USC
1500 San Pablo St
Los Angeles, CA 90033
PATIENT ROOM 800

The Hospital Show is new work by Dominic Quagliozzi made exclusively while inpatient (Artist In Residence) at Keck Hospital of USC. The new works range from drawings, paintings, limited edition prints and video art. He explores notions of health and well-being through visual, formal, and color arrangements. There are also drawings of people pissing and shitting.

Over the past 5 days, Dominic Quagliozzi has been making new works with limited materials, but an abundance of time. There have been some art materials, some medical stuff, some proper drug use, many minutes of thinking, looking, waiting, drawing, some coughing, nurses, doctors, flowers. Just come and see some art.

The Hospital Show explores the boundaries of what an alternative art space can be. Get a painting or limited edition hand signed print. It's on a Wednesday night, and visiting hours don't end til 10PM!

Dominic Quagliozzi lives and works Los Angeles, CA. He has had Cystic Fibrosis for 30 years and is currently listed for a double lung transplant. He has been a patient at Keck Hospital of USC for the last 6 years. He has been a patient at UMass Hospital in Worcester, MA, Boston Children's Hospital, Brigham and Women's Hospital in Boston, MA. Some notable medical procedures he's had are hernia surgery, partial left lung lower lobectomy, sinus polypectomy, and three pulmonary embolizations. In 2004, he was in a coma for 5 days after developing pneumonia from unknowingly inhaling a dime sized piece of steak. He is currently insured by GHPP and Medicare.

PARKING: Metered parking available on Norfolk St./ San Pablo St.

University of Southern California
1500 San Pablo Street , Los Angeles, California 90033 • Tel: 323 442 8522 • Fax: 323 442 8415

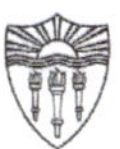

1.3 Press release from Dominic Quagliozzi's *The Hospital Show* at Keck Medical Center of USC, April 10–13, 2013.

Image description 1.3: An invitation to "The Hospital Show", new work by Dominic Quagliozzi. The invitation is printed on "Keck Medical Center of USC" letter head and formulated to look like a very formal letter.

in order to become an artist, he was also challenging the status quo of "artist" so that his identity as a patient with a lengthy medical history was centered in gallery and exhibition ephemera; the sick part of his identity informed the show more deeply than where he had exhibited before, or where he went to graduate school to get his MFA. Thus, Quagliozzi's hospital show became a recognition of that intertwined artist–patient identity that coexisted in his mind.

Quagliozzi saw the opening reception as a social action (see Figure 1.4). While visitors were coming to the event to see his drawings and paintings, which were hung in orderly fashion on the hospital room walls around his bed, they also had to go through a process to get to his room in the first place. This consisted of checking in at the front desk of the hospital, obtaining a visitor's badge, and snaking one's way through a labyrinth of hallways, rooms, elevators, and stairs to get to his room. Quagliozzi enjoyed the fact that, as a sort of psychological choreography, visitors had to negotiate the same process that he frequently has to deal with as a patient. He saw this as an equivalent of the hoops that an artist must jump through to become qualified, such as navigating art school bureaucracy and getting a degree.

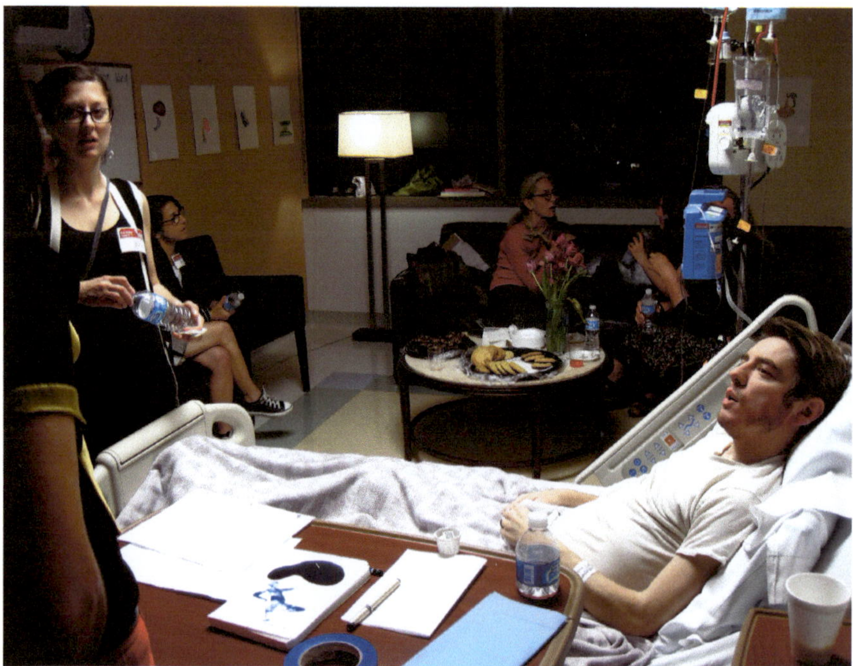

1.4 Dominic Quagliozzi engaging with visitors during the opening of *The Hospital Show* at Keck Medical Center of USC, April 10–13, 2013. Courtesy of the artist.

Image description 1.4: A man lays in a hospital bed at an incline talking to a small group of people.

Quagliozzi's desire to thrust his visitors into his shoes also stems from the natural feelings of alienation and otherness arising from being a sick person. While his peers from art school were experiencing success and recognition in the art world, Quagliozzi was in hospital waiting for a lung transplant. Further, Quagliozzi was professionally shunned for his artwork itself; this work, which centered around his medical experiences, was not considered suitable or palatable material by the for-profit art world. These experiences drove Quagliozzi's decision to show his work in a hospital rather than an art gallery. By virtue of being an unofficial hospital artist in residence, he was able to find an audience and a reception for this work, where fellow patients could intimately understand what it means to be sick. For nonpatients, his aim was for the process of navigating the labyrinth of the hospital to help contextualize and frame an understanding of his work, sans the trauma. When visitors finally found their way through the maze of hospital corridors, not only did Quagliozzi have artwork and catered food to offer them, but they were also confronted with the artist himself, who was propped up in his hospital bed, wearing his hospital gown, ready to say hello. This experience is different to what one might typically find after navigating the labyrinth of the hospital, where one would come upon a sick person and not much else.

Quagliozzi's work has a natural affinity with Bob Flanagan's work through the element of retrieving agency for the patient. Like Quagliozzi, Flanagan also had cystic fibrosis. He documented his experiences with his illness through his infamous *Pain Journal*, a documentary, and countless performances captured on video in partnership with his lover, Sheree Rose. One of the most recognized and memorable exhibitions by Flanagan and Rose was the 1992–95 retrospective *Visiting Hours*, which was held at the Santa Monica Museum of Art in 1992, followed by the New Museum in New York in 1994, and what was then known as the Boston Center for Fine Art in 1995 (see Figure 1.5). Similar to Quagliozzi's installation, with *Visiting Hours* visitors were invited to engage with Flanagan while he was a patient in a hospital bed. However, while Flanagan brought his literal hospital room into the gallery, where it functioned as if it were a real hospital room, Quagliozzi was bringing visitors directly to the source, ground zero – the hospital itself. Flanagan also brought more theatricality to his installation, and in some respects his was a more sanitized version of CF and the hospital experience than Quagliozzi's because Flanagan used a stage, while Quagliozzi used the real hospital. Nonetheless, Quagliozzi admits that Flanagan's work was a huge influence on him, and that he found his work powerful and transformative.

Performance artist Martin O'Brien, who has also noted that his work is greatly indebted to Flanagan's practice through his literally and symbolically baring all as a sick person, has written about the connection between Flanagan and Quagliozzi. Both artists commingle art and life as if they were one and the same, and both desire to show the body in pain, the body suffering, and

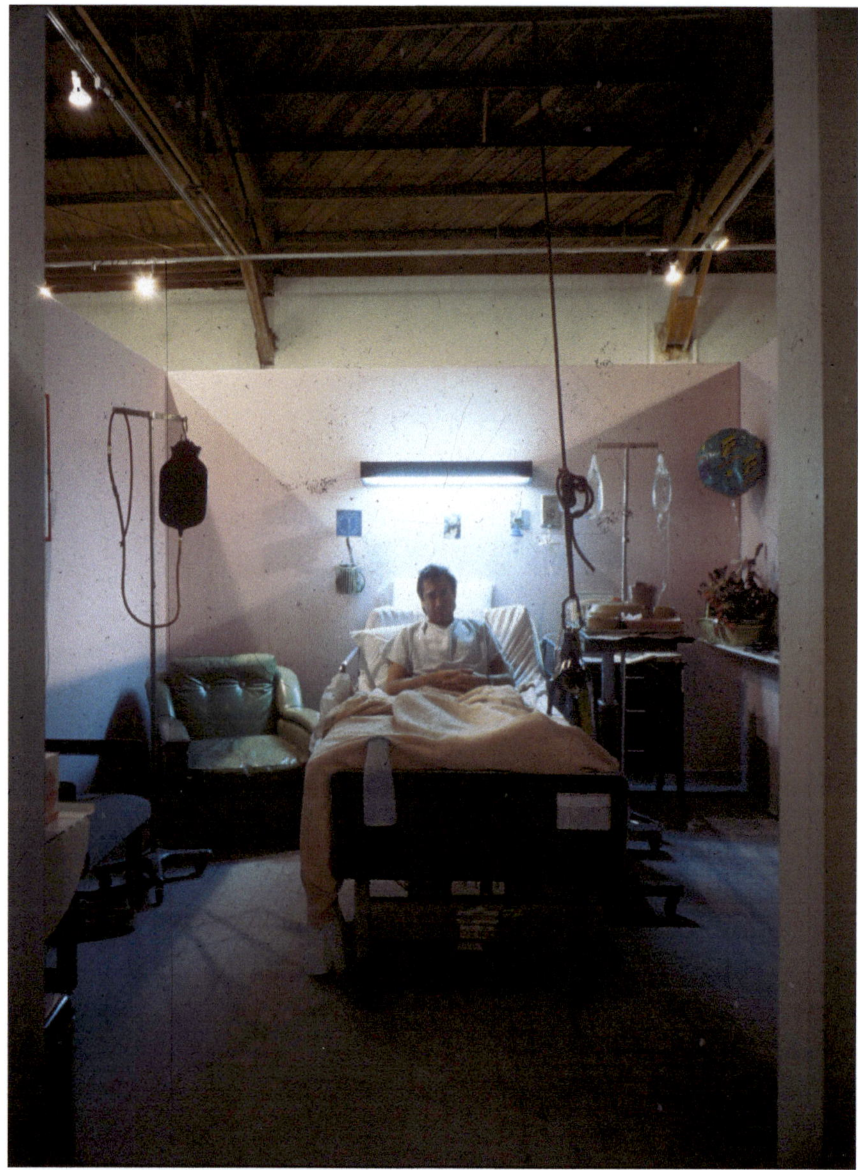

1.5 Installation view, Bob Flanagan and Sheree Rose: *Visiting Hours*, Santa Monica Museum of Art (now Institute of Contemporary Art, Los Angeles), December 4, 1992–January 17, 1993. Image courtesy of SMMoA. Photograph: Sheree Rose.

Image description 1.5: A man sitting up in a hospital bed with his hands folded on his stomach. Three walls surround him decorated to look like a hospital room.

the body enduring. O'Brien also pointed out that both artists explicitly play with the "relationship between the aesthetic and the medical,"[2] analyzing in particular the motif of the hospital bed and its semiotics of sickness, illness, and death. Flanagan and Quagliozzi are fully aware of these tropes of the hospital bed, and how the bed puts the patient in a position of submission and vulnerability where they must endure and wait for their treatment, "a role that is far from active."[3] The hospital bed is a tool with which to ensure the patient is under the full control of the medical establishment, and firmly places the individual within the strictures of the "patient" role. O'Brien discusses how both Flanagan/Rose and Quagliozzi draw attention to sickness, and "the ways in which our bodies are subjugated in the name of health. By presenting their body/life/experience as art work they are able to reclaim the hospital bed as a site of personal-political agency."[4] They reclaim the submission of their body so that they control whom they are submitting their body to, along with when and where. They change the context, the presentation, and even the destination.

Yet, interestingly, Quagliozzi has noted that his work is not a protest. To be sure, he still experiences challenges from time to time – a fight to access his life-saving medications each year, filing appeals to reinstate his insurance, etc. – but these are not the main impetus behind his art-making. He asserts that he doesn't necessarily have an antagonistic relationship with the medical industry, and that his work is not overtly political. Rather, he is fluent in the language of this industry because he is so used to it. This does not negate his desire to reclaim agency as a patient. To complicate this desire, I was struck by Quagliozzi's acute awareness of his white privilege within the medical establishment, including the fact that he was able to stage an exhibition of his work in his hospital room in the first place. (Indeed, Quagliozzi's "fluency" in the medical system and his awareness of that fluency also stems from his privilege.) He admits that not all patients would be able to stage exhibitions in their hospital rooms, and that he was able to maintain a relationship with doctors, nurses, and social workers over time, built on mutual trust and care. Not everyone has access to those relationships, let alone the healthcare itself. He notes his guilt at the knowledge that he has been treated very well in the medical system, and he's certain that this is because he is a young, white man who shows a high degree of compliance. Quagliozzi said he rarely challenges his care team, nor does he question their decisions regarding his health – attributes that he knows are favored by doctors. He speculates that perhaps he does this as a survival mechanism, but he also admits that he has an inherently high level of trust in the medical system, and he is privileged to have a support system and a network to help him. Perhaps it is this recognition of privilege that sets Quagliozzi apart from Flanagan.

In an in-depth interview I staged with Quagliozzi about his work, he explained to me that his childhood experiences during the 1970s and 1980s influenced his adult preoccupations as an artist. He recalls that doctors' discussions about people with CF tended to focus on life expectancy. He would overhear conversations between his parents and the doctors about how long he might have to live, and he experienced severe panic attacks when he was 6, 7, or 8 years old. Unable to sleep or awakened by nightmares, he would hop out of his bed and go downstairs to find his parents, screaming or bawling his eyes out. He would confront his mom and tell her that he had overheard her talking on the phone and telling someone he was not going to live, or that he had a shortened life expectancy. Another early experience that Quagliozzi continues to grapple with was the ableist expectation of being present. In the context of Quagliozzi's life, this meant a presence in school, something the artist found difficult to maintain given his constant stays in hospital. He recalls that his elementary school held an award ceremony for attendance – if you didn't miss one day of school, you received an award at the end of the year. The existence of this award imparted a sense that there was something inherent inside of him that wouldn't allow him to win it. Quagliozzi realized he had internalized these negative feelings; since that time, he has attempted to be present as much as possible, often to the detriment of his health. He would forgo or delay going into hospital for an extra week or an extra two weeks and become even sicker. His lungs would get worse but he would push through. CF is an invisible illness, and Quagliozzi was always trying to keep it that way.

In addition to how Quagliozzi's hospital aesthetics connects to his childhood experiences with sickness, his work also taps into healing, with all its complexities that the artist has dealt with as an adult. While his eventual lung transplant eight years ago gave him a new lung and a new chance at life, it also gave him a whole new set of health problems: he still needs to go to the doctor's office once a month, he has diabetes and chronic kidney disease because of the transplant, and he will likely need a kidney transplant in a few years, which will involve dialysis and a host of other challenges. Art-making, then, is about making his hospital experience more palatable and interesting, and is also tinged with an element of desperation and survival. Quagliozzi also enjoyed the limitations of using his hospital room like an art studio. The hospital room is not equipped with the same materials and tools as a conventional studio. He likens this to the limitations of his embodied condition, to CF itself. Thus, maneuvering within and overcoming challenges informs his artistic process, materials, and his hospital aesthetics too.

The evolution of a hospital gown

Quagliozzi has been using the hospital gown as a medium and a message in his artwork for ten years. For him, the hospital gown is a physical and emotional residue of bodies and transformational moments. It started when he came out of a four-day coma, upon which he asked his wife to remove the hospital gown that he had worn throughout the coma from the soiled linen bin. As the artist looked over the gown, he saw drips of blood, mucus, and many folds, rolls, and sweat marks, which looked like a drawing to him. He cut it up and mounted it onto 16 × 20 in. stretcher bars so the material became a substitute for canvas to be painted on. Quagliozzi has had mixed experiences with hospitalization: some very positive ones, and some very negative ones. He wanted to use the hospital gown to express this range of possibilities. He also treated the hospital gown as Japanese conceptual artist On Kawara treated his paintings, writing the date of every day as a measure of human existence. The gown would trace the days of his individuated existence in the hospital through the record of blood, sweat, mucus, and other bodily fluids.

Over the years, the artist has sourced a variety of hospital gowns. Most of the ones he reconstitutes into art he has worn personally, but others are mailed to him by friends who have spent time in hospital. At this point, he has a cross section of gowns from around the country. Most of them were manufactured by a small handful of companies, and the patterns are relatively similar. The color of the gown is usually a pale green or blue, and the small repeating patterns usually consist of dots, triangles, squares, crosses, stripes, flowers, or hearts. The design is no doubt meant to maintain equilibrium – no highs or lows or emotional outbursts in the gowns, just monotony and calm.

With its role as a material repository of his embodied experiences in hospital as a patient with CF, Quagliozzi also keenly understands the emotional aspects of the gown. It couldn't dissect him in the same way as scalpels and other intimidating medical tools, and it has no direct implications for his health. The gown also captures paradoxical qualities – on the one hand it becomes his security blanket, a thin layer of material that is the only thing between him and the doctors; yet, for this reason, it is also threatening, promising exposure to probing medical apparatuses, with limited barriers in place. The gown is also the most mundane representation of being a patient. Like the bed, the gown is a semiotic code for illness, and neither the bed nor the gown is threatening in and of itself, for they are not life-saving devices or diagnostic tests. But they embody gravitas nonetheless. The hospital gown is a uniform that you wear to indicate that you are now not able-bodied: you're not in society anymore, you're in this particular place, cut off from everything else. Given the disabling effects of the hospital gown and all its rich and heavy associations, it is reasonable that Quagliozzi would want to reciprocate, disabling its meaning from his own embodied perspective as a person with CF.

By turning the gowns into canvases and showing them in a gallery context, Quagliozzi allows audiences to look at the fabric in a new context. What stories and meaning does the fabric now hold outside of the hospital?

Is the gown still disabling owing to its symbolic properties and associations with sickness, or has it now become more benign, less sinister? No doubt people's reactions and their reception of the work, even in the gallery context, will be skewed by their own relationships to the gown, and whether or not they have spent time in hospital. Still, most people will have worn one, especially during regular physical exams at the local general practitioner's office, or during annual mammograms and other basic preventative checkups. Visitors may recollect experiences with a particular pattern on the gowns; for example, a pattern may recall the time their grandparent had a heart attack. For Quagliozzi, the gowns help to activate his own memory, but they are also a way to reclaim his life. The gowns can also capture both individual and collective experiences, and they can be reused over and over again by multiple bodies through multiple illnesses, carrying never-ending layers of stories. The hospital gown is a hand-me-down, albeit an institutional one. Quagliozzi cuts the gowns, layers them, and then sews them together, likening this process to quilting or grafting, where new skins are brought together to each tell its story under one uniform of being sick. Like the hospital bed, the gown is passive, but Quagliozzi makes it active and empowered. He shows us that there is power in its materiality to tell personal stories, and power in material relationships to weave and communicate those experiences outwardly. The artist uses the gown to disrupt the gown's psychology.

In 2019, rather than use the gown as canvases stretched on frames, Quagliozzi decided to turn gowns into a power suit (see Figure 1.6). He wears this suit at hospital conferences and medical events where he is invited as a guest to speak about his experiences as a double lung transplant recipient. By turning the hospital gown into a business suit, Quagliozzi disrupted the psychology of the gown as a uniform of sickness and subverted it into one of power. But the suit is also funny and jarring. At first, viewers may not recognize the familiar motif and patterning of the hospital gown, but within seconds it becomes obvious. Quagliozzi was also playing with the notion of rebellion. He broke a taboo by daring to appear in public in the gown, while knowing that he could get away with his transgression because the form of the suit causes confusion about his role and purpose. It creates ambiguity and uncertainty.

While Quagliozzi was certainly being playful in transforming the gown into a business suit, he also wanted to show that perhaps there is more malleability and flexibility in the business of medicine than we think, or to at least open up the possibility of questioning and transforming a medical policy or procedure from one thing into another. He explains that when someone has a chronic illness, this means they have been dealing with it for a very long time, which inadvertently makes them an expert on how their disease manifests in their own body. However, oftentimes the opinions

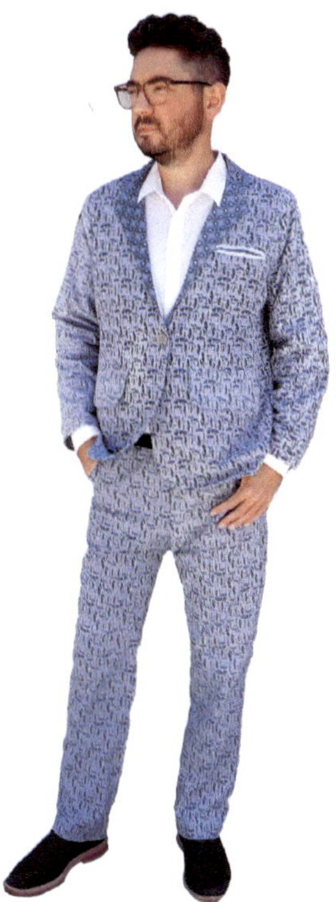

1.6 Dominic Quagliozzi, *Suit*, 2019. Used hospital gowns; a soft wearable sculpture for performances and patient experience speaking engagements. Courtesy of the artist.

Image description 1.6: A suave man stands with a relaxed pose and detached expression in his blue, tailor made suit sewn from recycled hospital gowns.

and thoughts of patients are negated by medical teams and doctors, who don't necessarily respect the individual's experience. Quagliozzi notes how he often hears stories from friends and fellow hospital patients who say they could have been spared so much pain and heartache had their doctor listened earlier to their grievances regarding their health concerns. The power dynamic between a doctor and a patient is clear and one-sided. Here, Quagliozzi wanted to don the power suit and use the fabric of submission to speak out to the medical establishment from his lectern at conferences. Wearing the gown as a suit was a different feeling – he no longer had an open back, cloth draped over him, with nothing underneath but cold wind passing through. One time he wore the suit in front of three hundred medical professionals. In addition to reclaiming the power seat, Quagliozzi wears the suit as a type of costume, with another message: I'm a sick person in the real world, and I'm functioning and surviving, despite the odds. Yet the fabric is a reminder that he is still tethered to the hospital.

At any moment, he could end up back there in an emergency, as that's the reality for people with CF.

In 2022, Quagliozzi's gown evolved into the *Transformers* series, described earlier in this chapter. Initially he made cabinet-sized structures that were wrapped in the hospital gowns; the doors of the cabinet would open up and there would be nothing inside. This action of opening the chest doors alludes to the opening up of his own chest for the lung transplant. The artist later decided to scale the structure down to toy size, like a transformer toy, because he wanted his toddler-aged son to be able to engage with them. Quagliozzi noticed that his son loved stacking blocks and moving blocks around, so he wanted to bring the same level of curiosity and interaction into a wall work. He bought the wood and started cutting it up into these different shapes: there was a main body or torso, and digits or ribs attached to each side with hinges to represent legs or arms. While the initial idea of these interactive wall works was to arouse curiosity and spark childlike imagination, the artist also wanted visitors to engage with the notion of a sick body. The work was to expose our hesitation to touch art (something that museums generally forbid) while simultaneously exposing hesitation over literally touching sickness and touching each other.

Quagliozzi was especially interested in instigating the sensation of touch, an important element in his life as a patient. For example, in the acute periods before and after his transplant, he needed people to take care of him. They had to administer his medications, insert his equipment, and move him around the bed. They had to transfer him from the bed to the toilet or prop him up in the shower. Nurses had to wipe his buttocks for weeks after his transplant, and he was not able to shower on his own for several months, which meant that he needed family and friends to help him once he was discharged from hospital. Thus, the transformers were a manifestation of Quagliozzi's ability to physically manipulate an object himself, where he was the one in control of its positions and its destination. One of the works includes the word 'Cyclops' in the title, a playful reference to the mythical monster of Greek lore that also connotes disability; the Cyclops has one eye, and evokes stereotypes of disabled bodies' supposed monstrousness and fearful appearance. Perhaps the artist also feels a bit monstrous, and wants us to shed our inhibitions and come close.

Thinking more about chronicles of health, medicine, and pain

The artwork described in this chapter has a long lineage. Before I discuss at length illness narratives and the act of chronicling one's health, medicine, and pain, I want to trace where the desire to resist the Western European and North American medical industry may have come from. Literature on the philosophical and historical origins of the medical gaze abounds. One of the foundational texts on the history of the medical gaze is Foucault's *The*

Birth of the Clinic (1963), which lays out the complex relationship between the medical gaze, the patient, and power. The patient became powerless and vulnerable under the gaze of medicine. The doctor was able to gain power through the acquisition of knowledge of the body and the study of medicine, which was considered factual. Any new information coming from outside of traditional and canonical texts on medicine was considered inferior and untrustworthy. If the new information happened to come from patients who were of a minority identity, especially disabled patients, then this information was trusted even less. Any knowledge that the patient has is lackluster compared to that of the professional knowledge of the doctor.[5] Laureanne Willems writes that the medical encounter is marked by hierarchy, and Anne Hunsaker Hawkins believes that this depersonalization in the exchange between doctors and patients is likely the impetus behind patients' desire to "speak back" to the establishment on their own terms. Catherine Kudlick discusses how the medical academy helped to fortify "bourgeois class standing by creating racial, gender, and sexual hierarchies," pointing to its unsavory history of privileging the white male of European origin.[6]

One of the first books I read when I started learning about the academic field of disability studies more than a decade ago was *Staring: How We Look* (2009), by the incomparable Rosemarie Garland-Thomson. I remember searching for the book excitedly among the stacks at the University of California Berkeley when I was a graduate student in Visual and Critical Studies at the California College of the Arts from 2010 until 2012. Garland-Thomson theorized and analyzed the many ways that disabled people are stared at, acknowledging that staring is physical, social, and cultural. Most critically, the scholar wanted to center the staree, rather than the starer, to give the reader a fuller picture of the staring encounter, or a full "anatomy of staring," as she states.[7] This was her way of empowering the disabled person, or in this case the staree.

Included in Garland-Thomson's text, and elaborated by Lisa Cartwright in her own book, *Screening the Body: Tracing Medicine's Visual Culture*, was a discussion of the medical stare or gaze, which she said initially evolved through medical apparatuses that improved natural human vision tenfold, such as the invention of X-rays, sonography, and genetic testing. Suddenly this technology allowed human beings to see the interior of our bodies. But this technology also aided in creating a barrier between human and human. The relationship was now between human and object, helping to build the aura of depersonalization so present in our perceptual encounters with the medical establishment. Garland-Thomson also mentions Foucault and his reference to the "clinical gaze" which is invasive, probing, and fragmented. She states, "Although the clinician may aim the clinician stare at many parts of the body, this kind of visual scrutiny seldom encompasses the whole person, but rather focuses on the aspects that are suspected of revealing pathology."[8] While the male gaze may also be characterized by staring that objectifies certain parts of a woman's body, such as her breasts, the medical gaze examines the breasts during a breast exam or a mammography, making the patient feel not sexually objectified but an impersonal object that has no name or feelings. This kind of stare is one I am personally keenly aware of – that most of us are probably aware of after getting our physicals every year, or getting our skin checked, or getting pap smear tests, but the medical gaze as it meets the disabled body is guided by the curative imperative, and this is what sets it apart.

Given the heavy shroud of the medical model of disability, it has long been the imperative of disabled people to resist it. For the artists in this book, their art – hospital aesthetics – is an act of resistance. In the Introduction, I noted that in the last few years I had witnessed a tidal wave of artist documentation of medical encounters on Instagram, commensurate with the illness memoir. This, combined with the visual culture that emerged from the pandemic, meant that the world was clouded with images of illness, sickness, death, and challenging access to healthcare. The content in this chapter was a natural place to start my investigations, given the plethora of images I have encountered documenting pain, medication, and illness. It was interesting to experience private chronicles of health and illness in such public ways. I see these images as a microcosm of sociocultural experiences with the medical industrial complex that seemingly continue to proliferate. Indeed, I want to reinforce to the reader how the work discussed in this chapter is just a very small portion of the incredible work being produced by contemporary disabled artists.

Historically and today, patients have sought to understand their sick bodies through art, writing, and memoir. They have tried to extricate themselves from the medical gaze which always already treats patients as objects for experimentation and resolution. The illness narrative comes in fictional and autobiographical forms across numerous literary genres; but I'm interested in narratives where disability is centered. This may sound like a paradox to some, given that disability and illness can be one and the same, but when authors and artists use the language of disability and explicitly identify as disabled in their writings and in their art, this is a choice, one that not all authors make. To use the language of disability is to also take on a political identity, and I know plenty of sick people and people who are atypical presenting who do not think of themselves as disabled. Editors G. Thomas Couser and Susannah B. Mintz certainly understood these complications when they compiled their important two-volume resource, *Disability Experiences: Memoirs, Autobiographies, and Other Personal Narratives* (2019). The collection offers over two hundred autobiographical accounts that center the experience of disability. The book's chronology spans from 1470 to 2018, evidence of how long human beings have been "disabled," but also of the personal narrative's role as a fixture in history and across cultures and geographies. In a review of the book, Claudia Gillberg mentions that oftentimes there must be a happy and trite ending in disability memoirs, and that journeys through illness should be accompanied by self-discovery and positivity.[9] Other authors who have also penned books in the illness narrative genre, such as Anne Boyer, Susan Sontag, and Leah Lakshmi Piepzna-Samarasinha, feel the same way.

This is noteworthy because hospital aesthetics doesn't attempt to do this; instead, the artwork discussed in this book is transparent and truthful about how things are. The artists ruminate on the good and the bad, the political and the apolitical, and express emotions, protestations, and critical reflections. But never is there necessarily a happy ending. Art critic Emily Watlington writes that Sontag, who wrote *Illness as Metaphor* (1978) after she discovered she had cancer, "makes the case that illness narratives have a profound impact on real life."[10] In the same vein, Anne Hunsaker Hawkins suggests that a motivation behind the illness narrative is to inform people of the illness journey in order to bring comfort and help to others.[11] When my late partner found out he had skin cancer in 2008, I recall checking out every book I could find on skin cancer from the local library to help assuage my anxiety and fear. While the medical books were scientific, factual, and informative, they were not calming (and perhaps only served to escalate my fear). Instead, it was memoirs that I read that calmed me – memoirs about how others in my partner's shoes coped with cancer and the many obstacles they bravely faced as their mortality was put to the test. There have been many other formats and vehicles through which other artists are deploying hospital aesthetics to effect a quieter activism.

Jo Spence, like Bob Flanagan, was an artist who recorded her experiences with illness, specifically breast cancer. She used her camera to photograph her body through surgery and recovery as a type of soothing exercise but also to critique the failures of the medical establishment. She felt that there was not enough information available on alternative therapies for breast cancer, nor were there efficient counselling services in place to support women through their health crises. Spence's defiance in reclaiming her body was pushed all the way to the point of incision, when she wrote in all caps with black marker pen above her breast, "PROPERTY OF JO SPENCE?" before doctors removed it in a mastectomy, the surgery of which was much to her disapproval. While Spence's powerful photographs acted as a visual diary of her experience (albeit perhaps more confrontationally than the other imagery considered in this chapter), she also created written illness diaries discussing her health regimes, which would eventually be the inspiration for other visual works of art. What is interesting about Spence's use of technology here – the camera – is that instead of acting as a technological apparatus that both enhances human vision and depersonalizes one body from another body, here the camera is a soothing and healing agent, and a permanent witness. Like Spence's work, Hannah Wilke's *Intra-Venus* series of photographs from 1992 chronicles the temporal progression of her cancer during her stay in a hospital bed over a period of eight months.

Perhaps the artist who must be most foregrounded in this chapter for his uncanny ability to chronicle illness is Félix González-Torres. Poetic and transgressive, González-Torres was a master at dramatizing the tension between presence and absence in his multimedia works, which draw on the legacies of both minimalism and conceptual art. His piles of candy canes and his pillows forever indented from the sleeping heads of lovers who have passed on through time and illness are haunting reminders of impermanence yet indelibility in material form. In *"Untitled" (Portrait of Ross in LA)* (1991), the artist has assembled a large pile of hard candies in colorful wrappers in a corner of a gallery space. A label on the wall adjacent to the pile instructs visitors to take some candy to consume. As each day passes, the candy "medication" slowly diminishes until it is gone completely – the artist's conceived metaphor for the inexorable wasting away of his partner, Ross Laycock, who was ravaged by AIDS and died in 1991. Visitors enjoy the candy, a bittersweet moment in which they are encouraged to think about the fragility of life and the finality of death while the sugary compounds slowly melt on their tongue.

In *"Untitled" (Billboard of an Empty Bed)* (1991), González-Torres erected a series of twenty-four billboards across New York City as part of an exhibition at the Museum of Modern Art. The billboard image depicts the top portion of an unmade queen bed with crumpled white sheets and two pillows lying side by side. The pillows show grooves where the heads of lovers lay the night before, leaving us to imagine their identities and their stories. In their absence, our minds are left to fill in their presence, and the work becomes "an abstract memorialization of loss."[12] While the works are quiet and poignant chronicles of illness akin to the artwork in this chapter, the work undoubtedly contributes to a sexual politics around gay identity and AIDS, that was greatly stigmatized during a time in which homosexuality was feared by the US government administration, which failed to act to support AIDS victims and their families. By drawing attention to these issues and to his own personal journey through loss and heartbreak, the artist makes public via a civic billboard the familiar tropes of grief and anguish.

The activity of journaling to document one's experiences with illness has been important for contemporary artists and scholars over recent decades. In 2000, the final year of his life, Flanagan developed his last finished work, *The Pain Journal*, before his death at age 43 of cystic fibrosis. The journal chronicles at once personal and universal experiences and emotions of someone negotiating the challenges of illness. It is a first-person written account of the artist's daily life chronicling his experiences with CF, an intimate portrait of someone who is aware that his own body will eventually kill him. Similarly, the feminist scholar and civil rights activist

Audre Lorde penned *The Cancer Journals* in 1990 to explore her breast and liver cancer diagnosis, treatment, recovery, and reoccurrence.

Especially notable among this group is Taiwanese American artist Yo-Yo Lin. Lin started to document her experiences of chronic illness and chronic health trauma through her *Resilience Journal*, which tracks what she calls "soft data" spanning seven different dimensions of her illness every day. These include chronic pain, logistical problems (e.g. instances when she has to ask for help), body image, social pressures, doctor's visits (she receives at-home care), future visions, and past memories. The journal was an opportunity for Lin to think about how to better put language to her chronic illness experience that wasn't coming from a medical framework. Excerpts and sections of Lin's *Resilience Journal* have been framed and displayed in numerous museum and gallery exhibitions over the past few years. She has also used performance and film to document her experiences with disability and chronic illness.

Carly Mandel is another artist who has turned ephemera into something comforting and empowering. Drawing on her personal experiences of becoming medicalized, her works highlight how we are augmented by medicine and synthetic objects. Mandel lives with several autoimmune diseases including Crohn's disease, and has had several traumatic experiences with medical intervention. In 2020, she created three custom medical-ID bracelets featuring a dove, which conventionally symbolizes hope, a rain cloud to show despair and gloom, and a biohazard symbol denoting danger. The practical function of medical-ID bracelets is to do just that – to provide an identification of a patient in hospital in the event that the patient is unable to communicate, whether because of emergency or some other circumstance. Mandel was struck by how these commodities held so much weight and importance in conveying the identity of someone within a medical setting. It is a practical, depersonalized, and somber system. Mandel's new iconography undoes the bracelets' original function and challenges their inherent detachment; instead, Mandel's bracelets offer a constellation of emotions – hope, despair, and danger, which come in spades in the hospital setting as filtered through patients, their families, and friends, in the face of uncertain futures. Similarly, Panteha Abareshi's moving image work *Not A Body* (2021) uses hospital bracelets to explore the semantics of naming and language from the perspective of a medicalized individual. Through this repetitive motif, overlapping with harsh industrial sounds, we are given insight into the depersonalized conditions of illnesses in a bureaucratic system.

In Jordan Lord's sixteen-minute video *After … After … Access* (2018), the artist considers questions of access by recording his open-heart surgery, including looking at medical imaging of his body with friends, and being admitted to the hospital. While the core of Lord's film is about issues of access, he nonetheless uses the recording of his own medical experience and encounter with the medical field to comment on more accessible healthcare practices for disabled patients.

Another excellent example of a new approach to illness memoir is the work of Korean American artist and author Johanna Hedva, who is based in Los Angeles and Berlin. They have garnered a profile for their important reflection piece "Sick Woman Theory," which was originally published in 2016, among many other writings and publications.[13] In it, they share frank experiences with their chronic conditions and mental health, political ruminations, a sick woman chant or rally call, and a series of recommended texts by fellow writers and scholars who have influenced them. Hedva critiques the simplistic binary of sickness versus illness, and capitalism's role in causing individual and collective illness. Hedva's work has become influential for scores of younger contemporary disabled and immunocompromised artists, and they have a strong following (over 10,000 followers on Instagram). Hedva's identity as both an artist and a writer is also emblematic of how they are establishing a new genre of memoir alongside other artist/writers such as Carolyn Lazard (more in the next section), Park McArthur, and Constantina Zavitsanos. This new genre falls squarely in the realm of hospital aesthetics, where even the traditional definition of "aesthetics" is troubled by these artists' investigations.

Support system

For more than a decade, contemporary Black disabled artist Carolyn Lazard has been making work about illness, disability, and the politics of access and race, where they consider illness as an aesthetic terrain. Lazard was born in California in 1987, and currently lives and works in Philadelphia and New York City. They completed undergraduate training in Film, Electronic Arts, and Anthropology at Bard College, and an MFA at the University of Pennsylvania in Philadelphia. Lazard has Crohn's disease and ankylosing spondylitis, which are both autoimmune diseases, attacking the intestines and the spine and joints. Considered one of the foremost artists of their generation to make work about these themes and subject matter, they won the MacArthur "genius" award in 2023 for their critical investigations and rich innovations in this field. Their work has been shown in solo and group exhibitions at such national and international venues as the Museum of Modern Art; Museum of Contemporary Art, Los Angeles; Walker Art Center; Institute of Contemporary Art, University of Pennsylvania; MoMA PS1; Museum für Moderne Kunst; Whitney Museum of American Art; and the Venice Biennale. Lazard deploys the language of minimalism and conceptual art using sculpture, installation, video, and performance, and often incorporates ready-made aesthetics into their work. One of Lazard's main preoccupations has been deconstructing the ableist expectations of individual productivity, labor, and efficiency, and they use the tools of access as material and subject matter for their art. Lazard is also a talented writer, and has authored several widely circulated essays including "How to Be a Person in the Age of Autoimmunity" (2013) and "The World is Unknown" (2019). Both writings engage in a critique of Western biomedicine by offering insights into Lazard's own journey with illness. In this section, I will discuss five different series of work by Lazard in chronological order: *Support System* (2016), *In Sickness and Study* (2015–16), *Pain Scale* (2019), *Pre-Existing Condition* (2019), and *Extended Stay* (2019). These next few paragraphs represent just a small portion of Lazard's varied praxis.

While the works by Lazard I have selected to discuss in this chapter are a good thematic fit because they provide a personal, minimalist, and unromantic chronicle of illness that represents the boredom and mundane reality of daily malaise, Lazard's work is incredibly complex. In their work, illness as critique is splintered into multiple political registers. The reasons for this are fourfold. First, Lazard appears to be a voracious reader, which is evidenced not just through their artwork (e.g. *In Sickness and Study*, which I will discuss shortly), but also through the many interviews they have given which can be accessed online, and in the many public lectures and talks they have delivered. Art historians and other humanities scholars have discussed how Lazard has been inspired by disability studies scholarship, particularly Alison Kafer's *Feminist, Queer, Crip* and work by Eva Feder Kittay and other thinkers who have written on the medical humanities, social justice more broadly across minority identity categories, and historical and contemporary cases of violence within disability and Black communities. For example, a ten-minute video entitled *CRIP TIME* (2018) animates the term coined by Alison Kafer, showing the artist compiling their daily sequence of colorful pills into many sets of small plastic vitrines so that they can keep systematic track of what is to be consumed to keep them alive and functioning. Through Lazard's interviews, we also learn that they are influenced by artists like Donald Rodney, Martha Rosler, and Adrian Piper. Lazard's depth of engagement with literature in the fields of art history, medicine, illness, and much more is evident in their art, which is strongly informed by current theoretical and philosophical discourses.

Second, Lazard expressly critiques the binary of sickness versus illness, and capitalism's role in causing individual and collective illness. In Lazard's world, each of these terms (sickness, illness, health, etc.) is broken apart, distilled, and reformed into new definitions that must be challenged over and over again. Lazard frequently calls on Marxist philosophy to frame the production of their work. In "How to Be a Person in the Age of Autoimmunity" (2013), Lazard introduces the reader to the Socialist Patients' Collective (SPK) which existed for a short time in 1972. They find inspiration in SPK's reframing of the typical patient/doctor relationship in Marxist terms. As Lazard says,

> For SPK, everyone is sick under capitalism. Their slogan was "Turn your illness into a weapon." They also wrote "sickness is the condition and result of capitalism." The chronically ill are often cast as victims of fate or genetics. Rarely are we politicized or allowed to relate our personal experiences to larger social or cultural phenomena. As far as doctors are concerned, our diseases are empirical facts and not much else.[14]

These sentiments continue to be harnessed in Lazard's overall politics and praxis.

Third, as I indicated at the beginning of this chapter, Lazard's work introduces us to a politics of disability, race, and the biomedical industrial complex that is critical to the argument of *Hospital Aesthetics*. In my discussion of Quagliozzi's work, I mentioned his admission that he was likely treated differently in hospital as a young, white, attractive male. In contrast, Lazard has commented on the poor and racist treatment of Black people in the medical field. While Quagliozzi's willingness to share his intimate encounters through his art and his stories is important for this book, his experiences must necessarily be counterbalanced by other encounters, which will always be different, and sometimes because of the color of one's skin. Fourth, Lazard's work is enmeshed in a support system, where literal support becomes conceptual support. All these complexities will be detailed in the upcoming paragraphs.

This fourth point is a good place to start. In October 2016, Lazard staged a one-day durational performance entitled *Support System (for Park, Tina, and Bob)* at Room & Board in Williamsburg, Brooklyn. While performance is part of the work, Lazard actually considers this piece their first socially conceived sculpture, where flowers become a proxy for the people with whom they engage in their performance. The venue was an experimental artist's residency and studio that took place in the apartment of Julia Pelta Feldman, which has since closed to the public. The title of the piece is a reference to Lazard's support system, namely the artists Park McArthur and Constantina Zavitsanos, whom Lazard has collaborated with for over a decade, and Bob Flanagan. The title also has multiple other meanings. Lazard certainly gestures to their friends and collaborators as a support system, and one can only assume the support system is one of friendship, care, and intellectual and artistic exchange. But Lazard also wants us to recognize that they are not making work in a vacuum. They have been, and will continue to be, inspired by the work of others (particularly those in the title of the piece), and this is how art is often conceived. Lazard is also paying homage to Flanagan through the performance itself. Lazard's one-day event consisted of lying in a bed from 9 a.m. to 9 p.m. and inviting visitors to come and sit with them in bed and hold a conversation, akin to Flanagan's *Visiting Hours* mentioned previously. The visitors were requested to bring a bouquet of flowers in exchange for time with the patient (see Figure 1.7). While the visitors were encouraged to help Lazard as they lay

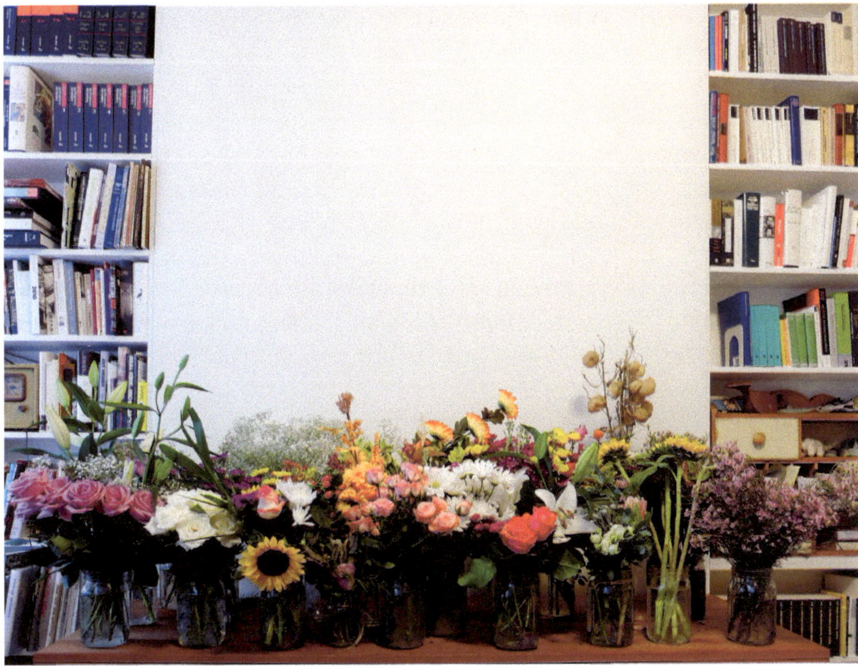

1.7 Carolyn Lazard, *Support System (for Park, Tina, and Bob)*, 2016. Documentation of twelve-hour performance and collectively produced sculpture. Courtesy of the artist.

Image description 1.7: Dozens of bouquets cover the top of a wooden credenza. These explosions of blooms include roses, lillies, sunflowers, and baby's breath.

in bed by perhaps retrieving an item such as food, or doing some laundry for them, or just engaging in conversation while propped up in bed with them, eventually Lazard switched the roles so that it was Lazard who was learning about the visitor and their needs in an important exchange of hospitality. This was the other level of support system, where Lazard points out that care is a mutual exchange, and that temporary and ongoing convalescence depends on a network of others.

In her essay documentation of Lazard's performance, Julia Pelta Feldman says that Eva Feder Kittay "has critiqued the disability rights movement of the 1990s for its insistence on independence for the disabled, for its embrace of an ideal that is not attainable – perhaps not even desirable – for the non-disabled."[15] Lazard's work in this instance draws on disability studies scholarship, pointing out the lived reality of the support system, and how that system should be acknowledged in more respectful and transparent ways. Oftentimes care work goes on behind closed doors in domestic spaces. Lazard opens the doors to their private space to not only expose the visitor to a mutual exchange of care and dependency, but to get them to engage in it too. Care work is therefore made more public to give it visibility and attention.

The many bouquets of flowers that Lazard assembled over the course of the day became one of the sole forms of documentation for the performances. They were a mandatory token for entering the room to be with the artist in their bed, but they also symbolize the most common material gesture gifted to someone who is unwell. Flowers, at least for me, give way to existential thinking – the cycle of life and death, beauty and decay, pleasurable variegations, smells, and textures, and relationships of love, intimacy, and care. The rows of many glass mason jars create a near garden of roses, carnations, sunflowers, and baby's breath, which also hold rich metaphors.

Books are just as plentiful as flowers in Lazard's next work, *In Sickness and Study* (2015–16). Here is the evidence that Lazard engages deeply with literature, as we are confronted with a grid of nine Instagram selfies, each showing Lazard's arm holding up a different book they are reading (see Figure 1.8). Lazard's choice to use the interface of Instagram in this work is what I think of when I reference a generation of artists who are using Instagram to document their individual experiences with healthcare in a hospital setting. Lazard's work clearly informs my definition of hospital aesthetics, but I believe it was also a harbinger of the many hundreds of other illness images that have flooded the visual culture of social media in the past decade. Given that the images are from Instagram, on the surface this may also suggest that perhaps Lazard is looking for gratification from their followers on their choice of book, in the same way that Instagram users like to share images of what they had for dinner. To be fair, I always find it fascinating to learn what other people are reading. It tells us something about the person's interests and intellectual curiosities and concerns. Indeed, I have learned a lot about Lazard based on what they read. But while it might seem that Lazard is enjoying a leisurely pursuit (for to have time to read for pleasure is something I never seem to accomplish), they are reading under punishing circumstances. Lazard is taking selfies of their arm holding up the books they are reading, but their arm is connected to a peripheral IV catheter for iron infusions. This gives us more context, so then we start to take more notice of the background. They are lying in a chair or a bed in a hospital room or a doctor's office. There is a privacy curtain in the background, a blue leather chair. There are waiting room chairs and desk chairs, and other pieces of furniture that are typical of medical spaces. What are they doing there? They must go often for their chronic illness. That must be boring, so it makes sense to read in those circumstances. Does the reading help ease the boredom and the anxiety that comes with being in medical spaces? It's hard to know. The title of the work appropriates the well-known line from marriage vows – "in sickness and in health" – suggesting there is no health as such, whatever that

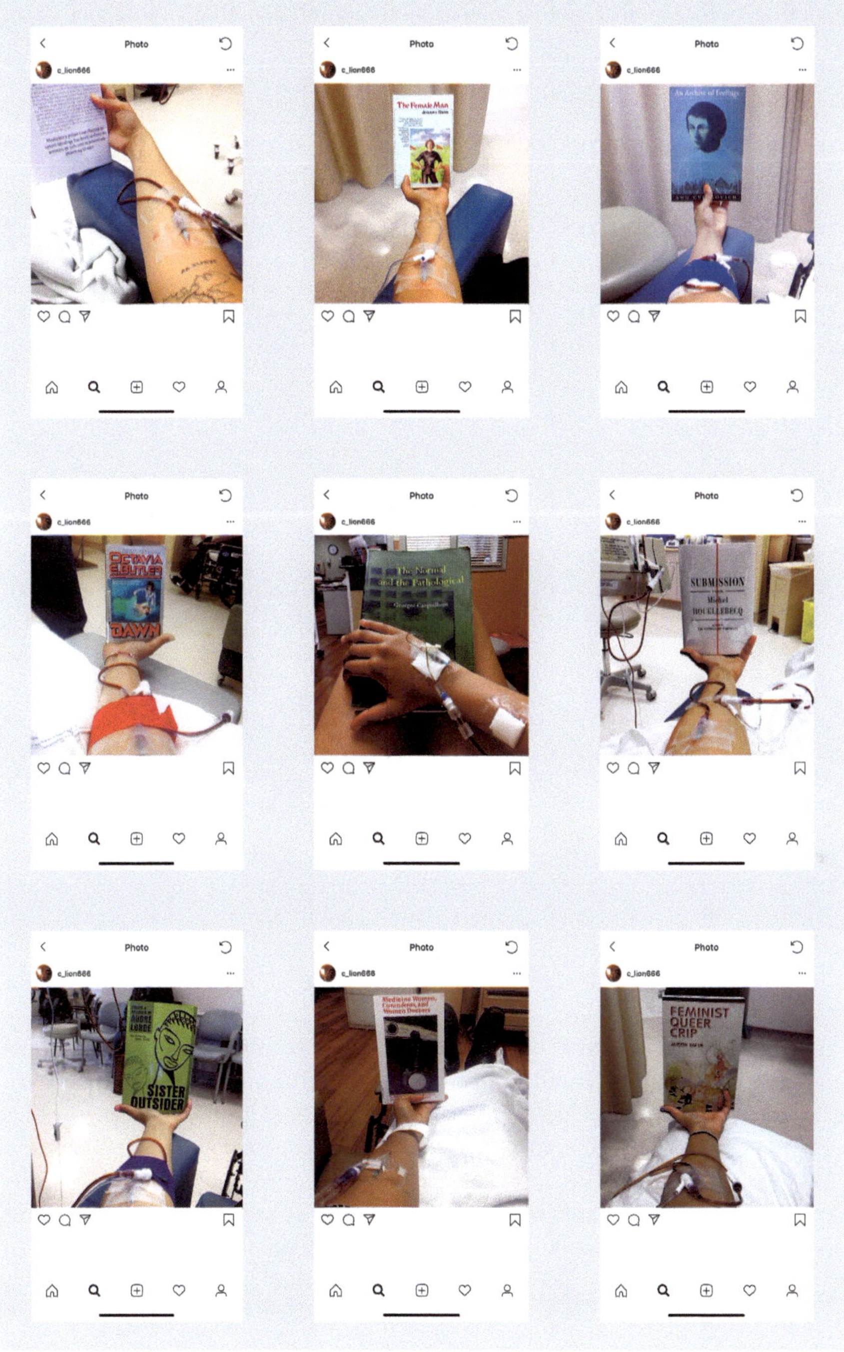

1.8 Carolyn Lazard, *In Sickness and Study*, 2015–16. Digital photographs, dimensions variable. Courtesy of the artist.

Image description 1.8: A grid of Instagram photographs, lined up in three rows of three. Each image is a selfie of the artist's light brown arm holding up a book while undergoing intravenous iron infusions. Titles include *Sister Outsider*, *Feminist Queer Crip*, and *Dawn*.

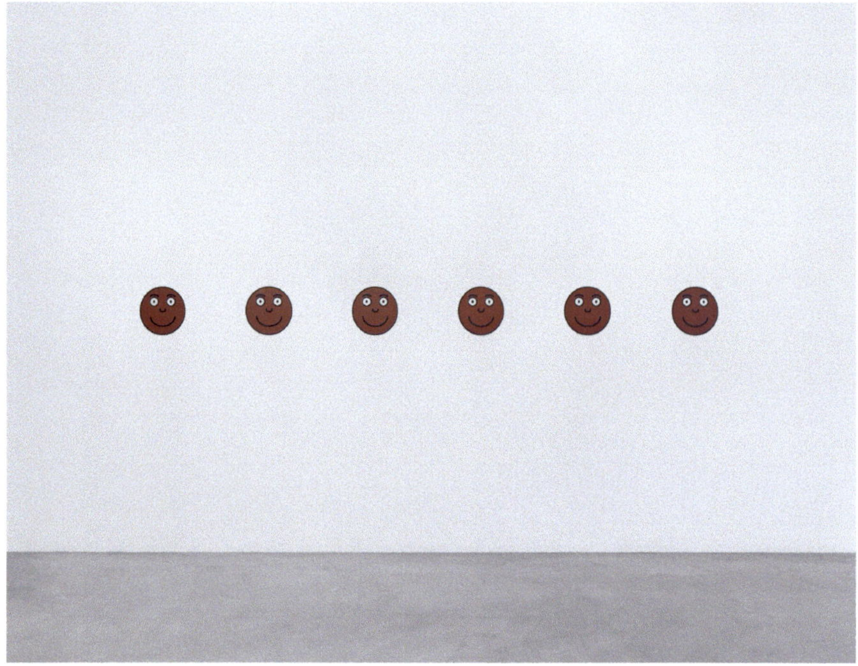

1.9 Carolyn Lazard, *Pain Scale*, 2019. Vinyl, overall: 148 × 12 in. (376 × 30 cm); six parts, each 12 × 12 in. (30 × 30 cm). Courtesy of the artist.

Image description 1.9: Six identical brown smiley faces hung in an even line on a white wall. The cartoon faces resemble the ones used to illustrate the pain scale, except their smiles stay exactly the same regardless of their placement.

means, and only sickness and study (of books) instead. Lazard also wants to break that binary again between sickness and health, and suggests that perhaps there is no health, but something else that we should all aspire to.

The next three works to be discussed were all made in 2019, at a time when Lazard's reputation was growing significantly, and they were receiving invitations to exhibit in high-profile galleries and museums. Their work became more political and even more layered. *Pain Scale* is a vinyl wall installation of six Black smiley faces (see Figure 1.9). At first, Lazard's pain scale seems like an enlarged version of the standard pain scale that medical staff hand out when one is checking into the doctor's office for an appointment, to give the doctor an indication of level of pain, from one to five (one being no pain, and five being the most pain). Lazard chose to use the Wong–Baker FACES Pain Rating Scale, which was originally designed for children and which has five faces with variations in color that move from happy on the left (0 – No Hurt, to very miserable on the right 10 – Hurts Worst). On closer examination, the smiley faces are just that – they are all smiling. If this was the Wong–Baker pain scale, the expressions on the round faces would show a sliding scale of emotion, from happy to sad. The skin color of the faces is also noticeable – they are Black, instead of, well, white, certainly, but also just blank, with no attributable color. Normally the smiley faces don't have a racial or ethnic identity, but in this instance they do.

What is Lazard trying to tell us? Why are all the Black smiley faces smiling at us? Black bodies are not meant to feel pain; at least, that's the stereotype that Lazard is pointing out, which unfortunately pervades the medical system. More pointedly, if Black bodies feel pain, that pain is dismissed or disqualified. Countless articles and publications point out the inequities that Black patients confront when they recount to doctors the battles they face with their bodies. Requests for pain medication might be rejected because Black people might be viewed as drug seekers, or the level of care they receive might be subordinate and certainly secondary to white patients, who might have exactly the same symptoms. Black people and Black pregnant women have higher mortality rates than white people. The white medical establishment does not listen and does not believe that Black people have an ontology of pain. In an interview published in *BOMB* magazine in 2020, Lazard said:

> I was thinking through the illegibility of Black patients' pain in the healthcare system. Black patients are overwhelmingly denied adequate pain management. Half of medical students believe that Black people feel less pain than white people. Pain is challenging to communicate in general, but some people are denied the kind of affective scaleability that's assumed in a medical setting.[16]

Lazard also said that people believe that Black people have thicker skin than white people and can therefore tolerate pain at a much higher level. By racializing the pain scale, Lazard is showing us how the pain scale has racist implications for patient treatment and well-being. Black people want to show the pain they feel, and they can't. Instead, they are meant to paint a smile on their face at all times; well, six times to be exact.

The spurious smiles also point to the problematic system of the pain scale itself. I've completed many pain scales myself, during visits to the doctor's office. I always wondered why pain was reduced to facial expressions on a smiley face. It seems like an inaccurate way to chart pain for the doctor, and also a shortcut to learning about patient pain without having to actually talk with them directly about it. Indeed, the pain scale is a tool to assist in the depersonalization of the doctor's visit, where little communication is needed, thanks to a piece of paper between the doctor and their patient. A thin veil of silence, and a wall of emoticons. No need for hello, as Lazard puts it.

Pain Scale is also important because it directly addresses racism in the medical industrial complex. Lazard has executed several other pieces that do this, especially *Pre-Existing Condition* (2019). This work includes a bench, reminding the visitor of the need for more places to sit in the art museum. But there is more here. In this important video work, the artist interviews Holmesburg experimentation survivor Edward Yusuf Anthony, as they take the audience through a sequence of documents acquired through the University of Pennsylvania Archives and the Philadelphia City Archives. The Holmesburg experiments and testings were undertaken by white male dermatologist Dr. Kligman at the Holmesburg Prison in Philadelphia from 1951 to 1974, and many of the scientific tests were unethically carried out on Black patients. In a repulsive statement by the doctor, he confessed that all he saw was "acres of skin," reinforcing the medical gaze as a fragmented gaze on body parts and no full person.[17] He would perform his experiments using detergents, soaps, and radioactive and hallucinogenic compounds, along with infecting his subjects with herpes, candida, and human papillomavirus. The interviewee in this film discusses the long-term detrimental side effects of having been victimized – by the experiments certainly, but Lazard focuses on Anthony's present-day struggles with the medical system, as he explains that he cannot trust medical workers owing to repeated failures and mishandling of his treatments. Thus, we understand that racism toward Black people by the medical industrial complex has been perpetuated across multiple temporal contexts, and is embedded in the foundation of so-called health and wellness.

In *Black Disability Politics* (2022), Sami Schalk examines how definitions of wellness and health vary greatly within Black communities. According to Schalk, spirituality must be figured into a more capacious definition of wellness, alongside emotional well-being, stress, and the dynamics in intimate relationships.[18] In Lazard's written piece, "The World is Unknown" (2019), they unpack concepts of healing and alternative medicine in contrast to Western biomedicine. They talk about their Haitian heritage (on their mother's side), and how health is assessed holistically in Vodou, a syncretic religion practiced in Haiti. Lazard states: "A person's sense of well-being or disease reflects their relationship to their environment, their community, and their ancestors. The body is a gateway to the spiritual world and illnesses are brought upon those who dishonor or disrespect the law, the spirits."[19] These rich, multifaceted, and diverse approaches to health must be considered by medicine, as they can deepen knowledges, relations, cures, and networks of care. These are some of the entry points that Lazard offers us through works that weave race into their many folds, imparting even more heft to the concept of hospital aesthetics.

Sami Schalk, Nirmala Erevelles, Christopher Bell, Moya Bailey, and Therí A. Pickens help us to understand that disability studies as an academic field of study has historically privileged white disabled bodies, while Black disabled bodies have been excluded from the narratives. Lazard's observations and artistic evocations make these racial occlusions and preferences vivid, both through lived experience and by sharing the experiences of others, historically and within their communities of friends, family, and allies. It shows that this is a legitimate and concerning experience of hospital patients that continues to go underacknowledged and should be urgently discussed. In his book *Vitality Politics: Health, Debility, and the Limits of Black Emancipation*, Stephen Knadler shows us how wide-ranging the discrimination regarding access to healthcare has been toward Black people; it has not simply been confined to the hospital. Racial violence extends to "unsanitary housing, polluted drinking water, unequal segregated healthcare, the absence of sewage lines, unsafe food, or traumatic and environmental stress."[20] Knadler argues that we must consider "the biopolitics of debilitation and medicalization," as seriously as the ever-growing problems of surveillance, police violence, and criminalization of Black people to understand why Black people have been made "not to matter."[21] Knadler further shows us the historical complexities of health and illness as they intersect with race, because this binary of health versus illness has been used as a tool for manipulation by a white majority. This is what the scholar calls a politics of "vitality," which means that even though the state may have taken an interest in the Black body, veiled as a "citizen patient," where the goal was to rehabilitate and emancipate the Black individual, ultimately the tactics were racist. Indeed, the politics of vitality was dubiously perceived by the Black population.[22] This is because this politics of vitality was actually a method to control Black bodies during cycles of crisis and recovery, and it was an effective means by which to exclude Black people from the dominant social and economic order.[23] In other words, to reference Jasbir Puar's work, "debility" and "maiming" were used as strategies to secure the injustices and inequalities of the racialized state.[24] Ultimately, the problems that Lazard is identifying belong to a broader historical and contemporary framework that must be considered when taking in their work.

Extended Stay (2019) was included in the Whitney Biennial at the Whitney Museum of American Art in New York (see Figure 1.10). (Lazard's work appeared in the Whitney Biennial again in 2024, with a work entitled *Toilette*, which comprises a group of ready-made medicine cabinets that store Vaseline instead of drugs.) Much has been written about *Extended Stay* and all its messages and possibilities. If any one work activated a section of this book's argument regarding how to make the art gallery and the hospital into more hospitable places, it might be this one. Accompanying a simple wooden museum bench is a small monitor intended for individual use, which extends from the wall attached to a moveable arm mount. Visitors are encouraged to sit down on the bench and watch a sequence of television programs. The scene before us has been appropriated from what one might see and/or experience as a hospital patient, providing entertainment, or at the very least distraction from hospital white noise. Giulia Smith likens this scene with televisions etc. to "the kind used in chemotherapy infusion rooms," and it reminds me of the setup in my dentist's office when I had

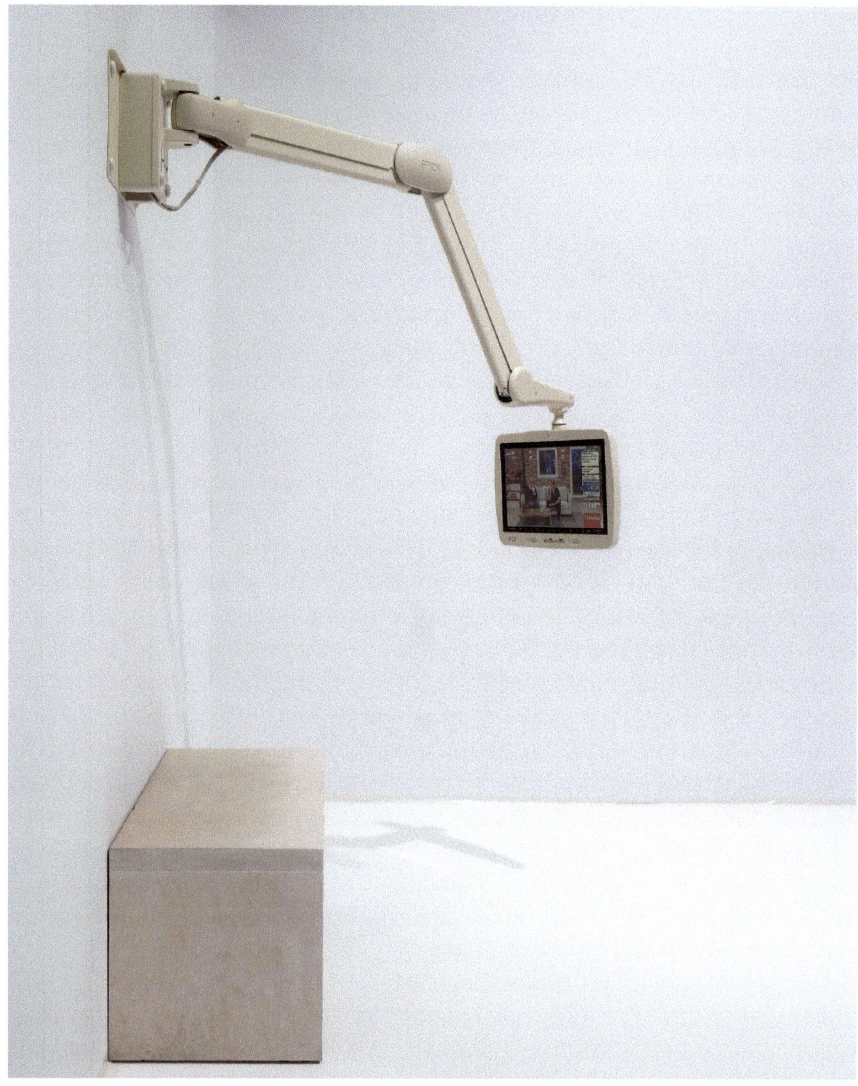

1.10 Carolyn Lazard, *Extended Stay*, 2019. Articulating medical arm mount, personal patient monitor, basic cable subscription, infinite duration. Courtesy of the artist.

Image description 1.10: A beige hospital TV monitor protruding from a white gallery wall and arching over a beige rectangular bench.

root canal work, and eventually a molar tooth extraction.[25] Lazard has often adapted furniture, props, devices, therapy aids, and other ephemera from the medical establishment in their work. Other examples include *Conspiracy* (2017), which is an installation of Dohm white noise machines; HEPA air filter purifiers (no official title, 2020); and from the same exhibition at

Essex Street Gallery entitled *Privatization*, two works entitled *Piss on Pity* (2020) (selected for the 2022 Venice Biennale) and *Lazy Boi* (2020), which are two leather recliner chairs, one in the upright position and the other in the reclining position. Richard Birkett writes that the loop implied by the upright and reclining positions offers a tension between leisure and idleness on the one hand, and an assistive device for sick and disabled people on the other.[26]

By inviting visitors to sit at the bench and engage with the television monitor, the work temporarily puts the visitor in the position of a patient inside of an art museum. The monitor was programmed to change television shows every one and a half minutes, similar to the experience of surfing through channels mindlessly when one can't find anything good to watch. This also reminds me of what walking through an art exhibition or a permanent collection hang can be like in the museum; I often find myself restless as I walk from room to room in an art museum, trying to find work that is stimulating. That movement back and forth through rooms or through channels evokes anxiety, boredom, and a hungry desire for more. Beyond this, the collision of the worlds of the art gallery and the patient as expressed through Lazard's installation raises many questions: what happens when the hospital is brought into the art museum, and what impact does this have on the individual and the museum as a whole? And vice versa, what happens when the gallery visitor is transported into being a patient? Including a bench in the installation is institutional critique work, because it is offering something to gallery visitors – an opportunity to sit down, which is typically and thoughtlessly withheld by galleries and art museums. But I'm not sure this is truly the point that the artist is trying to make to the Whitney's undoubtedly mostly nondisabled audience, who will take this opportunity to sit down as part and parcel of the installation. Granted, the opportunity to sit down is very likely welcomed after having endured a grueling journey through what is typically a demanding Whitney Biennial itinerary with hundreds of works on display to consume, but Lazard's point is about that bridge between the hospital and the art museum. What is to be gained by understanding them as bedfellows? In an interview with Lazard, they explained that they wanted the viewer to reflect on the spectatorship experience in the gallery, where visitors typically spend a very short amount of time engaging with a painting or a sculpture and a bit more time with work that is film- and/or video-based. When a sick person is in a hospital for an eight-hour infusion, they have to pass the time slowly as they wait; this is typical of crip spectatorship, in contrast to that experienced in the art museum. Hence, in this piece Lazard is not trying to create an experience of escapism through a large projected film, but rather wants it to be a work about how crip temporality rubs up against the temporality of the art museum, and how spectatorship in the art museum is a site of privilege unacknowledged by able-bodied audiences.

In a comprehensive 2021 article for *Art History*, British art historian Giulia Smith discussed Lazard's work in great depth, providing at the same time a robust Marxian political history of state welfare programs and their relationship to disability. Smith's historical and cultural framing has undoubtedly contributed to the means of production for a slew of disabled artists invested in these topics. In the past year, I noticed that Lazard had changed their website so that the thorough professional documentation of their work that used to be available is no longer. For a while, virtual visitors could typically truly spend time – crip time – with Lazard. But Lazard no doubt has plans for something new, generous, and foretelling for us to chew on. In their own crip time, we will get it.

The work by Dominic Quagliozzi, Carolyn Lazard, and the other artists mentioned in this chapter contributes to hospital aesthetics through chronicles of illness that subvert the romantic illness memoir genre. They confront audiences with pissing, shitting, boredom, surgery, infusions, and more, using journaling, hospital shows, furniture and materials from the hospital, and other avant-garde minimalist measures to convey complex concepts. Through these lived experiences of illness and disability, we also see a myriad of politics surrounding entanglements with racism, insurance, white privilege, institutional critique, and how the hospital and the art gallery might help each other through the generative state of sickness. Catherine Kudlick suggests that as a nuanced understanding of disability continues to grow based on more complex identifications with it, both individual and collective, it might become possible for us to have "the luxury of turning to medicine as something other than a villain."[27] While Kudlick's statement rings more and more true and this luxury might be one of the ultimate end goals, the artwork in this book proves that Western biomedicine continues to exhibit villainous qualities, as racism, sexism, ableism, and other 'isms' continue to exist.

The introverted chronicles of chronic illness in this chapter now lead us into a more extroverted focus on how the sick and disabled body receives tools that are engineered and designed according to the curative imperative. Contemporary disabled artists adapt and appropriate wheelchairs, canes, prostheses, X-rays, and more into creative crip critique.

Notes

1 Dominic Quagliozzi, interview with the author, December 19, 2023.
2 Martin O'Brien, "Lie Back and Take It: BDSM, Biomedicine and the Hospital Bed in the Work of Bob Flanagan and Sheree Rose," *Body, Space & Technology* 15 (2016). http://doi.org/10.16995/bst.18
3 O'Brien, "Lie Back and Take It."
4 O'Brien, "Lie Back and Take It."
5 Laureanne Willems, "On Caring Through Sharing and Reading When Seeing: Attending to Formal Potentialities of Illness Narratives," *Literature and Medicine* 40, no. 1 (Spring 2022): 38–54, https://doi.org/10.1353/lm.2022.0008; and Anne Hunsaker

Hawkins, *Reconstructing Illness: Studies in Pathology* (West Lafayette, IN: Purdue University Press, 1998).

6 Catherine Kudlick, "Comment: On the Borderland of Medical and Disability History," *Bulletin of the History of Medicine* 87, no. 4 (Winter 2013): 540–59. https://doi.org/10.1353/bhm.2013.0086

7 Rosemarie Garland-Thomson, *Staring: How We Look* (Oxford: Oxford University Press, 2009).

8 Garland-Thomson, *Staring*.

9 Claudia Gillberg, "Disability Experiences, Memoirs, Autobiographies, and Other Personal Narratives," *Disability & Society* 35, no. 9 (2020): 1527–29, https://doi.org/10.1080/09687599.2020.1744253

10 Emily Watlington, "Chronicling Illness," *Art in America*, September 2, 2021, www.artnews.com/art-in-america/features/chronicling-illness-guadalupe-maravilla-carolyn-lazard-1234602858 [accessed December 30, 2024].

11 Hawkins, *Reconstructing Illness*.

12 Thomas Folland, "Felix Gonzalez-Torres, *'Untitled' (billboard of an empty bed)*," Smarthistory, https://smarthistory.org/felix-gonzalez-torres-untitled-billboard-of-an-empty-bed [accessed January 22, 2024].

13 Johanna Hedva, "Sick Woman Theory + Get Well Soon (both 2020)," 2020, www.kunstverein-hildesheim.de/caring-structures-ausstellung-digital/johanna-hedva/ [accessed December 5, 2024]. A different version of this essay was previously published in *Mask Magazine*, edited by Hanna Hurr and Isabelle Nastasia, January 2016.

14 Carolyn Lazard, "How to Be a Person in the Age of Autoimmunity," *Cluster Magazine*, January 2013.

15 Julia Pelta Feldman cites Eva Feder Kittay, *Love's Labor: Essays on Women, Equality, and Dependency* (New York: Routledge, 1999); see Julia Pelta Feldman, *Carolyn Lazard, Support System (for Tina, Park, Bob): Sunday, October 30, 2016*. Brooklyn, NY: Room & Board, 2016. https://roomandboard.nyc/wp-content/uploads/2018/04/support-system-book-with-cover.pdf [accessed January 22, 2024].

16 Catherine Damman, "Carolyn Lazard by Catherine Damman [Interview]," *BOMB*, September 10, 2020, https://bombmagazine.org/articles/2020/09/10/carolyn-lazard [accessed December 5, 2024].

17 Joann Loviglio, "Albert M. Kligman, Dermatologist Who Patented Retin-A, Dies at 93," *Washington Post*, February 21, 2010, www.washingtonpost.com/wp-dyn/content/article/2010/02/21/AR2010022104116.html [accessed December 5, 2024].

18 Sami Schalk, *Black Disability Politics* (Durham, NC: Duke University Press, 2022), 90.

19 Carolyn Lazard, "The World is Unknown" [digital project], *Triple Canopy*, April 19, 2019, https://tc3.canopycanopycanopy.com/issues/24/contents/the-world-is-unknown [accessed December 5, 2024].

20 Stephen Knadler, "Introduction: Ill-Defined Emancipations," in *Vitality Politics: Health, Debility, and the Limits of Black Emancipation* (Ann Arbor, MI: University of Michigan Press, 2019), Kindle.

21 Knadler, "Ill-Defined Emancipations."

22 Knadler, "Ill-Defined Emancipations."

23 Knadler, "Ill-Defined Emancipations."

24 Jasbir Puar, *The Right to Maim: Debility, Capacity, Disability* (Durham, NC: Duke University Press, 2017).

25 Giulia Smith, "Chronic Illness as Critique: Crip Aesthetics Across the Atlantic," *Art History* 44, no. 2 (April 2021): 286–310, https://doi.org/10.1111/1467-8365.12559

26 Richard Birkett, "A Promise and a Practice: Carolyn Lazard," *Mousse Magazine*, October 13, 2020, www.moussemagazine.it/magazine/carolyn-lazard-richard-birkett-2020 [accessed December 5, 2024].

27 Kudlick, "Comment," 548.

2

Disabling medical assistive devices

A medical assistive device is defined as technology that helps to maintain or improve function. In this chapter, I show how medical assistive devices such as breathing apparatuses, prostheses, canes, and hearing aids can become personalized in revised forms that engage thoughtfully and critically with bodies – forms of engagement typically absent when the devices are issued in the cold and sterile environment of the doctor's office. Common assistive devices include a wheelchair, crutch, scooter, hearing aid, or even reading glasses.[1] The irony of the artwork in this chapter is that it is not interested in "assistance" in the conventional application or meaning of the word: prostheses, canes, and so on. Indeed, the artists aim to disable the function of the assistive device so that its materiality becomes fragmented, torn open, and reconstituted into a new shape and form, producing empowered conceptual meaning for the patient/artist. What else is bound up in the assistance device, and can there be more layers of meaning behind them than purely practical function? Medical assistive devices carry the weight of stigma, shame, marking, labeling, and a rigid semiotics of sickness, illness, and disability. They imply that the disabled body needs fixing so that it becomes closer to being "normal" and better integrated into functional society. But oftentimes these devices are designed by nondisabled makers who might lack intimate knowledge of disability or who are driven by the imperative to correct. The artists in this chapter aim to denaturalize the functions of medical assistive devices, and help audiences to look at them in more unfamiliar ways. They want medical assistive devices to be made strange, because they are strange. The artists push us to reflect on the purpose and intention behind these devices, and show us that it is possible to move away from the curative imperative. This is what the artists in this chapter aim to shake up and shake off.

I examine the work of two main artists in this chapter, along with many artists who cumulatively build on the visual culture and politics of medical assistive devices. Berlin-based, British-born artist Jesse Darling makes his props and braces comical, surreal, and bizarre. He draws from – and expands on – a long tradition of artists who use canes and prosthetic devices. In detailing this history, I will discuss the significant literature on the prosthesis and all its rich metaphors, as well as the work of other contemporary disabled artists who explore variations of the prosthesis. Bhavna Mehta turns to X-rays as a canvas for her textile and embroidery-based practice, adding intricate patterns with needle and threads directly onto the X-ray film. I contextualize Mehta's work by gesturing toward Katherine Sherwood's X-ray-based paintings, sculptures, and installations as historical precedent, along with work by Aminder Bindu Virdee and Donald Rodney. As I mentioned in the Introduction, I discuss these additional artists (Sherwood, Bindu Virdee, and Rodney) much less extensively than the two artists I have selected to focus on (Darling and Mehta). I wish to show how Darling's and Mehta's work is part of an array of work being developed across a complex constellation of praxis by contemporary disabled artists. Yet it is necessary to home in on several artists and their portfolios in order to convey what the work is trying to do, and how it demonstrates hospital aesthetics in powerful and evocative ways. These in-depth case studies are the backbone of my study.

This chapter builds on the argument made in Chapter 1, showing how impersonal medical tools become personalized and imbued with the stories and memories of the disabled user. Here, a more fervent and literal script/rescript is taking place.

Given my focus on how artists challenge the utility of medical assistive devices, it is important to briefly acknowledge here the importance of the politics of disability design, which emphasizes that design for disabilities must be disability-led, or that it should be developed in consultation with disabled communities and individual disabled users at the very least. Scholars such as Elizabeth Guffey, Bess Williamson, Sara Hendren, Gabi Schaffzin, Graham Pullin, Josh Halstead, David Gissen, and many others work at the intersection of disability and design in various ways. They all comment on how the design and engineering world would benefit from a dialogue with disabled users, just as I argue that the worlds of the hospital and art museum need to consult with disability communities. If these discussions took place more consistently, then the medical assistive device might have a different semiotics, aesthetics, and conceptual role to play in the work of contemporary disabled artists in the future. Ironically, much of the already existing scholarship at the intersection of disability and design centers on the importance of making assistance devices more aesthetically pleasing and fashionable so that the user can feel more pride and confidence in using them – and arguably, and perhaps controversially, to "fit" better into society. But scholarship on the ways in which the curative imperative is embedded in the medical assistive device is less well developed. By drawing some of these ideas into this chapter, I'm also reinforcing my argument that disabled artists must make medical assistive devices strange. As Lisa Cartwright's work has detailed, the visual culture of medicine aims to control, contain, and exert power and influence over patients. Part of the work of challenging this dominant visual culture is to offer imagery by contemporary disabled artists that helps us to question, and so transform, practices and access to healthcare.

Contemporary artists in this book aim to trouble the notion that a medical diagnosis, prognosis, or treatment should go unquestioned by patients, or at least unchallenged within the medical field. Similarly, the artists in this chapter aim to upset the function of the medical assistive device. They do this by first using medical assistive devices as materials and mediums for their work in innovative and dynamic ways, but they also flip the script on how those devices should be wrought onto disabled bodies and medical patients at large. Other artists and designers like Pernilla Philip and Aisen Caro Chacin make assistive device art where they hack medical assistive devices and engineer them into idiosyncratic new ones for self-care, scientific experimentation, and aesthetic purposes. Philip particularly works from lived experience with a chronic illness. Part of these artists' rejection of the curative imperative and their development of a hospital aesthetics, then, involves energetically flipping the medical assistive device on its head. Further, the artists I focus on in this chapter come from a diverse array of cultural and social backgrounds in different parts of the world, intersecting with a rich plethora of customs, rituals, and habits, both old and new. At the same time, I acknowledge how "dis-ability" is understood differently in cultures outside of Euro-America and that these contexts remain underdiscussed and undertheorized.

Cripistemology of the cabinet

Jesse Luke Darling is a British-born, Berlin-based transmasculine disabled artist who uses sculpture, video, text, performance, sound, and installation to explore the formation and reformation of bodily subjects and the socio-political forces behind these processes. Darling won the prestigious Turner Prize in 2023 and is lauded as one of the most brilliant artists of his generation. In this section, I will discuss several objects produced by Darling in the five years or so up to 2024, which are all connected by virtue of being prosthetic. Prostheses are a prime example of medical assistive devices and can range from a prosthetic leg or arm for an amputee, to a walking cane or crutch, to a white cane for someone who has low vision or no sight. Prostheses can also be nonmobile or nonportable human-made devices that help a person move from one location to another, such as grab bars in the shower or bathroom. After a discussion of Darling's engagements with the prosthesis, I will weave in much briefer discussions of other excellent prosthetic objects made by Constantina Zavitsanos, Jes Sachse, and Carmen Papalia to provide an overview of the landscape of contemporary artwork being developed on this topic. I will also outline the philosophical discourse around the prosthesis, and how it has been handled by the medical world and art world in controversial ways.

Darling has long been interested in exploring the vulnerability, imperfection, and inevitable decay of bodies. In 2016, the artist experienced a neurological disease after giving birth to his child, an outcome of which was partial paralysis and the loss of full use of his right arm. As a consequence, he had to learn how to make work with his left arm. While this life-changing event precipitated a focus on the signifiers of disability, damage, and the prosthetic body, Darling also notes that he was invested in topics of pain and malfunction prior to this moment. Darling modifies and adapts sculptural objects – including medical assistive devices – so that they become dilapidated, spindly, contorted, and wonky. Similar to the work by Sunaura Taylor discussed in the Introduction, in which a young boy is being fitted with and forced to wear an ill-fitting prosthetic device, Darling considers how the prosthesis is meant to impart a behavior of moving that is not necessarily automatic, but learned. He funnels these concerns through the larger frameworks of patriarchy, imperialism, white supremacy, ableist machismo culture, and the medical/psychiatric/diagnostic industrial complex. Bound up in the methodology of "cripistemology" in Darling's works is an inherent desire to resist the curative imperative and the cultural logic to repair, regularly deployed by the medical industrial complex, and to embrace the normativity of the broken. In Darling's work, the prosthetic device therefore allows us to consider how the state of the broken, or the wound, provides a new space for the production of knowledge.

Art historian Giulia Smith characterizes Darling's work within a broader framework of debility (as opposed to a narrower framework of disability).[2] I believe situating Darling's work in this way leaves it more open to broader and more complex conversations across numerous fields. Darling's work can also be read broadly across many philosophical themes. Like Lazard, Darling draws on a wide range of thinkers; his reference points range from Michel Foucault, Giorgio Agamben, Hannah Arendt, Naomi Klein, Jean Baudrillard, and Frantz Fanon to Cedric Robinson, John Berger, Claude Levi-Strauss, and Donna Haraway. Darling resists comparison with other artists, styles, or movements, but wants to make work about the current state of things and how the human body is implicated in issues of migration, land ownership, capital, health and wellness, and sovereignty. (Having said that, he acknowledges that he admires the work of Ryan Trecartin, Bjarne Melgaard, and Klara Lidén). He also resists being co-opted into more simplistic and easy categorizations of "disability artist" as an identity category, which museums are eager to deploy to demonstrate more inclusive policies. Instead, he prefers to embrace what David Serlin and Robert McRuer have called a "cripistemological" approach that, like hospital aesthetics, intends to undo the master narrative in the medical model of disability. "Cripistemology" heeds a call by disability studies scholars for a crip-based approach to method and methodology. In their essay, "Towards a Crip Methodology for Critical Disability Studies," Louise Hickman and Serlin ask:

> how might scholars develop methodological tools that are not only specific to critical disability studies but also anchor and apply perceptual, sensorial and experiential dimensions of what it means to be a disabled subject in the first place? ... In short, how might we embody both our knowledge *and* our methods? As crip scholars, how do we insist on being the ones who not only "talk back" to researchers but who develop, or co-develop, the research questions that animate research methods?[3]

Darling's praxis takes up "cripistemology" as methodology.

In 2017, Darling presented a solo exhibition at Chapter NY gallery entitled *Support Level*, during the stage in his life when he was experiencing his neurological crisis. Some of the pieces produced for this exhibition included *Collapsed Cane* (2017), *Comfort Station* (2017), and *Cut Curtain* (2017). All these works convey an irony around levels of support, as the pieces illustrate a more accurate or truthful representation of support levels in the hospital and medical setting, and how so-called support is typically rife with indecent and impersonal conditions. While Darling creates these works from his own lived experience, he also hopes to make strange everyday objects that are immediately recognizable and obvious to a broader public. Indeed, Darling's familiar objects become anthropomorphized. Instead of an upright stiff cane or walking aid that is intended to hold a body steady, *Collapsed Cane* more closely resembles the crumpled-up body it is meant to support (see Figure 2.1). The top portion of the white cane with its gray handle unfurls slowly down the side of the steel-based bottom in snake-like fashion, appearing as if heavily used and worn out, or radically defying the engineering of its original function and purpose.

In *Comfort Station*, Darling similarly twists up a commode, which is a collapsible and mobile piece of furniture containing a chamber pot. It is typically stationed at the bedside of convalescent hospital patients who want the convenience of using the toilet without having to move very far. Commodes can also be found in assisted living facilities. Once again, Darling's version of a medical support is anything but comforting or comfortable, as the legs of the commode are contorted, while one armrest is fastened tightly against the toilet lid, rendering the commode entirely unusable. *Cut Curtain* is a thick PVC plastic curtain suspended on a metal rod which juts out horizontally from a gallery wall. While visitors can easily walk around one side of the curtain to see both sides, Darling wants us to notice the gash in the center of the curtain's material, a metaphor both for the cuts and injuries sustained by the human body and for the body's own transparency within the confines of the hospital. Indeed, the cut in the curtain is similar

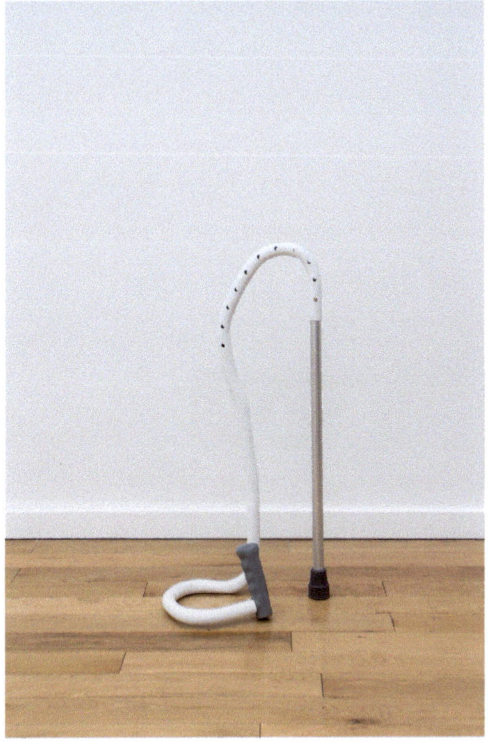

2.1 Jesse Darling, *Collapsed Cane*, 2017. Steel, aluminum, rubber, and lacquer. Courtesy of the artist and Chapter NY.

Image description 2.1: A sculptural white cane. Its sturdy metallic base stands up straight before abruptly slumping back down to the floor like cooked spaghetti.

to the "cut" in the hospital gown. The hospital room, with its curtains and gowns, lacks total privacy, and the patient is never truly alone. The irony of the hospital is that it is meant to be a place of support for recuperation and recovery of bodies that are unwell; in the end though, it can be a place of great stress, anxiety, and discomfort. Other architectures from Darling's *Support Level* exhibition showed further distress and pain from the care industrial complex, including a back brace, a cool pack, waiting room posters vandalized with graffiti, and a grip bar, among other things. Collectively, the work in this exhibition seems both constrained and free: constrained by being literally broken, yet free from the burden of laboring under the conditions of the capitalist regime. As Heather Holmes says, "sometimes the arm does not fling up from the ground because it cannot; sometimes the arm does not fling up from the ground because it would rather not."[4]

Darling's eerie modified sculptures bring to mind the work of Robert Gober vis-à-vis Marcel Duchamp, who also uses found objects such as sinks, drains, urinals, cots, playpens, doors, and windows as metaphors

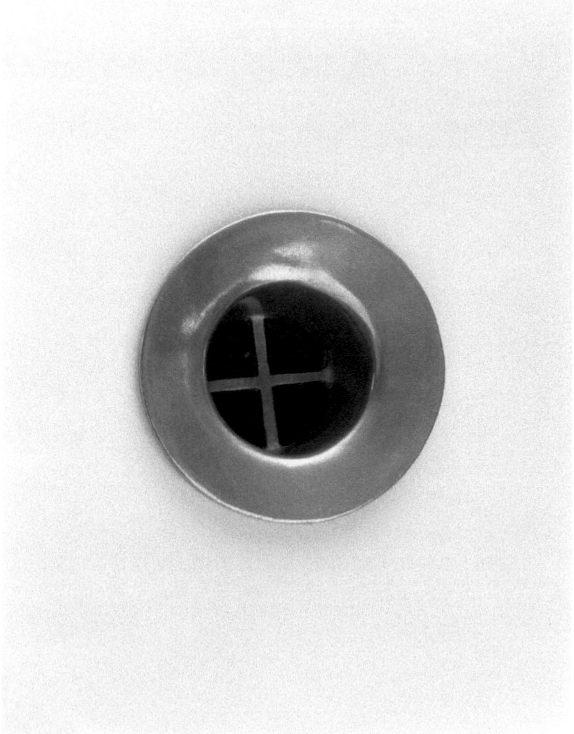

2.2 Robert Gober, *Drains*, 1990. Cast pewter, 3.75in. (9.5cm) diameter × 1.75in. (4.5cm) deep. © Robert Gober. Courtesy Matthew Marks Gallery.

Image description 2.2: A circular metallic drain.

for pathology, pathos, grief, spirituality, longing, identity, and alienation. Like Darling, Gober renders everyday objects and furniture with new meaning, making strange the quotidian and the mundane. Similarly, Gober anthropomorphizes his sculptural creations with a rich poetics that aims to denaturalize that which is deemed natural, including homosexuality and heterosexuality. Gober's objects, especially his drains (see Figure 2.2), operate as windows into other worlds that one might seek to inhabit, where otherness might be possible. On the other hand, Darling's work shows us that which is antithetical, as objects that might be full of possibility are closed off, or conversely, exposed. Darling's poetics comprises a language of dysfunction and debility. Both Darling and Gober manage to evoke trauma in both familiar and disturbing tones at once.

While Darling's work incorporates the trauma, vulnerability, and failure of the body, he also considers his objects as expressions of resilience and resistance, full of life and agency. From a state of brokenness, the body is brought into a generative state, similar to the idea that the artist is creative

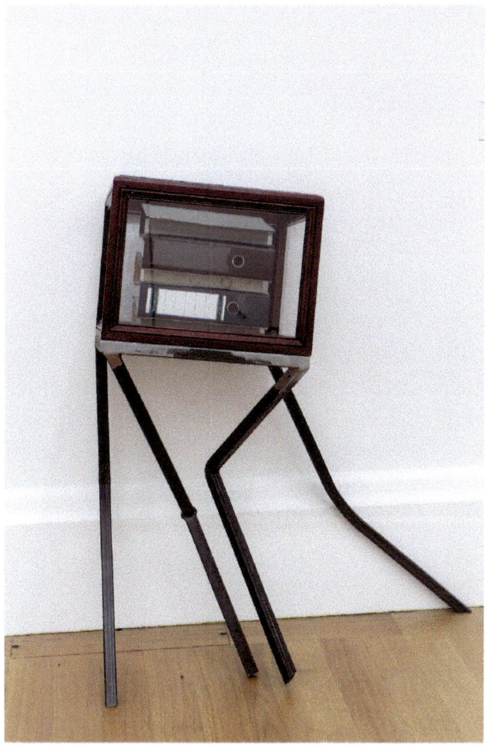

2.3 Jesse Darling, *Epistemologies (Shamed Cabinet)*, 2018. Mahogany, glass, steel, linen, archival binders, concrete, 49.2×43.3×19.7 in. (125×110×50 cm). Photograph: Matt Greenwood. Courtesy of the artist and Arcadia Missa, London.

Image description 2.3: A small box, made from a wooden frame and glass panels, holds a small stack of books. The box rests on four bent and wobbly metallic table legs.

through illness. This sentiment parallels the argument in disability studies that the disabled body contains new ontologies and epistemologies that can expand our definitions and understandings of embodiment in most generative ways. *Epistemologies (Shamed Cabinet)* (2018) by Darling is a work that seeks to complicate definitions of conventional epistemologies (see Figure 2.3). (*Epistemologies (Shamed Cabinet)* is part of a series that also includes *Epistemologies (Limping Cabinet)* (2018) and *Epistemologies (Collapsed Cabinet)* (2018). This work was also originally part of another solo exhibition by the artist for Tate Britain in 2018–19, entitled *The Ballad of Saint Jerome*, which was subsequently displayed in the Venice Biennale in 2019. The artist offers an adapation of the legend of the Christian saint Jerome, who supposedly tamed and healed a lion by removing a thorn from its paw. Jerome was able to tame a wild creature of nature through his superior knowledge. In cripping the story, Darling wanted to raise questions about the position of dominion and control that Jerome held over the lion, that might resemble the tense relationship between doctor and patient. The patient is held captive by the wiser and more knowing healer, a subjugation of otherness that Darling calls into question.

Epistemologies (Shamed Cabinet) is a typical museum glass cabinet, animated by bent legs that suggest ambulatory motion. Despite the cabinet's apparent desire for motion, however, it is unable to move freely owing to its injured form. What, the work asks, could be destabilizing its typically stable form? Inside the glass cabinet, archival binders containing historical medical records are piled up on top of one another and, on closer inspection, evidently filled with concrete. The sharply angled legs of the cabinet are not so much moving as bending from the weight and heaviness of its contents. The weight of the concrete in the cabinet mimics the 'cultural' weight of the precious and fragile relics and objects typically found inside museum cases. In Darling's act of filling their contents with concrete, he shows the true weightiness of medical records, which clinicians have asserted as an essential tool of scientific progress. From a contemporary perspective, however, such progress might be viewed differently, these records offering proof of the construction and production of white medical knowledge that is skewed, narrow, and prejudiced. This, the work claims, is an epistemology that must be shamed. By pouring concrete into the cabinetry, Darling rejects the white medical heteronormative imperative to collect and collate, and by association he also rejects, crips, and shames the archives of Western knowledge in museums, which have been acquired through the extractive, violent measures of colonization. Indeed, the legs of the cabinet no longer supply adequate support, buckling under the weight of oppression. Thus, similar to how Mehta, Sherwood, and their peers reject the reduction of their disabled bodies to the logic and vocabulary of an impersonal X-ray. As will be discussed in the next section, Darling is rejecting medical knowledge collected and collated in binders of medical notes. It is in this work that we find another bridge between the art gallery and the hospital, similar to Lazard's *Extended Stay*.

The title of the work also references Eve Kosofsky Sedgwick's *Epistemology of the Closet* (1990), a defining book in queer theory troubling binary oppositions between heterosexuality and homosexuality.[5] Darling's shamed cabinet is also a cabinet that shames closeted homosexuality, disability, and debility, especially given the museum's long and problematic obstruction of centering queer knowledge, or of putting identity positions on display in an egregious manner. This point was made in James Luna's *Artifact Piece* (1987), in which the artist put his own Indigenous body on show to imitate standard museum practices of display at a time when wax bodies of Indigenous people were commonly fixed within static tableaux that ran contrary to the contemporary realities and lived experiences of Indigenous communities. Such falsifying systems of representation foreclosed agency for the communities in question. Similarly, Darling shows how the communities to which he belongs are literally being foreclosed by the strictures of the display cabinet, with the weight of concrete literalizing this oppression. When visitors, often startled by his moving chest, realized that Luna was a living and breathing person inside the cabinet, the idea that the cabinet must contain legible knowledge, or should be an artifact of an objective 'truth' was disturbed. The work created a visual taxonomy no longer controlled by the museum, asserting that a seeing and knowing body can no longer be viewed and reviewed in the museum's sanitized conditions.

Darling's cabinet does this same work, using a cripistemological framework. In the cabinet's decapacitated state, however, there is an opportunity to consider what generative new knowledges may emerge. While the concrete may weigh down the cabinet's contents, hanging heavy in our history and in our hearts and minds, Darling empowers it with an agential discontent that suggests its mobility or lack thereof from a different point of view. It can still function as a prosthesis in its own way and in its own time, which is ultimately its premise for freedom. In their 'Introduction' to *The Matter of Disability: Materiality, Biopolitics, Crip Affect*, the editors David T. Mitchell, Susan Antebi, and Sharon L. Snyder state that disability is an active participant in meaning-making, and it is not just about looking at disability through positive and affirming terms; it is more about how disability evidences embodiment's tendency to shift and unfold. Darling's cripistemology makes this apparent for us. In his literal reassemblage of support structures such as cabinets and prostheses, he is also reassembling what it means to support, and how bodies can be carried, or in turn how they can carry us. Indeed, while metaphors of the prosthesis have been deployed ad nauseum by scholars as a signifier within technoculture, or trauma-informed narratives, Darling fleshes out his cabinetry limbs with mobilizing form so that the work becomes a vehicle for new and empowered knowledge production and epistemologies in art history, disability studies, and the critical medical humanities.

Darling's work has influenced a slew of other contemporary disabled artists interested in cripping the aesthetics of the medical industrial complex, including Park McArthur with her stacks of disposable ventilator filters and text from an incentive spirometer device, Berenice Olmedo, Ezra Benus, Alex Dolores Salerno, Hayley Cranberry Small, R. A. Walden, Carly Mandel, and many others. Among these is Constantina Zavitsanos, a conceptual artist who works in sculpture, performance, text, and sound. Their work elaborates what is invaluable in the (re)production of debt, dependency, and other shared resources. In *Specific Objects (Stack)* (2016), a vertical stack of grab bars are evenly spaced and mounted to the wall, yet another iteration of a dysfunctional medical assistive device (see Figure 2.4). Zavitsanos titled the work after an essay of the same name by minimalist artist Donald Judd, as their grab bars are presented in a manner which evokes Judd's vertically stacked wall pieces. Displayed in this way, the grab bars also lose their function so that the visitor can think about them from a new framework. Grab bars are typically used as an assistive aid for disabled

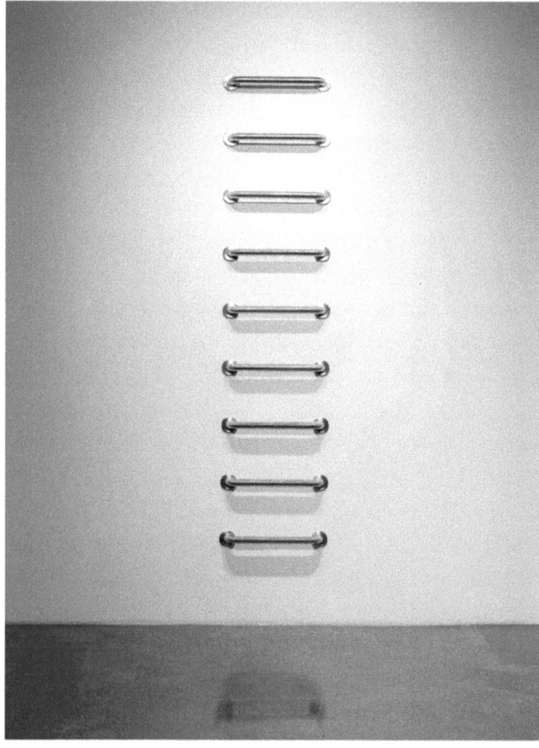

2.4 Constantina Zavitsanos, *Specific Objects (Stack)*, 2016. Disabled access grab bars mounted on wall, dimensions variable. Photograph: Clare Gatto. Courtesy of the artist.

Image description 2.4: Nine iconic stainless steel grab bars are mounted at various heights in a tidy continuous vertical line on a white wall from low to high. The vibe is very minimal and yet still somehow excessive. The repetition of stacked bars every foot or so appears to take the form of a ladder.

people who may use them to get in and out of the shower, or to get on and off the toilet in the bathroom. They are engineered and manufactured using specific measurements to meet the requirements set by the Americans with Disabilities Act, and they frequently appear in public spaces and places to ensure compliance. In this work, the artist critiques these standardized measurements by pointing out that they were actually designed and based on the metrics of a disabled veteran's body (and no one else's). Yet they purport to apply to disabled people at large according to what is deemed "universal design."

In yet another iteration of the grab bar, disabled artist Jes Sachse attempts to revise the praxis of indexing through an installation entitled *Undeliverable* (2021). The work consists of one thousand metal plaques arranged in a grid-like formation in the shape of a column going up one length of a wall. The plaques are an index of donors who conventionally supply funds to a gallery. Depending on how much is donated, they may be given certain status and perhaps even naming rights to particular galleries in the museum. In this appropriation by Sachse, the plaques are engraved with the word 'permission' and are accompanied by aluminum shower grab bars. The work is ironic because, while the recognizable grab bars are suggestive of giving permission – access even – they become a decorative accessory as they don't ultimately function well to support the weight of a body – any body – that desires to climb them to get a view from up top. Sachse critiques the institution that is oftentimes more interested in the funds and donations it will receive from wealthy patrons than it is in the needs of its disabled audiences. In short, Sachse's project highlights the unfortunate truth that access is also frequently treated with tokenizing gestures rather than with the care it requires. Is making it to the top of the donation ladder all that it's cracked up to be if the climb is arduous and elitist? As Sam MacPhee-Pitcher says in their review of the exhibition, "Accessibility should be community-building, life-affirming, and expansive, but what is the cost of insisting upon it?"[6] Access, then, in this instance, is obscured and dismissed, as it is commonly considered too complicated by the museum world. Museum and gallery administrators often complain of feeling weighted down by the administrative and material hurdles they must overcome to comply with state and federal regulations and provisions for disabled audiences. Sachse is indexing how some bodies are prioritized over others within the spaces of museum culture (rich abled bodies of benefactors versus disabled bodies). Sachse's work, then, embodies a crip approach to institutional critique. In this work, Sachse also succeeds in showing how the world of the hospital meets the world of the art gallery, as the hospital also indexes, stores, and archives bodies.

Darling, Zavitsanos, and Sachse have theoretically and methodologically stumped the prosthesis, grinding it to a halt, while giving it new support for continued learning. In the next section, I provide a detailed reading and history of the prosthesis, a metaphor I have long been interested in alongside other disability studies scholars, particularly David Mitchell and Sharon Snyder through their iconic "narrative prosthesis" analysis. The discussion that follows is intended to provide further historical and artistic framing for Darling's work against a much larger backdrop of fragmentation, modernity, and metaphor.

Thinking about the prostheses

The prosthetic symbolizes disruption – it is the body in chaos, the body fragmented and broken. The prosthetic is a symbol of loss. A limb – a leg, or an arm, or even an ear or an eye, a finger or a toe – that is lost is surely indicative of a gap, a space for something that is missing. In her seminal essay, *The Body in Pieces: The Fragment as a Metaphor of Modernity*, art historian Linda Nochlin writes that while she does not wish to propose some "grandiose, all-encompassing theory of the fragment," she still believes that it should be grounded "on a model of *difference*."[7] She also acknowledges the dual marvelous/horrific function that the fragment continues to have in artwork, and traces its lineage in different periods and movements in art history, starting with paintings, drawings, and sculptures from the French Revolution, through Impressionism, Surrealism, and the more modern art practices of Louise Bourgeois, Robert Mapplethorpe, Robert Gober, and Cindy Sherman. Even though Nochlin argues that the fragment assumes new transgressive forms in the practices of these contemporary artists, in which the body is hardly unified or unambiguous, she does not discuss this rupture's intersections with – and impact on – disabled subjectivity.

Amputee, prosthesis user, and scholar Steven Kurzman brilliantly captures how ableism shapes the metaphor of the prosthesis: "Artificial limbs do not *disrupt* amputees' bodies, but rather reinforce our publicly perceived normalcy and humanity ... Artificial limbs and prostheses only disrupt ... what is commonly considered to be the naturally whole and abled Body."[8] In other words, using the prosthesis as a metaphor to connote loss, trauma, or abjection indicates ableist thinking in an ableist world.[9]

It is worth here briefly turning to the origins of the word "prosthesis." Emerging from ancient Greek, it was imported into the English language in the sixteenth century. Its root "pros" translates as "adding, furthering, advancing, giving additional power" and so emphasizes the prosthetic as an addition to, rather than the extension of an existing word.[10] Therefore the prosthetic gives power to that which is missing, so it is possible that the literal definition of the word lends itself to a suite of metaphorical constructions that have little or no basis in the everyday experience of an amputee. Indeed, the root implies that losing an arm or a leg is considered traumatic, and thus the prosthesis is a kind of "savior" that is endowed with a power in its ability to fill in the gap or loss. Like the word "disability" itself, the word "prosthesis" is also freighted with certain connotations in Western discourses. The dominant culture may wish to assign prostheses and their so-called grotesque associations to anyone with physical and mental "handicaps." But given that so many people from a wide spectrum of ages, classes, and ethnicities have many visible and invisible impairments, either congenital or acquired, it is hard to affix "prosthesis" to any one defined signifier or experience. In other words, meanings associated with prosthesis are varied and cannot be permanently defined and located in any one individual experience. Ultimately, the status, value, and significance of prosthetic metaphors are absolutely reliant on entrenched cultural perceptions that must be destabilized.

Tiffany Funk has sought to break down what she calls a "prosthetic aesthetic," asserting that "much of current art historical theory depends upon predominantly psychoanalytical readings of the prosthetic to illustrate certain trends in contemporary artworks"; she feels that such writers largely ignore the "common usage [of prosthesis] to denote the physicality of technological devices and cybernetic body augmentation and its social effects" and make no mention of the day-to-day, real-life embodied experiences of amputees.[11] Curator and scholar Katherine Ott writes that "prostheses usually perform cultural work unrelated to the practicalities of everyday life ... Prosthetic devices, as social objects with a complex set of meanings in the daily lives of people, have rarely, if ever, been understood as part of vernacular material life."[12] Ott and Funk, along with several other scholars who fully or partially work within a disability studies context, such as Sarah S. Jain and Vivian Sobchack, try to provide alternative historical, cultural, and embodied perspectives as a corrective to the vogue for prosthetics as found in psychoanalytic theory (Freud, Lacan, Silverman) and contemporary cultural, science, and technology studies. Ott makes particular mention of how the prosthesis is used reductively as "a synonym for common forms of body–machine interface," most explicitly in conversations around the cyborg and Donna Haraway's scholarship.[13] The fusion of technology (in the form of prosthesis) and body is one that ends up displacing the material body. Ott argues that these discussions "hardly begin to comprehend the complex historical and social origins of prosthetics."[14] Jain concurs, suggesting that little work has been done on the "everyday social, economic, and semiotic mediations that occur between persons and objects in the technologically infused spaces of life ... ."[15] Jain is particularly interested in the deployment of the prosthesis trope as it applies to broader human–technology relationships, especially in factory labor practices, mass production, and marketing.

All of these scholars ask: what does it mean to be a prosthesis user? Vivian Sobchack is a single above-the-knee amputee and scholar formerly working in film studies at the University of California in Los Angeles. She provides a more intimate, practical tale of her experiences as an amputee and prosthesis user in her essay "A Leg to Stand On: Prosthetics, Metaphor, and Materiality." Sobchack questions why so many scholars find the prosthesis such a seductive object. As the prosthesis has become "extraordinary," she endeavors to "both critique and redress this metaphorical ... displacement of the prosthetic through a return to its premises in lived-body experience."[16] Sobchack is not interested in intervening in any flights of the artistic or scholarly imagination and denying artists freedom or mobility to explore the prosthetically enhanced body. Sobchack says that "perhaps a more embodied 'sense-ability' of the prosthetic by cultural critics and artists will lead to a greater apprehension of 'response-ability' in its discursive and artistic use."[17] In other words, it would be nice to see more creative metaphorical and literal constructs of disability that are explored from within, for example the spatial experience of an amputee, or that examine what it is like to use a prosthesis or to feel a phantom limb.

Part of the challenge with dismantling the reductive use of prosthetics is addressing the binaries through which its representation is mediated, including self/other, body/technology, Global North/Global South, beautiful/ugly, perfect/grotesque, male/female, global/local, West/East, and so on. Sobchack claims that the literal and material ground of the metaphor of prosthesis has been largely forgotten, if not disavowed, although I would go further to question whether any direct, personal interaction with the materiality of the amputee/prosthetic experience is very common in the first place.[18] Apparently the prosthesis has hidden powers in artistic discourse that elide any complex and logical ground for their real users. Ultimately, Sobchack claims that the true scandal of the metaphor is that the prosthesis becomes fetishized and "unfleshed-out," an uncomfortable "floating signifier" or catch-all word for a broad discourse on technoculture or the abject, obscene, and traumatic.[19] It is here that the work of Darling helps to "en-flesh" the narratives of the limbs. I argue that the discomforting effect of "immobilizing" disability in art history is the product of an *uneasy fit* of narrative prosthesis itself. In other words, the prosthesis can be used as an apt metaphor for how disability, as a subject worthy of consideration in the canon of art history, has never truly been taken up; indeed, it has never truly been a comfortable fit. Art history has always been uncomfortable with disability and the fit has not been seamless.

For example, Matthew Barney's symbolic use of prostheses – an important practical tool that assists amputees with mobility and therefore independence – demonstrates how an everyday tool for amputees is used in an uninformed way in contemporary art as a metaphor for interior emotional and psychological states. Matthew Barney is an important contemporary American artist who is known for producing grand, elaborate film works and sculptural installations combined with performance, photography, and drawing. One of Barney's most ambitious works is his Cremaster Cycle series. Barney has worked with model and double amputee elite athlete Aimee Mullins in *Cremaster 3* (2002), and literally turns her prostheses into an artwork. I was drawn to this work as I wanted to learn why Barney was interested in working with Mullins in particular. Barney had offered to work with her as he wanted her to wear special prosthetic legs as part of her costume for her various characters in the film. These prostheses included a pair of transparent glass legs designed by Alexander McQueen (as an "extension" to the fairy tale of Cinderella's glass slippers), cheetah legs, and transparent glass man o' war tentacles. Barney was also interested in the symbolism that Mullins's body could evoke. Specifically, he wanted her to appear in a scene in the film where she was not wearing prosthetics at all. Like Marquard Smith, who has written about Mullins's role in this film, I believe Barney was engaging in metaphorical opportunism by working with an amputee.[20] Barney's request seems dehumanizing and fetishistic, given his fixation on having impractical prosthetic legs fabricated for her, recalling Vivian Sobchack's amusement that prostheses are somehow now magical, and endowed with power.[21] Barney has gone one step further here than simply rehearsing the magical properties of the prosthesis, given the prosthesis now takes on a similar presentation and function to that of a relic: it becomes a sculpture/artwork in and of itself, and sits on a pedestal in a museum, to be admired and prayed to.

Where Mullins's prostheses became literal works of art to be reified and considered as precious objects, her embodiment as an amputee was considered by Barney as fragmentation, symbolizing "loss." Even if Mullins's loss was going to symbolize sacrifice according to Barney's narrative in the film, the artist obviously wasn't attuned to how this might affect Mullins in real life – both physically and emotionally. Even though Mullins and Barney negotiated and compromised on what would work for the film, I argue that Mullins still ultimately made a sacrifice for Barney's vision and made herself vulnerable and exposed in a way she may not have been entirely comfortable with. Mullins has also often talked about how difficult it is to stand still while wearing impractical prosthetic legs, and in the film we can observe her tottering around, seeming unbalanced and on the brink of toppling over. Such instability is the antithesis of the seeming gracefulness of her glass "Cinderella" legs, which are meant to evoke romance, fantasy, and eroticism. But her instability is the shared reality of daily life for many amputees. This is likely not obvious to the regular lay person watching the film unless they have had direct experience with amputees.

Ideally, Barney's narrative trajectory would have taken a different path or integrated added layers of complexity with Mullins's own personal narrative to give the model some agency. In her interview, Mullins reveals how vulnerable she feels in real life without her prostheses on.[22] Such insight is rarely a part of the discourse around prostheses, if not in visual art representation then especially not in rehabilitation, where amputees are expected to be determined and strong to "overcome" their "deficiencies." Mullins's comments shed light on the gray area between the inanimate and the animate – the moving flesh, as well as the wood, metal, leather, plastic, and other materials that make up the prostheses. Aside from giving Mullins more agency in expressing her true attitudes around the phenomenology of her prosthetic legs, her intimate insights around what being an amputee feels like could powerfully inform art practices in the future.[23] While Barney employs the prosthesis in his work, a lived experience of the prosthesis, such as Mullins's, is not incorporated directly or explicitly into his narrative. Representations of disabled people and their contributions exist throughout art history, as disability is an integral part of the human condition; yet disability is still not fully integrated into mainstream art historical discourse. Surely a prosthetic visualized on Mullins's body in this vein, beyond just a marker of fetishism and eroticism, will provide us with other kinds of worthwhile prosthetic practices.

Barney's opportunistic use of the prosthesis as a metaphor for abjection and absence exemplifies an approach that Darling and other contemporary disabled artists like Zavitsanos keenly avoid. Instead, in their work, the prosthesis is a medical assistive device that is disabled through a robust cripistemology and disability activism, demonstrating the generative qualities of being vulnerable, and falling down and getting up, over and over again. Darling tells the counternarrative from frank lived experience instead of sensationalizing it, and nor does he rely on heavily overused tropes of otherness. In Darling's world, the prosthesis is most certainly not the savior; rather it morphs into the body of its user, providing a new perspective on the interconnectedness and intimacy that a disabled user can have with their prosthesis. While Darling's engagement with the realities of the care industrial complex at large reveals the levels of support are actually at an all-time low, from an individual perspective, the prosthesis grows and transforms in symbiosis with the flesh of its user in loyal and consistent fashion.

In Chun-Shan (Sandie) Yi's work, the artist challenges notions of a "complete" body by suggesting that the body can reinvent itself through new wearable art, footwear, and other objects that she calls "crip couture."[24] Yi has been influenced by members of her family who for generations, like her, were born with variable numbers of fingers and toes. Indeed, Yi's work often revolves around memories of familial interactions that were focused on the appearance of her body. The process of making her adornments and objects taps into the artist's hidden emotions and distress when confronted by the medical establishment in its quest to fix her body.

By using metals, fabrics, and found objects in combination with heavily handcraft-oriented techniques like metalwork, crochet, felt-making, and sewing, Yi examines the stereotypes and values placed on physical "deformity" and their impact on a person's well-being. For Yi, making art about her body becomes a process of redefining embodiment itself. In *Dermis Leather Footwear* (2011) (see Figure 2.5), Yi uses latex, cork, rubber, and thread as she focuses on the reconfiguration of the wearer's body through mapping the memories of medical and surgical intervention. Altering the purpose of conventional prosthetics and orthotics, which aim to create more-or-less standardized body form and function, Yi blends prosthetics and jewelry-making to make this unique, personalized footwear, in this case for a female friend. The artist likens this process to jewelry-making, as the body is adorned with materials that function in both practical and aesthetic ways to empower atypical features of the body. The wearable item is designed based on the individual's medical experience, physical posture, and state of mind. Ultimately, this work questions what it means to expect a "complete" body. Rather than reject the notion of physical alteration, Yi provides intimate and empathetic bodily adornment as a tool for remapping and engaging with a new physical terrain, one imbued with personal standards of physical comfort and self-defined ideals of beauty. Viewed as a collection of wearable works, the objects – along with the wearers – have helped to create space for the new field of disability fashion,

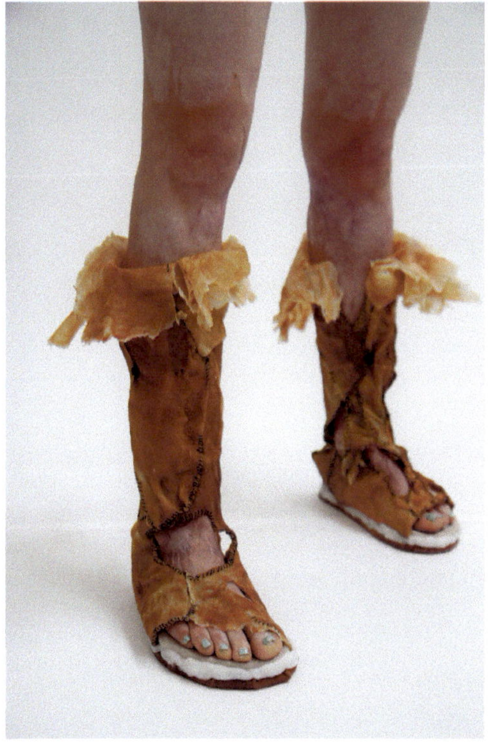

2.5 Chun-Shan (Sandie) Yi, *Dermis Leather Footwear*, 2011. Latex, cork, rubber, thread. Courtesy of the artist.

Image description 2.5: A pair of legs, seen from the knees down, model a pair of tattered boots. The boots mimic yellowing dead skin flaking off the model's peachy colored legs and feet.

which has emerged prominently in the past few years through artists such as Sky Cubacub and Rebirth Garments.

Carmen Papalia's *Long Cane* (2009–11) takes the prosthesis in a new direction (see Figure 2.6). This work addressed the visual meaning ascribed to the walking cane. *Long Cane* involved a comically long mobility device – a walking cane – that, when used, draws attention to the user as an obstacle, as a kind of intelligent practical joke. Papalia developed the idea for what he calls his "performance object" in 2009 because he didn't feel comfortable with the institutionalization of the white cane as a symbol for blindness or blind people, although he also acknowledges the cane's power in offering him personal access. He speaks of his ambivalence toward the cane in the following passage:

> On one hand, it was a tool that promoted my access and mobility. It showed me things and made my map a whole lot bigger. On the other hand, it institutionalized me. It was a symbol that was connected to an institution that

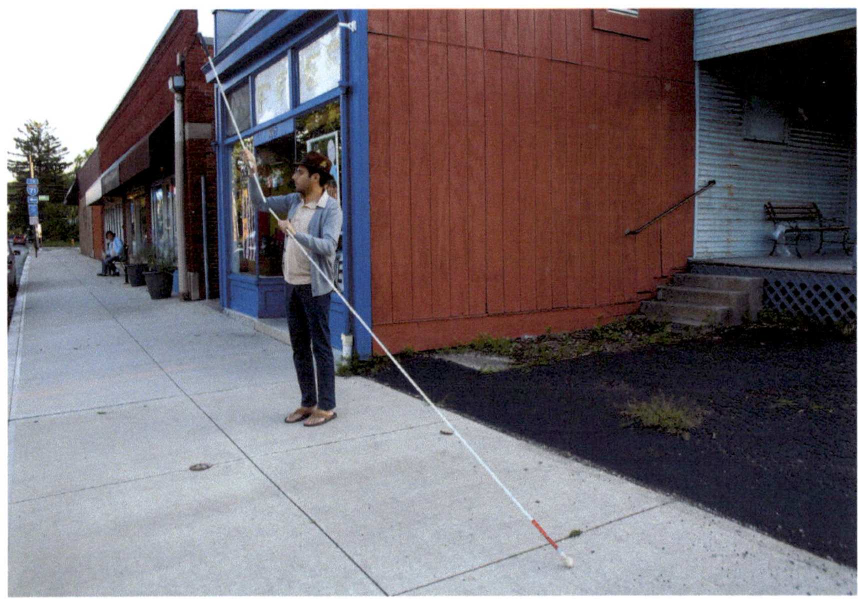

2.6 Carmen Papalia, *Long Cane* performance, 2009–11, Columbus, OH. Courtesy of the artist.

Image description 2.6: A man stands at a distance assembling an absurdly long mobility cane on an empty side walk.

> wanted me to be a certain kind of blind person – the kind with huge sunglasses. The kind that was either a piano tuner or a masseuse. The kind that walks a certain way on a predetermined route, and that talks a certain way about his blindness ... But the white cane, with all of its problems, did promote my access. I was guaranteed a seat on the bus. I had the power to make dense crowds of people part like red seas. I could pass for a Paralympic athlete. I could talk my way into museums and movies. I was a focal point.[25]

Papalia further remarked that the white cane was a lightning rod for attention, separating him from his peers and identifying him as different, therefore creating a hierarchy, reinforcing the binary of ability and disability, and marking and organizing bodies. The artist recognized the distance that the cane was creating between his body and other bodies on the street – the cane tended to push people away, as they would often jostle to scurry out of his way and avoid bumping into the cane. At the same time, Papalia recognized that he enjoyed the power he had in wielding the cane on public streets, and that he controlled the cane that caused his fellow pedestrians to act in a certain manner. Papalia's *Long Cane* project was his response to the revelation that he felt about the power to be had as a blind person. The artist's manipulation of and emphasis on the length of the white cane is what makes this project distinct and interesting. According to the National Federation of the Blind, while the length of a white cane varies from person to person and can be adjusted to individual preferences based on the length of stride, walking speed, and reflexes, a general recommendation is that it should reach somewhere between the armpit and the nose. Papalia's *Long Cane* is 12 feet in length, more than double the height of the artist. When one observes images of the artist as he walks along Commercial Drive in Vancouver, it is very obvious that the cane is too long. As Papalia describes, his reach is now of Herculean proportions, "extend[ing] across an entire span of sidewalk."[26]

In the documented images of Papalia's various sojourns with this *Long Cane*, people are conspicuously absent from the sidewalk. It is difficult to tell whether this is due to the nature of the areas or the time of day, or because the *Long Cane* was actually working at getting people well and truly out of the way (at least out of reach of the camera lens). Nonetheless, the images show Papalia confidently concentrating on his gait and his route, the *Long Cane* held sturdily and defiantly ahead of him on deserted streets. The goal of the *Long Cane* was to make the force field bigger, exaggerating the distance between his and other bodies in order to occupy public space with more agency. The exaggerated length of the cane also meant an exaggeration of the space that Papalia's body occupied on the sidewalk. It also then exaggerated the dramatic reaction of other bodies on encountering the extra-long cane attached to Papalia's now empowered body, which the artist characterized as a 40-foot monster of sorts.[27] Indeed, the artist was now a "real force to be reckoned with."[28]

Although Papalia enjoyed reveling in his newfound power through *Long Cane*, he also recognized that his work literally had a "pointed" antagonistic quality. He says, "I wanted to become an obstruction for others because I was faced with so many obstructions."[29] Papalia's everyday experience with both habitual and new routes through cities typically involves extensive negotiation of other bodies, objects, and architectures. Oftentimes, when carving out routes in a new place, or when something different appears in his regular environment, such as a fallen branch, Papalia bumps or trips into things that make contact with various parts of his body, such as the tips of his toes inside his leather shoes, or his calf, his shins, knees, his waist, hands, elbows, arms, and knuckles, even his head. Sometimes, as with inanimate objects and surfaces, this contact is forceful and painful, while other times the contact is a soft brush or a slight twinge. Of this frequent experience of pain, Papalia has said that he "learn[s] to navigate the city by simply bumping into it. It [is] a long and painful game of pinball that end[s] with the high score of me gathering a sense of place."[30] Through Papalia's physical translation of space, synesthesia is literally a painful process. Papalia's accidental contact with other bodies is affective in nature; reactions elicited from both himself and others range from the embarrassed to the empathetic to the nonchalant to the rude.

I have often walked as a personal guide with Papalia through many different environments and international cities, including Vancouver, San

Francisco, New York, and Dublin. Papalia is comfortable with asking for an arm or an elbow to guide him through a space as a substitute for his white cane, especially if his relationship with a person is familiar. Given my short stature and Papalia's 5 foot 8 inch height, I usually jut my elbow out at a particular angle so that Papalia can reach it at the point where his hand naturally falls to the side of his torso. Sticking my elbow out in this way is not very comfortable for me, but I enjoy the relationship that our bodies inhabit side by side as we walk together. In a sense, Papalia is offering me a window into his ambulatory world, which is often enlightening. Indeed, from this point of view, I am able to observe Papalia's encounters with objects, other bodies, and buildings. Papalia's use of my body as a replacement for his cane in no way guarantees an elimination of his bumping or tripping, but it does offer a new constellation of insights as our differently scaled bodies move side by side.

Through *Long Cane*, Papalia enacted his desire to obstruct the pathway of others, as he himself was constantly obstructed. After some time, he realized that the antagonistic intentions behind the *Long Cane* were not necessarily useful to furthering a dialogic relationship with his audience – he was pushing people, literally, further away, rather than offering them a safe space in which to engage in productive conversation about the causes he was passionate about, including the negative significations associated with the cane. To add to Papalia's later thoughts about his antagonistic approach, the artist also wanted to challenge the standardizing of any prosthesis attached to a disabled body, such as a cane for blind people, arguing that a prosthesis can be personalized, radical, and powerful (instead of just antagonistic). Papalia hoped that his fellow pedestrians would become more aware of any discomfort they might express toward disabled people through their body language and gestures.

Donald Rodney was another important Black British artist who incorporated his own medical devices into his art. Rodney was of African Caribbean descent; his parents were immigrants to the UK from Jamaica, and he had sickle cell anemia throughout his life. Sickle cell anemia causes blood cells to become irregularly shaped so that they become sticky and thus block the flow of blood throughout the body. Rodney often incorporated images of his illness into his artwork and used it as a metaphor to speak of the illness and injustices of broader society and culture, particularly issues of race and racism, slavery, the African diaspora, and police brutality toward BIPOC (Black, Indigenous, and people of color) groups. In the 1980s Rodney was part of the BLK Art Group, which included fellow artists Eddie Chambers, Marlene Smith, and Keith Piper. They were all preoccupied with the marginalized place of the Black individual in British society and the prejudice and discrimination that they regularly experienced.

Rodney's work also incorporated sculpture and installation. In *Psalms* (1997), Rodney used a motorized wheelchair accompanied by computerized technology. The wheelchair became a stand-in for Rodney at the art opening of one of his solo exhibitions, as he couldn't be there in person owing to a hospitalization for his sickle cell anemia.[31] The wheelchair moved and circled around the gallery, and the cameras fixed to the sides of the chair were substitutes for Rodney's eyes. The wheelchair as another prosthetic tool or medical assistive device shows how being separated from the disabled body in this instance is a symbol for disabled embodiment. In a manner reminiscent of Park McArthur's *Ramps* (2014), Rodney plays with the tension between presence and absence of disabled bodies, and the work reveals ableism and racism when minority bodies are both pathologized and made invisible. Sinéad Gleeson states that "the chair refutes the gaze of strangers who stare at disabled and non-conforming bodies; it is also a stand-in for a body of color in the overwhelmingly white space of the art institution."[32]

Sickle cell anemia has been dubbed a "Black" disease as it appears to only impact people with African, Caribbean, Eastern Mediterranean, Middle Eastern, and Asian ancestry. Individuals who have sickle cell anemia experience pain and may end up requiring hospitalization. Rodney spent extensive amounts of time in hospital when he was alive, and he decided to use much of the medical ephemera from this time in hospital to educate the public on sickle cell anemia. He also used this autobiographical data as a framing device for broader issues of identity politics across Great Britain. In *The House that Jack Built* (1987) (see Figure 2.7), Rodney created a profile outline of a house on the wall which was then filled with a collage grid of his X-rays. Jareh Das writes that "societal stereotypes are challenged by the artist who takes ownership of his body as it is inhabited by illness, the X-rays serving as a metaphor for looking below the surface to discover how overarching power systems operate."[33] Black hands and arms painted over the X-rays peek out from the frame of the house, along with numerous pairs of white painted scissors and text that reads as though from a journal entry by Rodney. In front of the collage is a tree trunk that is dressed up in men's clothing, a self-portrait of the artist as part of a literal family tree. As with Lazard's critique in Chapter 1, Rodney comments on how medicine and its attendant treatments show a lack of care for his body simply because it is Black. The Black body is treated more forcefully and violently as it is mistakenly assumed that it is tougher and less sensitive than white bodies. Rodney also depicted some of the scarring on his body following numerous procedures and operations. In *The House that Jack Built*, Rodney shows how the family tree is often riddled with literal and metaphorical scars, sadness, and imperfections.

Electromagnetic journey through embroidery

The X-ray is a dominant feature in the work of several contemporary disabled artists. Bhavna Mehta lives and works in San Diego, California,

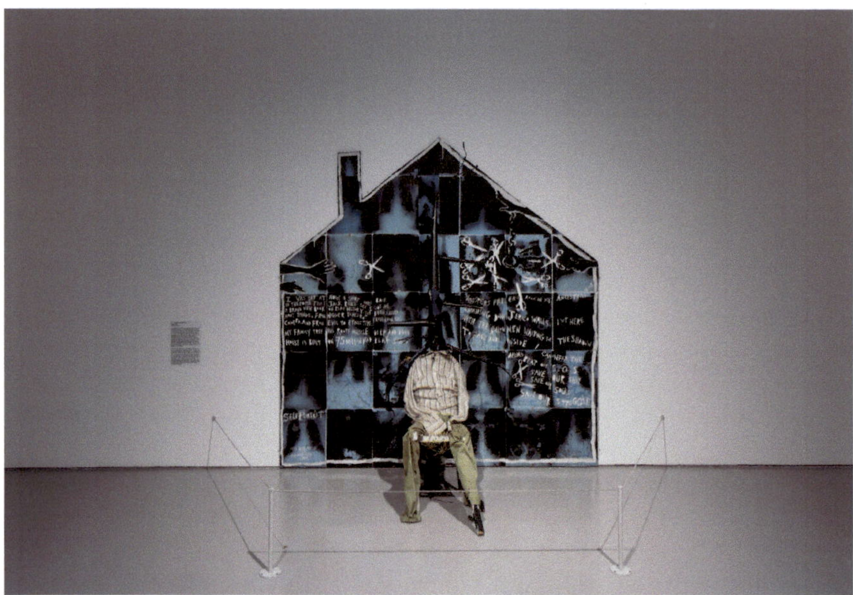

2.7 Donald Rodney, *The House That Jack Built,* 2024. Installation view at Spike Island, Bristol. Photograph: Lisa Whiting. Artwork courtesy the Estate of Donald Rodney.

Image description 2.7: A headless torso sits in front of a collage of x-rays arranged into the shape of a house with a pitched roof.

and is originally from India, where a majority of her family are still based. Mehta has long worked with paper, cutting, sewing, embroidery, and other craft-based practices that she inherited from the female relatives in her family and from Indian folklore traditions passed down to her as a child. As an immigrant living for over forty years in the United States, Mehta is also interested in common stories, memories, and narratives. A wheelchair user born with both polio and scoliosis, Mehta has recently produced work exploring the politics of her embodiment as a disabled immigrant woman, while still drawing on the craft-based praxis that is critical to her artistic production. Polio is a virus (poliovirus) caused by an infectious disease that infects the spinal cord, sometimes resulting in paralysis. Scoliosis is a condition that causes curvature in the spine. While most of the time the cause of scoliosis is unknown, in some cases it develops because of disc degeneration in the spine, hereditary genes, arthritis, or osteoporosis. Mehta sees how these conditions of her body have been captured in her X-rays and chooses to utilize the X-rays' visual and transparent qualities.

Mehta's family was not traditionally in the business of craft education and making. They worked as businesspeople selling food items such as groceries, spices, and grains. They did not sell any of the embroideries they did make. In Mehta's generation, the women had to go to school and learn

English. English was going to be the language of the future – the language of commerce, trade, law, and medicine – when Mehta was growing up in the 1970s in India. Further, India's constitution was established in 1950, seventeen years before Mehta was born. In the context of India's young democracy and changing economy, people used education as a way to advance. Although rural families were still practicing crafts and keeping the family skills alive, many other families in cities started to move toward more academic and professional careers.

Mehta developed her skills in embroidery with her female relatives, mostly during the summer break, which was several months long. The first step in the embroidery process would be to transfer a design from tracing paper onto the fabric using carbon paper. Colors would then be selected, along with hoops, needles, and threads, and somebody would start the embroidery. If the stitch was something new that everyone was learning for the first time, they would use a little scrap to practice the stitch on. The embroideries were not very big. There might have been three or four pieces; people would work on their hoop for a while and then exchange with somebody else. Mehta notes that embroidering was a way to be together more than anything else.

For a long time, Mehta regarded the Indian embroidery she learned from her family as traditional, and she was unable to translate those traditional forms and designs into something that she could make contemporary and connect with her own ideas. But then she started looking at other artists' works, in which they would develop repetitions that could be transformed into new forms. Mehta wanted to translate a traditional design and a texture and a pattern into a more contemporary version of those same forms. She was excited to realize that she could develop her own language with embroidery, that the stitches of her past could be depicted anew. Embroidery could reflect the subjects she wanted to talk about.

Mehta states that she can feel her mother's presence and her hand when she is embroidering: "It's a deep connection to my mother. It's a deep connection to India's ancient history."[34] She discovered that to the Greeks and the Romans, the word *India* meant cotton, including textiles, threads, and embroidery. Textiles from India were fine and rich, and included cotton, silk, and wool, all integral to India's status as a superpower thousands of years ago. This is a deep connection and history that Mehta feels very fortunate to have in her pocket. With these profound historical and personal connections to embroidery, Mehta realized that she could say something further about her experiences as a disabled woman, which had little place in discussions during her childhood. Mehta was the only visibly disabled person in her family and in her school. She used crutches and braces to walk in India. While she was not able to use her wheelchair anywhere outside the house, she notes that she was fortunate to have a wheelchair in the first place: "that was one difference between me and other people who were disabled in India."[35] Mehta experienced a great deal of isolation as a young person, only meeting others who were disabled when she was in hospital. She notes that the world seemed to relate to her through the medical model of disability in India, perceiving disability as an individual problem to be fixed rather than within a social context: "the idea of the social model of disability would have never entered our minds."[36] Even talking about disability was shunned in India, as the notion of drawing more attention to oneself (even more than the attention one would already receive by virtue of being physically disabled) was considered taboo. Mehta said that these ideas were further reinforced and complicated by the fact that women were not expected to talk about their bodies at all, let alone a disabled body.

Embroidery offered Mehta a canvas through which to express herself and speak of her disability. Mehta felt that the role of her disability in her identity often got hidden away and forgotten, but her embroidery allows this crucial element to be revealed. When Mehta left India for the USA, she stuffed medical X-rays of her chest, ribs, and spine into a suitcase, only to find them again decades later. The X-rays were taken when she was a teenager and showed scoliosis in her spine, caused by the poliovirus that disabled her at the age of 7. She looked at her X-rays as she never had before – through the eyes of an artist. She compares finding them to finding her body "buried beneath layers of silence. Just like an X-ray reveals the unseen architecture of a body, a story can unearth the shifting language of our experiences."[37] Mehta wanted to focus on how she could connect her body of the past and present with nature, which is often inaccessible to her as a disabled woman. She sought to find nature within her own body instead.

Mehta used the black and white X-ray as her canvas and embroidered a colorful silk landscape of rivers, plants, mountains, and valleys in the middle of her chest to create her piece *I Found a River in My Body* (2022) (Figure 2.8). The canvas is a rectangular piece of silk fabric with a printed X-ray of chest, ribs, and curved spine in black and white. Two metal rods can be seen in the center of the print; they are attached to the spinal vertebrae. The embroidery is on the bottom left ribs on the X-ray canvas, done with silk thread in a variety of colors. It forms a circular topographic map, its colors corresponding to those commonly used on maps to represent plants, mountains, valleys, deserts, rivers, etc. There are many rivers running along in the circle, but the main river runs alongside the two rods shown in the X-ray. There are a few threads which just leave the primary circle of the map, representing features such as rivers, plants, deserts, etc. spreading to different parts of the body. By combining the body (the X-ray) and the topographic map (representing the land and the environment), Mehta asks the viewer a thought-provoking question: "How does the discovery of a disabled body relate to the discovery of land and what value does that have?"[38]

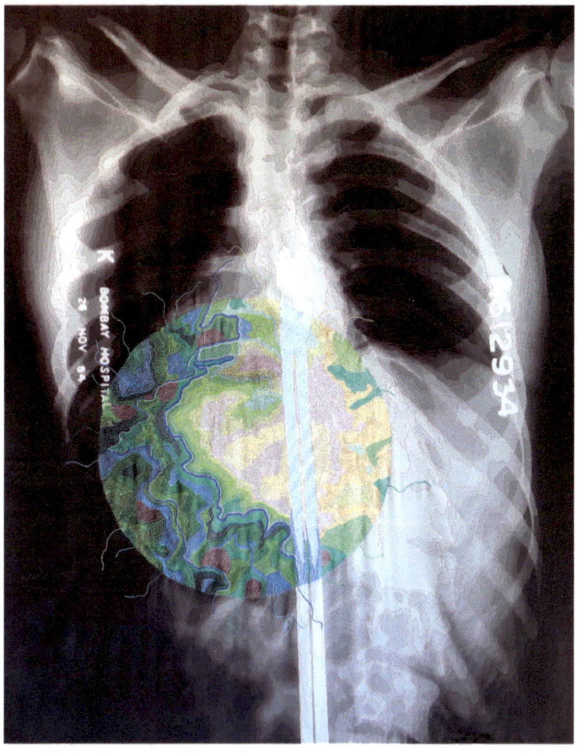

2.8 Bhavna Mehta, *I Found a River in My Body #1*, 2022. Hand embroidery on printed silk, 60 × 51in. (152.5 × 129.5cm). Courtesy of the artist.

Image description 2.8: An x-ray of a torso with scoliosis where the spine is being supported with metal rods. A circular topography map overlaps with the rods like an oasis floating within a rib cage.

Through this artwork, Mehta rescripts the perception that disability is unnatural. By using her old X-rays to make the prints on fabric and then embroidering into these, Mehta has found a way not only to look inside the body and gain clarity about what the architecture of the body is, but also to consider how the body has tenderness; the fabric is like skin and can absorb different kinds of marks, both intended and unintended. While Mehta acknowledges the feminist political discourse surrounding embroidery as women's domestic work, she also connects strongly to how embroidery is tied to the flesh. Like flesh, embroidery has the ability to take the shape of something, both literally and metaphorically. Mehta asks, "what is the story we can tell through the colors and designs of embroidery?"[39] In answering her own question, Mehta comes back to her Indian notion of embroidery as a kind of abundance: you might have a plain piece of fabric and then suddenly there are marks and there's an abundance of form. The

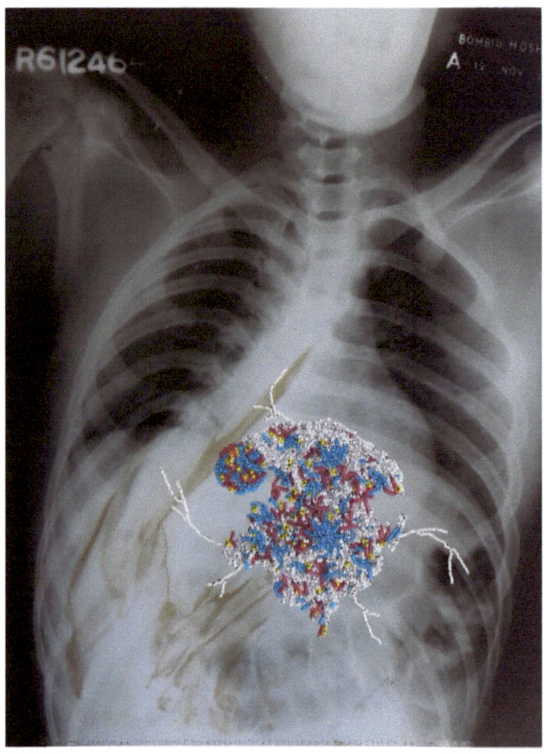

2.9 Bhavna Mehta, *Throughlines: Poliovirus #4*, 2020. Glass beads embroidered on X-ray, 16 × 13in. (41 × 33cm). Courtesy of the artist.

Image description 2.9: An x-ray of a torso with scoliosis. Beads of blue, yellow, red, and white have been embroidered onto the torso to resemble the polio virus.

X-ray literally makes transparent that the body has many different things happening inside, and by embroidering over the top of the X-ray and into the fabric-as-skin, Mehta adds to the layers of flesh and the layers of meaning.

Mehta has made other related work using her own X-rays. In her piece *Throughlines: Poliovirus #1*, she illustrates a single virus by embroidering colorful beads directly onto her X-rays. She interprets a virus as the beginning of a story. *Throughlines: Poliovirus #4* (Figure 2.9) depicts how the multiplication process of the virus progresses, which she describes as an attack on her neurons, affecting muscle function.

In an interview with Mehta, I asked her what her family in India thinks of her artwork, particularly regarding how she has reconstituted her embroidery into new form through the X-rays of her disabled body. She said it was hard for them to understand it, not least because for them embroidery is not art, but simply embroidery. While there are clearly major cultural differences between Mehta's native country and her country of residence, the artist has successfully weaved together a story of her identity that combines old traditions from the fabric of India's history with layers of feminist politics, alongside newer notions of disabled embodiment. This makes for a unique and textured contribution to disabled approaches to craft.

While Mehta's praxis is critical work that simultaneously intervenes in and contributes to a history of textile politics and feminist production, I acknowledge how histories from the Global South are also woven into these revised traditions. Mehta is part of a diaspora in which a culture of disability politics is still repressed; instead, the economy and politics of textile labor comes with other forms of radical activism that must be accounted for. In the introduction to her book *The Necessity of Craft*, editor Lorna Kaino offers insights into women's craft production in the Asia-Pacific region.[40] In this part of the Global South, craft production is a matter of survival, so crafts are commodities that are not afforded the luxury of being displayed in an art gallery. While women are the makers of these craft objects, often, ironically, they have to rely on men to sell them. So on the one hand, while women have a direct and important role in the production of the means of survival for a community, on the other hand they are cut off from being able to represent themselves and their literal craft in an exchange of goods for currency. Within this problematic, disability doesn't even enter the conversation, as craft production is understood rather as an issue of feminist politics and survival. For the women in Mehta's family, this work is not necessarily a matter of survival. However, I argue that their relationship to textiles sits between the notion of craft as necessity, and craft as women's work (and therefore solely belonging in the domestic sphere). Having grown up making crafts alongside her female relatives, Mehta comes to this work understanding the politics attached to craft and her place as a woman within it, on both micro and macro levels. And yet Mehta also had to contend with her body and identity as a disabled woman while growing up, and eventually when she immigrated to the United States. Mehta endows her craft-based practice with these additional layers of meaning, which bring to life her unique intersectional stories and identity as a disabled Indian woman. Her work demonstrates that the role disability craft has to play in representing minority subjects is critical, both inside and outside the museum.

As a way to theoretically frame Mehta's work and approach, it is useful to look at Leigh Gruwell's *Making Matters: Craft, Ethics, and New Materialist Rhetorics* (2022). In the book, Gruwell discusses the historical figure Ada Lovelace, a woman who is known as the "mother of computer programing."[41] Lovelace had discovered a mathematical breakthrough that enabled calculations on an analytical engine machine far more advanced than had previously been possible. Gruwell informs us that a key aspect of Lovelace's discovery (of which few people are aware) is that it was in fact the Jacquard loom, which stores data for creating patterns in weaving, that inspired Lovelace in her calculations. Gruwell writes that Lovelace faced many obstacles in her career, juggling motherhood and work, and facing additional barriers as a woman. Gruwell notes that she had poor health, including asthma attacks, and used a crutch for walking. She states: "Navigating the world through her ill, female body and the expectations that followed it, Lovelace faced the intersection of power and materiality every day."[42] In her recounting of Lovelace's story, Gruwell establishes not only the connection between weaving and the birth of digital technology (showing that materiality intersects with the digital), but that ultimately these worlds were fused together by someone with an intersectional identity as a disabled woman – someone who understood power imbalances intimately, as Mehta also does. Lovelace paved the way for creating a more equitable future for disabled women.

Gruwell's work develops a new materialist rhetorical framework, pointing out how relational entanglements of actors are the true engine of what produces work either at the loom or in programs through a keyboard. She writes, "new materialist rhetorics ... productively orient the field toward an understanding of agency as distributed among assemblages of human and nonhuman actors ... ."[43] Craft as a medium shows how materiality is very much entwined with power and politics, and we must recognize the ethical implications within it. Craft is produced by many hands in a class system where its actors have different levels of power within a community, and the ways in which the fabric is woven and unwoven can directly impact the assembling and disassembling of those same power relations. Craft, then, has the capacity to carry agency, otherwise called "craft agency." Gruwell goes on to argue that through craft agency, we can observe how power circulates and even stagnates, and that craft can even provide tools to challenge the "uneven distribution" of power and resources.[44] Mehta demonstrates craft agency through her art practice based on her identity as a brown disabled woman from the Global South, and shows how models of relationality between human and nonhuman things can help to enact social justice. By literally interweaving her own X-rays into the politics of craft and identity, Mehta brings a new stitch to the pattern, namely the politics of medicine and the diagnostic gaze.

As Gruwell emphasizes, the materiality of relationality itself is the glue that makes textiles the communal activity that it is, a reality that is acknowledged and felt deeply by Mehta. The familial entanglements bound in textile-making within cultures and countries around the world are also connected to contemporary thinking in disability justice. Western concepts of care and dependency focus on how access is formed through social relationships. In the field of disability studies, concepts of care have been theorized by feminist activist scholars, particularly Eva Feder Kittay through her groundbreaking work on "ethics of care" and how care work is often cast as "feminine."[45] All these philosophical frameworks coalesce around Mehta's work. Through this work, we can envision a different future in which alternative embodiments can not only shape our fabrics and X-rays, but also ensure that these same fabrics, in turn, reshape the world too.

Bhavna Mehta is contributing to a growing and evolving disability arts and craft praxis that adds a rich and generative layer to the medium of craft itself. Her work showcases how craft traditions from India that have been shaped by unique cultural and sociological forces can be woven into the fabric of disability studies discourse in the United States. Mehta shows how the dynamics of intersectional identity can be unraveled, recontextualized, and retold, using ancient and revered textile traditions. She brings a rich constellation of politics and metaphors to her work, including the connection between flesh, skin, and material form; the connections between interior and exterior environments; and tactility as a zone for challenging the hierarchy of the senses. Mehta's stories from her childhood and her work's reception in the United States and in India also remind us that the medium of textiles and their philosophical, epistemological, and methodological treatment are still contested ground around the world. In carefully parsing out these stories and traditions, we have much to learn.

The penetrating radiance of X-ray art

Mehta's interest in using X-rays as the foundation for her crafts and her politics has a long lineage. Many contemporary artists have been drawn to using X-ray ephemera over the past few decades. One of the most significant and earliest precursors to Mehta's work is that of California-based painter Katherine Sherwood, an artist of Riva Lehrer's generation who has also made crucial contributions to the representation of disabled embodiment. Yet rather than focusing on external appearances, Sherwood has been intent on revealing the interior workings of her disabled body. Mid-career, at the age of 44, Sherwood had a cerebral hemorrhage which paralyzed the right side of her body. Turning back to her painting afterward, she was drawn to the MRI images and scans of her brain taken in the hospital. She started to use the brain imaging as a basis for her art – a conceptual and literal ground to work upon. Indeed, the scans served as the catalyst for new gestural shapes and forms that emerged from the necessity of working flat and pouring paint directly onto the canvas.[46] Sherwood has been especially interested in challenging images produced by the medical industry, which are used as diagnostic tools. Sherwood prefers to interpret the images of her own body with paint, collage, and other materials that transform the portrait of her brain into an empowered one. In several early works from this period, Sherwood overlaid her scans on canvas with painted symbols drawn from *Secrets of Magical Seals* by Anna Riva.[47] According to Sherwood, medical imaging technology has made the artist's role as a pictorialist of anatomy obsolete; she seeks new means by which to participate and intervene in the process of depicting the body.[48] This move mirrors the historical shift that followed the invention of photography, when artists

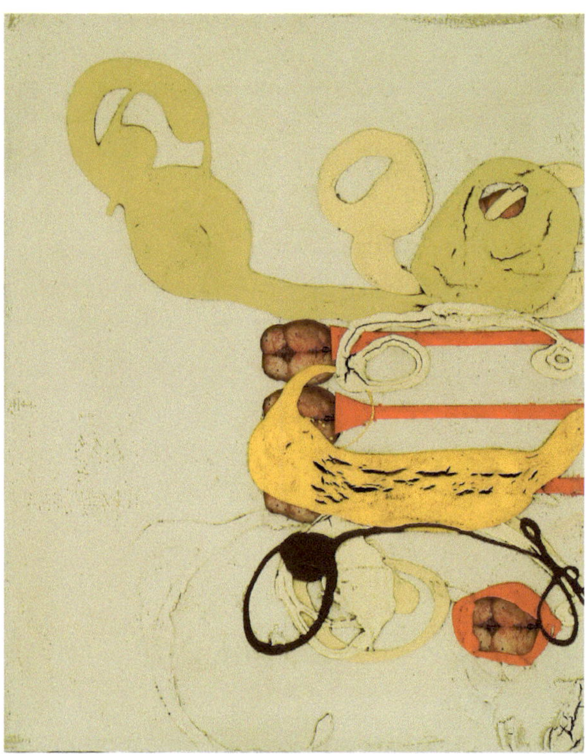

2.10 Katherine Sherwood, *Ladmiral's Brain*, 2005. Mixed media on canvas, 32 × 26in. (81 × 66cm). Courtesy of the artist.

Image description 2.10: An abstract mixed media painting on a vertically oriented rectangular canvas. Thick fluid swirls crowd the right side of the painting, loosely layering muted oranges, yellows, and browns on top of each other over a pale yellow background.

were no longer limited to realistic depictions of landscapes, portraits, or still lives. Technology precipitated the emergence of new artistic genres and movements at the turn of the twentieth century. Ultimately, Sherwood's work also contributes to the larger tradition of disabled artists reclaiming images of their body (see Figure 2.10).

Aminder Bindu Virdee is a British South Asian multidisciplinary artist, writer, access consultant, and social justice activist. In several series of works from the past few years, she has actively used X-rays taken of her own body to articulate lifelong pain and to subvert rampant racism, ableism, sexism, and classism in the medical industries. One such work is *KaleidoSkeleton Ti* (2020), a digital new media artwork that subverts the diagnostic gaze to instead amplify the beauty of the brown, chronically ill, female body. In *KaleidoSkeleton Ti: The Desi Cyborg* (2020–21), Bindu Virdee created a colorful, X-ray-generated audiovisual video through transmedial programming and computational code art. As with the first work from this series, Bindu Virdee seeks to disrupt the diagnostic gaze, challenging Western beauty ideals and normative performativity and labor under a capitalist regime. Bindu Virdee has had lifelong exposure to medical imaging, which has urged her to rescript these images into ones that center her autonomy instead of erasing her identity. Similar to Mehta, Bindu Virdee has integrated a reclamation of her diasporic identity and her Indian Punjabi heritage into her activist politics regarding disability, health, and illness. These Indian Punjabi aesthetics are evidenced through the vivid, opaque colors in her video that echo the visual culture of Indian fashion, religion, rites of passage, festivals, and other traditions. By weaving her identity as an ethnic immigrant disabled woman into all her work, Bindu Virdee points out not only the threat of erasure of her body as a disabled person, but that all the other elements of her intersectional identity are oppressed as well. In the artist's most recent series, *Eco-Crip, Cybotanical Futures* (2021–22), she uses biodigital images, data art, artificial intelligence, and manipulated public domain photographs of indigenous South Asian flora, Punjabi scripture, and the artist's personal archive of hospital-generated X-rays. She mounts these on the wall in twentieth-century X-ray lightboxes. The Punjabi script in the images translates to "Disabled bodies are sites of resistance," "Disabled bodies transcend mobility," and "Disabled bodies are the future" – lines that act to crip both the botanical and medical material. Bindu Virdee has coined the term 'cybotanical' to describe both the work and the form of a disabled cyborg body as it intermingles with botanical art – a body now unburdened of both the colonial and clinical gaze.

Both Mehta and Bindu Virdee are creating X-ray-based art steeped in the politics of disability and medicine from the perspective of immigrant BIPOC women of the diaspora. They also share an impulse to bring traditional cultural and artistic influences from the Global South into their work. Their identities as immigrant women also suggest how the X-ray can be read on other levels as, historically, human chest X-rays were collected from long-term visa applicants in different parts of the world, to ensure the immigrant was not sick prior to crossing a border. The X-ray becomes a frontier and a divider all at once, presenting numerous binaries: insider versus outsider, internal versus external, legal versus illegal. The X-ray is an embodiment of being able to see what is on the other side of a divide, and is thus used not only as a tool of control by the medical establishment, but by governments as well. As Kasia Ozga states, "the border-as-process of inclusion and exclusion [is] linked to regulative authority in social relations, nation-building, political sovereignty, as well as personal identity formation."[49]

Lisa Cartwright discusses the complexity and power of X-ray imagery in her previously mentioned book, *Screening the Body: Tracing Medicine's Visual Culture* (1995). Cartwright points out that, beyond the well-understood fact that the X-ray is used for surveillance and control of all bodies in the medical industry, who gets to be X-rayed in the first place indicates a hierarchy and privileging of bodies based on gender, race, and class. Cartwright states that "though medicine may control the bodies and communities it images, it also offers imaging as a class and cultural privilege."[50] Minority bodies do not always have access to X-ray technology, just as minority bodies do not always have access to adequate healthcare. Cartwright uses the example of how men and women were frequently X-rayed to uncover tuberculosis infection from the 1930s to the 1950s, but X-ray imaging of women's breast tissue for cancer was sorely lacking. Women's bodies were not accorded the same optical scrutiny or investment by the medical establishment. While the X-ray is used as a reclaiming device by the contemporary disabled artists in this chapter to thwart and retool the curative imperative of disability that motivates the white medical establishment, access to the X-ray is also a privilege. Bearing in mind the politics of race, disability, and medicine discussed throughout the book so far, we must view the X-ray as a complicated medium that mixes power and privilege, authority and control, elitism, and access (or lack thereof). Access to the technology of the X-ray becomes even more fraught if we compare it to the accessibility of craft as an economic necessity, particularly in the Global South. Combining craft, artistic praxis, and the X-ray thus not only blends disability empowerment in medical worlds, but it also reveals the conflicting worlds of access that exist across the diaspora.

The work of the contemporary disabled artists discussed in this chapter shows us how hospital aesthetics encompasses a zone where medical assistive devices can be dismantled through a radical new cripistemology, where counternarratives do not shy away from vulnerability, and diagnosis equals resistance. While Mehta's work blends craft activism from the Global South and privileged access to X-ray technology to weave new scripts regarding her body and polio, Darling's canes, grab bars, back braces, and other prosthetic equipment make transparent the insufficiencies of support available in the medical industrial complex. Both Mehta and Darling demonstrate how the wound – and the recording of that wound – can have an empowered voice. Rather than leaning on supportive objects such as X-rays and prostheses, the viewer instead becomes destabilized as the artists unravel assumptions about what the sick body is capable of. While the sick body is capacious, these artists also show that debility is not to be feared. Quite the opposite: it is the space and place where new definitions and understandings can be acquired.

Notes

1 Technically, an X-ray is an electromagnetic imaging test that doctors use as a tool to determine prognosis and treatment, so the "assistance" of this medical tool is for the doctors rather than the patient. One might say then that the X-ray offers

indirect medical assistance to disabled people, while a cane or a prosthetic device offers direct assistance to help the body move and function.

2 Giulia Smith, "Chronic Illness as Critique: Crip Aesthetics Across the Atlantic," *Art History* 44, no. 2 (April 2021): 286–310, https://doi.org/10.1111/1467-8365.12559

3 Louise Hickman and David Serlin, "Towards a Crip Methodology for Critical Disability Studies," in *Interdisciplinary Approaches to Disability: Looking Towards the Future*, ed. Katie Ellis, Rosemarie Garland-Thomson, Mike Kent, and Rachel Robertson (New York: Routledge, 2019), 131–41.

4 Heather Holmes, "On Jesse Darling," *Journal of Visual Culture* 19, no. 2 (2020): 272–76, https://doi.org/10.1177/1470412920944482

5 Eve Kosofsky Sedgwick, *Epistemology of the Closet* (Berkeley, CA: University of California Press, 2008).

6 Sam MacPhee-Pitcher, "Undeliverable and What it is to Care," Akimbo website, https://akimbo.ca/akimblog/undeliverable-what-it-is-to-care-by-sam-macphee-pitcher/ [accessed February 21, 2024].

7 Linda Nochlin, *The Body in Pieces: The Fragment as a Metaphor of Modernity* (London: Thames and Hudson, 1994), 56 (italics in original).

8 Steven L. Kurzman, "Presence and Prosthesis: A Response to Nelson and Wright," *Cultural Anthropology* 16, no. 3 (August 2001): 374–87. www.jstor.org/stable/656681

9 This history is also very similar to the social construction of Blackness in art history. Kobena Mercer says, "the social construction of Blackness creates a condition of polyvocality in which visual signs of identity and difference are invested with a multitude of contradictory meanings and antagonistic values … once 'black' is understood not as a category of identity given by nature, but as a subject-position historically created by discursive regimes of power and knowledge in the social domain of 'race,' then the goal is to explore how art produces a signifying difference in the cultural codes of collective consciousness and thus has the potential to alter or modify prevailing consensus in the symbolic construction of reality." Kobena Mercer, ed., *Pop Art and Vernacular Cultures* (Cambridge, MA: MIT Press, 2007), 138. The one-sided, limited use of "grotesque" across Black and disabled subjects shares a similar history and a similar desire for disruption and to "talk back."

10 Tiffany Funk, "The Prosthetic Aesthetic: An Art of Anxious Extensions," https://digitalcommons.wayne.edu/macaa2012scholarship/1/ [accessed January 20, 2025].

11 Funk, "The Prosthetic Aesthetic."

12 Katherine Ott, "The Sum of its Parts: An Introduction to Modern Histories of Prosthetics," in *Artificial Parts, Practical Lives: Modern Histories of Prosthetics*, ed. Katherine Ott, David Serlin, and Stephen Mihm (New York: New York University Press, 2002), 2.

13 Ott, *Artificial Parts*, 2.

14 Ott, *Artificial Parts*, 2.

15 Sarah S. Jain, "The Prosthetic Imagination: Enabling and Disabling the Prosthesis Trope," *Science, Technology & Human Values* 24, no. 1 (Winter 1999): 31–54, www.jstor.org/stable/690238 [accessed December 5, 2024].

16 Vivian Sobchack, *Carnal Thoughts: Embodiment and Moving Image Culture* (Berkeley, CA: University of California Press, 2004), 206.

17 Sobchack, *Carnal Thoughts*, 207.

18 Sobchack, *Carnal Thoughts*, 208.

19 Sobchack, *Carnal Thoughts*, 209.

20 Marquard Smith and Joanne Morra, eds, *The Prosthetic Impulse: From a Posthuman Present to a Biocultural Future* (Cambridge, MA: MIT Press, 2005).

21 Consider the film *Avatar* (2009), where the main character's avatar replaces his paralyzed legs and gives him power and superhuman abilities.

22 Smith and Morra, *The Prosthetic Impulse*.

23 There is no shortage of detailed insight on Mullins's experiences as an amputee, as can be seen and heard in countless interviews, including her TED talks from 1998 and 2009.

24 Chun-Shan Yi, "From Imperfect to I am Perfect: Reclaiming the Disabled Body Through Making Body Adornments in Art Therapy," in *Materials and Media in Art Therapy: Critical Understanding of Diverse Artistic Vocabularies*, ed. Catherine Hyland Moon (New York: Routledge, 2010), 103–17.
25 Carmen Papalia, "A New Model for Access in the Museum," *Disability Studies Quarterly* 33, no. 3 (2013): http://dsq-sds.org/article/view/3757/3280 [accessed December 5, 2024].
26 Papalia, "New Model for Access."
27 Papalia, "New Model for Access."
28 Papalia, "New Model for Access."
29 Papalia, "New Model for Access."
30 Carmen Papalia, "Bodies of Knowledge: Open Sourcing Disability Experience," *Journal of Cultural and Literary Disability Studies* 9, no. 3 (2015): 357–64, https://muse.jhu.edu/article/596373 [accessed December 5, 2024].
31 Keisha Jacobs, "Motifs of Social Maladies Abide: Remembering the Artistic Legacy of Donald Rodney," Arts Help website, www.artshelp.com/donald-rodney [accessed February 10, 2024].
32 Sinéad Gleeson, "A Different Kind of Healing," *Frieze*, September 7, 2020, www.frieze.com/article/different-kind-healing [accessed December 5, 2024].
33 Jareh Das, "Illness as Metaphor: Donald Rodney's X-ray Photographs," *Nka: Journal of Contemporary African Art* 45 (November 2019), 95, https://muse.jhu.edu/article/738989 [accessed December 5, 2024].
34 Das, "Illness as Metaphor," 95.
35 Das, "Illness as Metaphor," 95.
36 Das, "Illness as Metaphor," 95.
37 Das, "Illness as Metaphor," 95.
38 Das, "Illness as Metaphor," 95.
39 Das, "Illness as Metaphor," 95.
40 Lorna Kaino, *The Necessity of Craft: Development and Women's Craft Practices in the Asian-Pacific Region* (Perth: UWA Publishing, 1995).
41 Leigh Gruwell, *Making Matters: Craft, Ethics, and New Materialist Rhetorics* (Denver, CO: University Press of Colorado, 2022), 3.
42 Gruwell, *Making Matters*, 5.
43 Gruwell, *Making Matters*, 5.
44 Gruwell, *Making Matters*, 7.
45 Eva Feder Kittay, "The Ethics of Care, Dependency, and Disability," *Ratio Juris* 24, no. 1 (February 2011): 49–58, https://doi.org/10.1111/j.1467-9337.2010.00473.x
46 Katherine Sherwood, "How a Cerebral Hemorrhage Altered My Art," *Frontiers in Human Neuroscience* 6 (April 2012): 1–5, https://doi.org/10.3389/fnhum.2012.00055
47 Anna Riva, *Secrets of Magical Seals: A Modern Grimoire of Amulets, Charms, Symbols and Talismans* (New York: International Imports, 1975).
48 Sherwood, "Cerebral Hemorrhage."
49 Kasia Ozga, "The Internal Frontier: How Art at Once Problematizes Borders and Draws Us Closer to Them," *Contemporaneity: Historical Presence in Visual Culture* 6, no. 1 (2017): 1–18, https://doi.org/10.5195/contemp.2017.186
50 Lisa Cartwright, *Screening the Body: Tracing Medicine's Visual Culture* (Minneapolis, MN: University of Minnesota Press, 1995), 146.

3

Sensual hospital aesthetics

A nude white man lies on his side, his back facing the viewer (Figure 3.1). He is resting on what could be construed as a medical uniform, "scrubs," a blue wrinkled hospital sheet stretched over a mattress, which is resting on wooden floorboards. The room is dark, but the man's body and the mattress he is lying on are well lit, showing every hair, crease, curve, mole, and freckle on his skin. His brown hair is shaved short, and his legs are bent at the knees. It looks as though he has empty IV bags strapped to each of his legs, and a long, deep indentation of his spine travels from the base of his buttocks up to the back of his neck. We also see a hint of the man's scrotum peeking through the back of his thighs and buttocks, where it dares to engage in a cheeky game of reveal versus conceal, taunting the viewer with its implied sexuality. The work is *CripFag* (2021) by queer disabled contemporary artist Robert Andy Coombs, part of an extensive photographic series that the artist has been working on for several years since receiving his MFA from Yale University in 2020. The man in the photograph is Coombs, and this could be classified as a self-portrait, and an appropriation of the classic Greek statue, only disabled. I argue that this work displays an evocative new element of hospital aesthetics. When I look at this photograph, I see hospital aesthetics because it provides layers of complex information that are both aesthetic and political. At first look, Coombs offers us a straightforward image of a nude lying in a posture made famous by a long lineage of portraits of (mostly female frontal) bodies posing for artists throughout art history since the Renaissance. Given that the work is plain, and bare even, with the only visual elements being Coombs's body, the mattress, and the black background, the work may more closely resemble what a real hospital looks like, and what a sleeping and/or resting patient might look like. Coombs also gives direct hints of the hospital and the possibility that he is a patient through the blue mattress

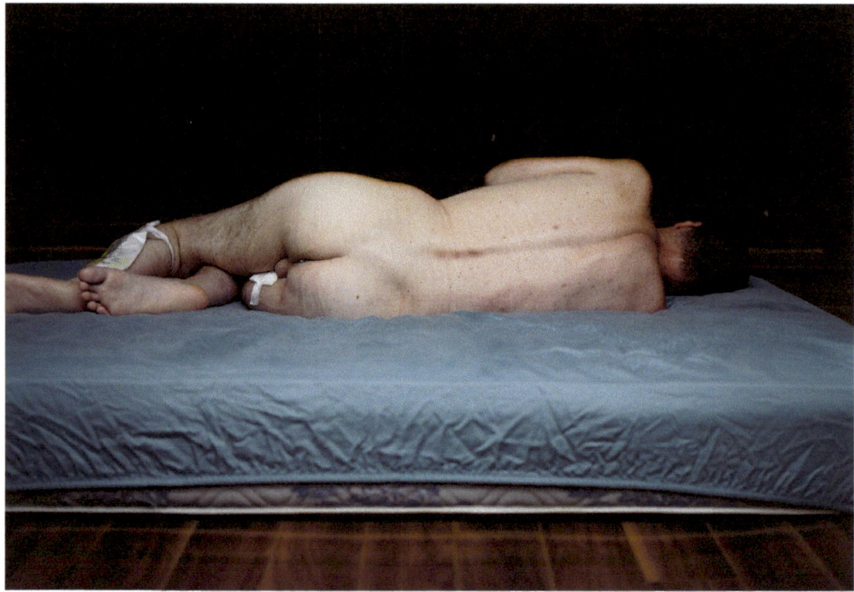

3.1 Robert Andy Coombs, from the series *Cripfag*, 2021. Courtesy of the artist.

Image description 3.1: A naked disabled white man lays on his side with his back facing us. He lays on teal colored sheets and has a catheter bag attached to his left shin.

cover and the empty IV bags encircling his calf and thigh. The unusual nature of Coombs's spine is also noticeable. But what is unusual here is that it is Coombs's scrotum that the eye travels to first after the initial recognition of his overall form. Then, as the eye continues to travel, we see the IV bags. Coombs's hospital aesthetics offers a reboot of the aesthetics of the hospital on his own terms, which also incorporates the politics of queer disabled identity, and the politics of queer disabled sexuality. I will return to this artwork again.

This chapter focuses on arguably the most overt and bold expression of hospital aesthetics. I analyze the work of several artists who explore sexuality and sensuality using the hospital as an interface for encountering sex that would otherwise be taboo. They work to debunk the assumption that disabled people do not and cannot have intercourse, and they focus on the medical system's inability to see disabled people as whole people. The artists I examine here include Robert Andy Coombs and Panteha Abareshi, with supporting discussion on the performance collective Sins Invalid and other contemporary disabled artists who challenge assumptions about the disabled body's sexuality or asexuality. The work by the artists in this chapter uses the mediums of photography and performance to explore eroticism, fetish, intimacy, and intensity. I argue that their work is contributing to a new form of hospital aesthetics that is a far cry from the docile and monotonous patient life that is the foundation of the hospital. Instead, these artists strip the hospital of its unrealistic views of sex and disability by being disruptive, playful, and uncompromising in both their sexual desires and a larger desire to overturn stereotypes. Additionally, the topic of disability and sex is not a new one. Later in the chapter, I spend time framing the work of the artists with theoretical material that has been critical in helping to shape the politics of disabled sexuality, focusing particularly on how this politics has arisen within visual culture and contemporary art.

Intended to be at the center of the book, this chapter acts as somewhat of a climax. While the sexual pun is imbricated in this structure, the climax is also meant to indicate a bright spot, or a moment, that separates itself sharply from the rest of the content. This is because this chapter not only takes a new direction, but also shows a hopefully unexpected quality of hospital aesthetics. In this chapter, hospital aesthetics earns its rainbow-colored stripes. Indeed, this chapter is meant to be colorful and fun, while also offering lessons, even if those lessons are somewhat rubbed in our face, amidst genitals and other body parts. The main takeaway is that disabled people are sexual people too, contrary to the stereotypes that disabled people are not only sexless, lack interest in sex, and cannot have sex, but that they are unsexy and undesirable. Of course, none of this is true, and if one is not convinced of this fact prior to reading this chapter, the work of Coombs and Abareshi will shatter these misconceptions into a thousand pieces. While Coombs's and Abareshi's work is (arguably necessarily) confrontational in its use of nudity and the fact that the nudity belongs to disabled nude bodies (Abareshi is also queer), it is equally refreshing, playful, and serious. While their praxes may evince tongue-in-cheek wit and humor (particularly in Coombs's work), it is critical that the reader realize how mainstream bias around disability and sexuality must be broken apart. A sexless disabled body or a disabled body with a limited or no sex life should not be assumed to be part of post-hospital life.

This is not simply a rant about how disabled people are sexy too. Rather, I seek to point out how the specific lived experiences of the contemporary disabled artists discussed in this chapter have provided us with a particular perspective on the medical industrial complex that is in dialogue with their sexuality, or assumed lack thereof. Both Coombs and Abareshi draw from the lengthy periods of time they have spent in hospital as patients, and they use these experiences as impetus for their art and to project a politics that expands our understanding of hospital aesthetics. They have both been victimized and subjected to dehumanizing treatment, and they both react to this treatment through their work; they have both been told that they would not be able to have fulfilling sex lives, and they were not instructed or guided on how to attempt to do so; they have been treated like 'pounds of flesh' instead of people with feelings and valid life experiences. These demoralizing encounters have driven them to make the work that we are about to experience.

Eroticizing the hospital

In 2020, the popular art critic Jerry Saltz wrote a story about Coombs's photographs for *New York* magazine in which he called Coombs's work some of the most "unshakeable" new work about masculinity and sexuality that he had seen in a long time.[1] Coombs also brings the rarely considered perspective of a queer *disabled* man into that mix, and he has acknowledged that he regularly experiences ableism within the queer community too. He has been prolific in the last four to five years, producing many different styles and genres of work, including the *CripFag* series; *Polaroids* taken between 2008 and 2023 in various cities, ranging from Grand Rapids, Yale, Fire Island, and Miami; *Portraits* (people); and *Street* photography. Throughout his work, Coombs records both his own sexual experiences as someone who is queer with a disability, and the sexual experiences of others. His work also provides a record of queer life, city life, and the aging process.

Coombs turns the conventional patient look on its head. For starters, one doesn't typically encounter a hospital patient in the nude; he completely abandons the hospital gown that Quagliozzi so fastidiously explores (see Chapter 1). Coombs doesn't care for it; he is far more interested in what is underneath the gown. He wants to be completely freed from it. Coombs is not one to be inhibited, and he demands that his body be both viewed and treated as sensorial. His work comes from the lived experience of spending a great deal of time in hospital as a patient. Earlier in his life, Coombs was an avid gymnast, but when he was 21 years old he broke his neck during training. He completed a double backflip on a trampoline and landed incorrectly. His body became paralyzed from the shoulders down, and he is now quadriplegic and a wheelchair user. At the time of the accident, he had to spend one month in the intensive care unit, a part of the hospital that provides care to patients who are critically ill. Coombs then spent another month on a ventilator, followed by six weeks at the Spinal Cord Rehabilitation Center at the University of Michigan.[2] When he was released from hospital, he moved back into his parents' house. His mother is a physical therapist, so she was able to help him, and to this day, ten years later, he has a regular rotation of caregivers who help him bathe, eat, use the toilet, and perform other daily physical tasks that he cannot complete independently. To make his art, he controls his digital camera with a joystick which he operates with his mouth. His art takes time to produce, and he has assistants who help him create his impressive portfolio of images.

While Coombs was in hospital and later during rehabilitation workshops, he found that the medical professionals he came into contact with would rarely want to talk with him about sexuality. Instead of being direct with him about what his body might be capable of sexually, including ejaculation, they were dismissive and glossed over the topic in a superficial way. They told him to go watch very dated VHS tapes about disability and sex that he found unhelpful and irrelevant to his lived experience. (Coincidentally, in Panteha Abareshi's video, *Methods of Care for the Precarious Body* from 2020, the artist draws loosely from the government-subsidized medical videos produced for education purposes between the 1950s and 1970s, and critiques how the silent educational video depersonalizes the imaging and handling of the disabled and chronically ill body.) Coombs realized that he would have to pursue his own research on the topic by looking up disability porn or wheelchair porn so he could understand what might be possible with his newly acquired body. He feels that the medical professionals could really improve their engagement with patients who have acquired disabilities by researching what a fulfilling sexual life might look like for their patients. Medical professionals mistakenly assume that this is not a topic they need to know about or cover because people with acquired disabilities like those Coombs has will not be able to engage in sexual activity. This is certainly part of the overarching ableism that still pervades the medical system. Coombs states:

> There are people with disabilities who have no idea how their body even works sexually because healthcare professionals don't cover sexuality as part of their practice. People with disabilities are left to go figure out everything on their own. Society doesn't view us as sexual human beings. My work is just scratching the surface of whatever "disabled sex" looks like. We need to start shifting the conversation from "How do you have sex?" to "What sexual acts do you enjoy?"[3]

Coombs has been answering this latter question through his bold images. The title of the *CripFag* series already captures Coombs's confrontational style. He uses derogatory slang words for queer and disabled people – *faggot* and *cripple* – but reclaims them. By putting both terms together, Coombs is going for the jugular; society is still getting to grips with how minority communities are wielding each of these terms to empower themselves, but on a separate and individual basis, not together. The implied intersectionality of the portmanteau word "cripfag" is progressive, truthful, and important, but almost ahead of its time because he puts two slang terms together for more punch. Coombs is one of a few artists who meaningfully show us what intersectional identity looks like in a very bold manner. Some artists may choose to highlight or make a case for one identity category over another in their art-making, but for Coombs, his layered identity is spelled out clearly for us, each part taking up equal space at the table.

In Figure 3.2, we are confronted with an aerial view of Coombs's white, outstretched torso which is cut off at the neck along the top, and at the

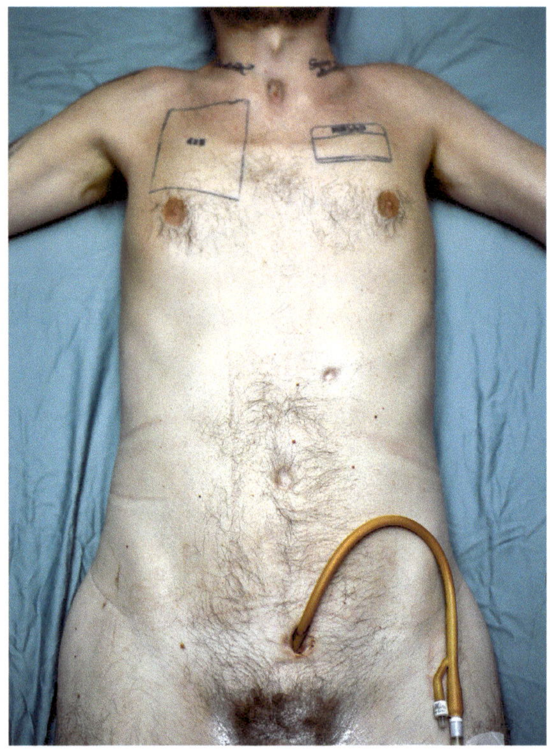

3.2 Robert Andy Coombs, from the series *Cripfag*, 2021. Courtesy of the artist.

Image description 3.2: A close up of a white man's torso. A rubber tube protrudes out from the man's lower abdomen, just above his unpictured genitalia.

top of his pubic area along the bottom. We can see his shoulders and the top half of each arm stretched out to the sides, and his ribs are showing through taut skin. He looks as though he is lying on the same scrubs-blue mattress cover as in the first image discussed in this chapter. A suntan line created by a shirt or a tank top is visible along his neckline, and the skin is noticeably pink above the line compared with his chest below. As in the first image, the body is well lit and almost looks as though it is about to undergo a surgical procedure, and we, the viewer, are the doctors who are examining him with our scalpels, ready to splice him up. Of course we *are* examining him, and Coombs gives us permission to do so.

The lighting picks up every detail on Coombs's body, including lines that may have been impressed on his waist area from pants and other clothing. We can also see hair, freckles, moles, and especially the holes or pockets in his skin that have been created by the incisions from all the tubes that are fed in and out of his body to keep him alive. One of these sites is in the center of his neck, which is used for his breathing tube.

Another is on the left side of his torso, above his belly button. The most visible opening is in his abdomen, where a phallic yellow tube slithers out from the somewhat bloodied incision and furls downwards. We can see the hint of a bandage at the bottom of the image, suggesting that the tube is taped to his leg. This is a medical assistive device called a suprapubic catheter, which is a flexible tube that drains urine from the bladder. Below the incision site, we can see a patch of Coombs's brown pubic hair, and along the creases on each side of his genital area we see what looks like a lining of white baby powder. While I am not sure why the powder is there, I do know that doctors sometimes use powder during surgical procedures to prevent and control troublesome bleeding in a variety of situations. Another standout component of the image is the tattoos on Coombs's body: he has two small handwritten scripts on either side of his neck, and one square and one rectangle with small writing inside each shape above his nipples on either side of his chest. The rectangle on the right-hand side (our view) of Coombs's chest mimics a name tag, which further reinforces the aesthetic of a hospital, where the patient is just a name and a body to be dissected. The fact that Coombs has cut off his face in this image reinforces the anonymous and cold feeling that we might have toward this body, but he is also forcing the viewer to focus hard on the lesions, cuts, and cords in his body, things that we typically do not encounter in an artwork. While we therefore might read "disability," "hospital," and "patient" in this photograph, Coombs is giving us an implied eroticism by once again playing with the reveal versus conceal visual tactic that we witnessed in Figure 3.1. By showing us just a hint of his pubic hair, without allowing us to see the full glory of his genitalia, he teases and torments the viewer. Further, the image is paradoxical, because while we understand that this is a person who is vulnerable, we are also experiencing surprising visual pleasure at what he proudly puts before us. This body is sexy.

Coombs draws from works by many artists, particularly photographs by Robert Mapplethorpe, Cindy Sherman, Erwin Olaf, and Catherine Opie. Mapplethorpe's work provides an obvious connection through queer nude photography of Black and white male bodies that are frank, slick, and highly sensorial. Additionally, the way Mapplethorpe approached formalism in his work, with great dedication and commitment to the beautiful, contributed to his unique aesthetic oeuvre; this approach is also evident in Coombs's work. And like Mapplethorpe once did, Coombs works meticulously under controlled studio conditions that likely surpass Mapplethorpe's own scrupulousness, given that Coombs relies on many other people to create his work.

Some of Catherine Opie's earlier portraits also present matter-of-fact depictions of homosexual desire, with a twist. Like Coombs, Opie mines art history in creating her classical compositions, drawing from canonical baroque and old master paintings for inspiration. In *Self Portrait/Cutting*

(1993), the artist's back faces us, covered with a bloodied scar drawing of two female stick figures holding hands; as with Coombs's self-portraits, our eyes are drawn to another point the artist is trying to make about identity, sexuality, and normalcy. In *Self Portrait/Pervert* (1994), Opie faces us, but this time she wears a leather mask. She is topless and across the top of her breasts the bloodied word "Pervert" has been carved into her skin with a scalpel blade. A decorative pattern also outlined in blood is evocative of angel's wings, a jarring contrast to Opie's nude-chested, leather-faced appearance. Her arms have orderly, military-like rows of pins threaded, apparently painfully, through the skin, emphasizing her sadomasochistic sexual predilection. Lastly, in *Self Portrait/Nursing* (2004), Opie is breastfeeding her infant son, proving that butch lesbians can not only be pregnant, but they can be mothers too. Her body still bears the scar of the inscription, "Pervert," from her days as a sadomasochism practitioner. Both Coombs's and Opie's bodies have undergone transformation, self-inflicted or not, and they both use similar visual tropes to convey these major transitions. While Opie reveals layers of complexity around lesbian identity, sadomasochistic sexuality, and motherhood, Coombs explores disabled queer sexuality that defies medical and mainstream stereotypes.

Coombs also draws from other great paintings in Western art history, particularly with baroque theatrical embellishments as evinced through both color and lighting. One work that Saltz previously highlighted in his writing is Rembrandt's well-known painting, *The Anatomy Lesson of Dr. Nicolaes Tulp* (1632). In this painting, a group of white men in black suits with white collars are witness to a doctor performing an autopsy. The painting embodies the same aesthetics that are present in the two Coombs photographs discussed so far. All the light shines on the body, which is the main and central focus point in the image, while the viewer – the observing men and us – gazes upon the form. Both of the images exude a quality of grotesqueness, telling us that we shouldn't look. In Rembrandt's case, the stigma of looking at a dead body is keenly felt, and in the case of Coombs's work, looking at a disabled body comes with just as much stigma. Indeed, the observing men in Rembrandt's painting don't look at the dead body directly. Instead, their eyes roam to different parts of the room, either because they are embarrassed or ashamed to look at the corpse, or because they are too involved in the procedure of autopsy to consider the actual body of the dead person. Saltz astutely points out that the men not looking is part of what Coombs is trying to upend, as he is keenly aware that people do not want to look at disabled bodies.[4] In fact, people go out of their way to avoid disabled bodies out of fear that in the act of coming into contact with a disabled person, they might "catch" the contagion/disability too. Coombs gives us no choice but to look and to stare. There are many details to pore over, and through Coombs's generosity in giving us so much, perhaps the viewer will realize that this is just another body too, and we can learn something from it.

I would now like to return to the photograph discussed at the beginning of this chapter, as this one also urges me to think about art history and how the nude body has been presented to us over time. Of course, feminist art historians like Linda Nochlin, Griselda Pollock, and others have unpacked the various nude poses of the female form, and those poses either are submissive to the male gaze and painted by men for men, such as Ingre's *Grande Odalisque* (1814), or feature women who are more empowered, returning the gaze back to the viewer, as per bell hooks's oppositional gaze, or as depicted in Manet's *Olympia* (1863). By having his back to us, Coombs deflects the gaze; we are unable to make eye contact with him, and instead he cheekily shows his back and his peek-a-boo scrotum in a gesture of simultaneous playfulness and defiance. It is almost as if he is saying, "You can't have me, but look at how desirable I am." At the same time, Coombs appears as though he is shielding himself from the obtrusive medical and nonmedical gaze; perhaps he is more comfortable showing this side of himself because this side is safer and, ironically, far less revealing after all. This complexity in how Coombs interacts with and investigates the gaze is made manifest in the third photograph which I would like to discuss.

In Figure 3.3, Coombs introduces a new protagonist apart from himself; there are now two men who look like they might be preparing to engage

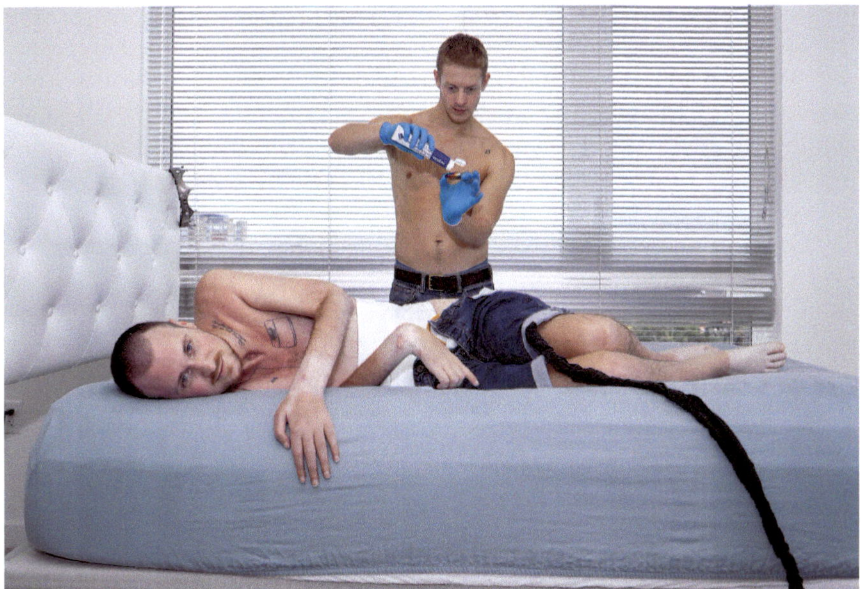

3.3 Robert Andy Coombs, from the series *Cripfag*, 2021. Courtesy of the artist.

Image description 3.3: A thin white disabled man lays on his side facing us, with a sly smile on his face. He is shirtless and has his denim shorts pulled down below his butt. A second white man stands behind him lubricating a small object carefully held in his gloved hand.

in a sexual act in this erotic scene. A white man stands behind Coombs in a bedroom. He is shirtless, and he wears blue plastic gloves. He has a serious-looking expression on his face as he pours lubricant on an unspecified object from a white bottle in his right hand. One can assume that he is going to insert this object into Coombs's anus to arouse sexual pleasure. Coombs is lying on his side on the bed again, and his denim shorts are unzipped, pulled down around his hips. A hint of his yellow suprapubic catheter can be seen amidst his unzipped pants, and a long black leash emerges from one of the openings in the pants, which one assumes is the catheter with a black fabric cover on it. Once again, Coombs is lying on the baby blue mattress cover, but now we can see more of the room, which is filled with white light. The bed headboard is white, the walls of the room are white, and the opened blinds at the window behind the standing man are also white. The starkness of the white components of the image against the flesh of the two men and the blue mattress once again evokes being in a hospital or sterile environment. The portrayal of the men is matter of fact and straightforward. Coombs's skin once again shows tan lines, this time on his feet and hands. But the most titillating part of the photograph is Coombs's gaze itself. This time, he stares back into us; indeed, he sees *into* us, and even stares *through* us. But there is a glint in his eye; not only is he looking back at us looking at him, but he is looking at us with an expression that can be read as sultry, sensual, and seductive. He seduces us with his eyes while the male behind him is about to do the same to him with his unidentified object. Coombs also looks quite smug. No doubt he is showing off his excessive pride at being able to engage in this sexual encounter despite what the world at large may think of disabled people and their sexuality. He is saying with his eyes, "Look at me, getting some ... I am so hot and sexy and desirable." I'm really quite taken by how Coombs wields this art historical gaze to develop layers of disabled identity and sexuality that have not been encountered before.

This work then takes us further in dissecting the gaze. I already mentioned Manet's *Olympia* as one of the great works of art to return the gaze to the viewer, where the subject of the gaze is empowered and is prideful of their appearance and their situation. Coombs is certainly a contemporary Olympia, but he is a queer, disabled Olympia. Katherine Sherwood, discussed in Chapter 2, has also taken it upon herself to appropriate and literally disable Olympia's image by giving her a prosthetic leg, a cane, or a crutch. But Coombs is interested in making his embodiment a highly sexual one too, foregrounding the fact that he is a queer disabled man who has a sexual appetite. While the philosophy of the gaze and the semiotics of embodiment are important in this work, so too is the language we use around embodiment. In his important essay, "How to Teach Manet's *Olympia* after Transgender Studies," art historian David J. Getsy explains that we can no longer teach or write about the nude in art history in the same way, because we cannot assume female or male designations for the bodies we see portrayed and illustrated in visual works of art.[5] Instead, we must question these interpretations and be sure that more room is made for how these different bodies may or may not be perceived by a broader range of individuals, in the classroom context, but also in the gallery or by the reader of the art history textbook. Situated within transgender studies, Getsy argues that the doctrine of the binary that we employ in our art historical writings and teachings is too simple, and that art historians must account for a greater diversity of bodies. Of course, as a disabled art historian, I have been arguing this point for over a decade, specifically that we must also come to recognize the nude disabled body. The ideal, then, extrapolating from Getsy's point, is for art history to include disabled nude bodies in its discourse, for their ability to challenge the aesthetics of bodies that have been elevated in the canon since the ancient Greeks, and for their ability to show us a hospital aesthetics that reveals and confronts.

Another critical component for understanding Coombs's work is photography history and discourse. Photography theory has begun to prize open the legitimacy of the dominant/subordinate power dynamic in photographic representations. John Tagg argues we create this very space of the photographic image for acknowledging that power is no longer uniform, unified, general, and only "emanating from one privileged site."[6] The criticality of this space therefore "exposes a rift … in the general conceptions of representation" and Coombs shows us this rift most powerfully. Other important theorists of photography include Abigail Solomon-Godeau and Jordan Reznick. As both a photographer and an art historian, Reznick uses his trans feminist lens to depict trans subjects and their affective relationships with themselves, the photographer, and the viewer. In his important series, *Gallery of Illustrious Queers* (2016–20), Reznick offers large-scale portraits that show gender deviants of various sizes, colors, and disabilities. In his scholarship, Reznick has written an important essay on the photography of French surrealist Claude Cahun, an important artist well ahead of their time, who created compelling self-portraits demonstrating gender nonconformity in the 1920s. Reznick argues that Cahun and their partner Marcel Moore "deliberately opposed the medical and psychological discourses of their era," and instead used the camera to wield a "stridently misfit corporeality" which was "politically engaged with broader struggles for liberation."[7] Reznick asserts that they developed their own visual alternatives to debunk scientific discourse, and to capture an embodiment that was self-determined and self-possessed. Like Getsy, Reznick centers the specificities of trans subjecthood in his essay, and there is great value in considering how trans and queer art history scholarship brings generative meaning to Coombs's portfolio of photographs.

Having situated Coombs's important work in these broader discourses, I want to underscore how bereft the artist feels about his career and life aspirations at the time of this writing. In 2023, Coombs had to move from Miami back to his parents' house in Alabama because he was unable to find employment owing to discrimination and ableism in the workplace. Potential employers did not want the burden of hiring Coombs. Further, he has been using Instagram over the past few years as the primary means by which to circulate his work and gain followers and interest, but he has been consistently censored by the social media platform because of its sexual content and nudity. Coombs has often publicly spoken of how frustrated he feels with this ongoing censorship. He believes that the company is ultimately being hypocritical, as they promote themselves as a free place for individual artistic expression while banning and silencing individuals and images that convey an uninhibited sense of BIPOC and disabled identity. In February 2024, Coombs posted on Instagram about how he does not have the luxury to be autonomous like other artists, and that hiring assistants to help him make work costs time and money. He noted that he is not marketable or digestible for a cis, heteronormative, able-bodied general public because of the nature of his work, and acknowledged how the public prefer to see "inspiration porn" from disabled artists. "Inspiration porn" refers to representations of disabled people that are "inspirational" and show them overcoming all odds despite their disability. The term is likened to pornography because of the gratification that able-bodied people get from looking at these images; thus the disabled body is objectified within this limiting trope.[8]

I write about Coombs's current circumstances because it is important to understand the truthful context in which the artist is making his work. While hospital aesthetics focuses on the empowering imagery being produced by contemporary disabled artists, it encompasses this work's politics too. For Coombs, the politics of censorship and erasure is something he must fight against every day. He will continue to be outspoken and rally against the normative art world until things start to change, and institutions start to welcome him and his lush work instead of fearing it. The highly offensive measure taken by Meta (which owns Instagram) of repeatedly erasing Coombs's account has deep historical roots. In the Introduction, I discussed how some of the earliest egregious medical acts performed on disabled bodies were forced sterilizations of disabled women in the nineteenth century, when the state believed it to be a crime against humanity for disabled people – especially developmentally disabled people – to reproduce, and thus to have sex. Clearly the state had to scrutinize and contain disabled bodies given that they were a strain on normalcy. As Henri-Jacques Stiker powerfully put it, "An aberrancy within the corporeal order is an aberrancy in the social order."[9] In 2005, the British sculptor Marc Quinn unveiled his sculpture, *Alison Lapper Pregnant*, in Trafalgar Square in London. The sculpture depicted the real-life figure of the artist Alison Lapper, who was born with phocomelia, which is a congenital condition where she has no arms and shortened legs. She was eight months pregnant with her now deceased son at the time that Lapper sculpted her likeness. The work was praised but it was also greatly reviled. People protested at the so-called obscenity of the subversive work, because they were insulted by the image of a disabled woman who was pregnant and who was therefore having sex. In 2007, Margrit Shildrick wrote that "the call for sexual citizenship for people with disabilities is fraught with difficulties."[10] The historical and contemporary treatment of disabled people who want and have sex is deeply problematic.

Given there are few queer disabled artists exploring male sexuality, I want to devote some space to discussing Wes Holloway's work. I am especially drawn to his beautiful collages that interrogate male body ideals, vanity, and the tension between pleasure and pain. Holloway uses the medium to deconstruct beauty and pathology to create new compositions that generate reflection and contemplation. Like Coombs, Holloway acquired his disability through an accident, when a spinal cord injury left him paralyzed at 18 years of age. While Holloway's work is not as confrontational in his exploration of male sexuality, he nonetheless creates witty commentary regarding beauty and the so-called flawed disabled body in a manner akin to Coombs. Holloway uses magazine clippings and overlays these with drawings made from ink, acrylic paint, or charcoal, interspersed with other materials like foil, sequins, and even Viagra pills. In one collage entitled "Doctor Recommended: Why Settle for Less, When You Can Get the Very Best!," we see the torso of a male bodybuilder overlaid with a pound of red meat, a frontal view of a fish with a hook emerging from its mouth, Superman "Kapowing!" through clouds as he shoots through the sky, and what looks like surgeon's gloved hands kneading a red fleshy body organ in a bowl, among other elements. The work reads as a medically prescribed and unattainable male ideal; it says nothing else will do. With his blend of sarcasm and surprising juxtapositions, Holloway is an invaluable peer to Coombs and another strong voice contributing to a sensorial hospital aesthetics.

Bondage, performance, and the patient

Panteha Abareshi is a Los Angeles-based contemporary disabled artist originally from Montreal, Quebec, Canada. Abareshi has sickle cell zero beta thalassemia, a genetic blood disorder that causes debilitating pain and bodily deterioration that increases with age. They have acknowledged that their work is informed by gender, race, and sexuality, and they hope to fill a void in the representation of these marginalized identities. They state:

> In my practice I am warping concrete, physical forms into highly disembodied abstractions. … I aim to discuss the complexities of living within a body that is

> highly monitored, constantly examined, and made to feel like a specimen. Taking images that are recognizable as human forms, and reducing them to gestural forms is a juxtaposition of my own body's objectification, and dissection.[11]

While Abareshi's work encompasses a broad range of media, including sculpture, performance, and video, I am particularly interested in examining their work focused on performance documented on video. Abareshi's performance work engages with sexuality, bondage, and other sadomasochism practices, and it is closely connected with Robert Andy Coombs's work discussed in the previous section. Taken together, these two artists' bodies of work establish a dimension of hospital aesthetics based in the medium of performance art, but their work also extends the parameters and definitions of performance itself, and what constitutes so-called normal movement and normal form. In my book *The Agency of Access: Contemporary Disability Art and Institutional Critique* (2024), I spent time discussing the Capitol Crawl that occurred in 1990 on the steps of the Capitol building in Washington DC, a moment, I argue, when disabled activists established the beginnings of disability performance art. Disability performance artists today get to define and redefine embodiment and movement intertwined. There is more on this in the next section.

The first video performance piece I would like to discuss is Abareshi's *Unlearn the Body* (2020) (see Figure 3.4). In this film, we witness Abareshi acrobatically interacting with a walker and crutches, using them as a prop to contort their body into a series of yoga positions. The video plays as a series of scratchy clips interlaced with distorted medical diagrams that kaleidoscopically swirl together into unreadable patterns. As the film progresses, Abareshi uses cords and crutches, but rather than propping the body up, they become constraints that seem to limit further movement. Toward the end of the video, the artist's feet are constrained by a yellow cord that is affixed to the wall, and while trying to balance on two crutches, Abareshi dramatically falls. The work speaks to the oppressive ideal body that calls for us to adhere to specific medical protocols that ultimately break down and limit the body's ability to function. Abareshi wears nothing but thick white medical bandages that are strategically wrapped around their breasts and genital area as if they were a bra and underwear or a bikini swimsuit. By sensorially engaging and moving with the constraints of these medical assistive devices in their provocative bandage/bondage garments, Abareshi also prompts us to imagine this as a sadomasochistic activity. While they are showing us how the medical industry contains and limits them, they turn around and use the same tools to pleasure themself instead.

In an interview by art critic Emily Watlington entitled "Between Bondage and Bandage," Abareshi discusses their solo exhibition *Invalid Pleasures*, which was held at Kunsthall Trondheim in Norway in 2023.[12] The exhibition explored sexuality and sensuality in the context of disability, and how the

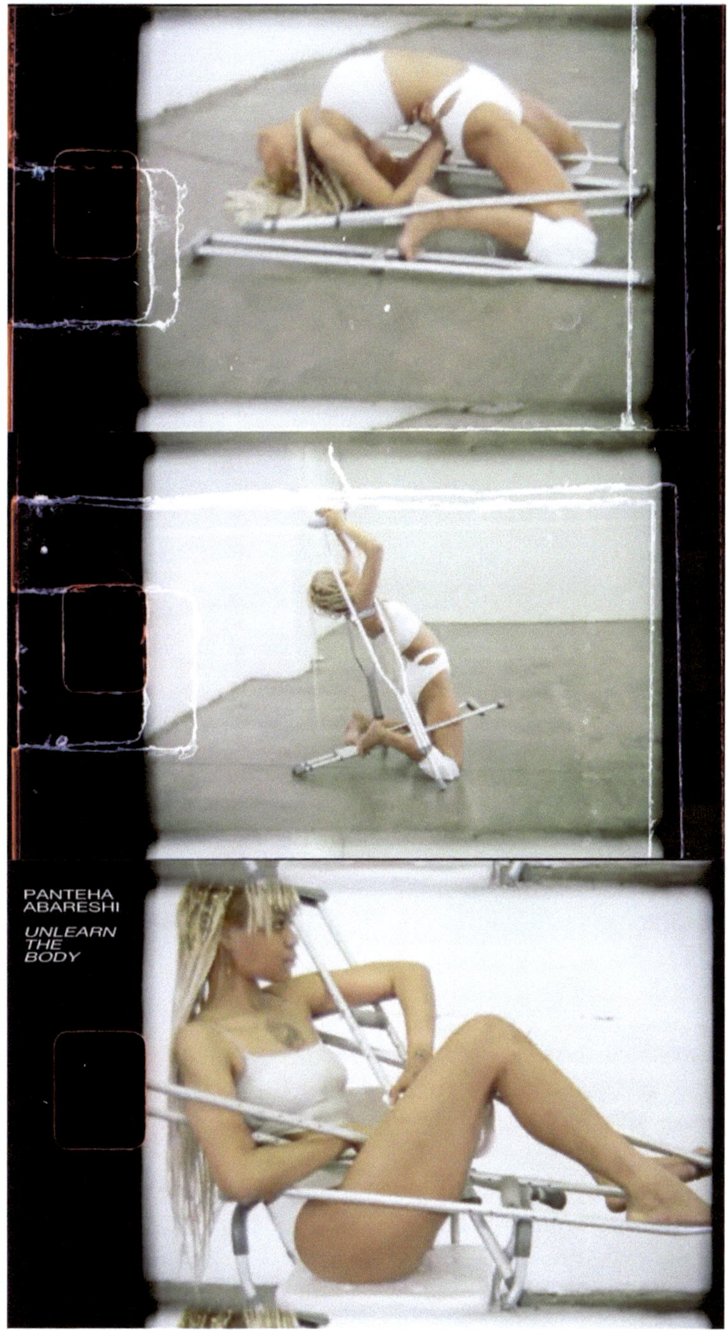

3.4 Panteha Abareshi, *Unlearn the Body*, 2020. Courtesy of the artist.

Image description 3.4: Three stills from the video, *Unlearn the Body*. Each still features a mixed race worman with long bleached blonde box braids and light brown skin. She wears a white two piece and does artful poses with a pair of underarm crutches.

disabled body and mind are treated as fetish objects. Some of the video-based work in the exhibition depicts Abareshi performing for the camera, as in the eight-minute VHS video *An Exercise in Logic (If you Put the Bodies in the Fire)*, and *Fetish Material*, an almost ten-minute VHS video. Both were produced in 2023. In the interview, Abareshi discusses the symbolism of their choice of medium – VHS video – and defunct forms of analog media representation. Abareshi wanted to set up a barrier between their body and its own representation, and the barrier was the medium of VHS. Not only was using the videotape an interesting artistic and practical challenge, but the medium also became the message. In this case, it was a symbol for how the medical record often represents a barrier for disabled people, where it is most often withheld from individuals or otherwise difficult to access. It's only through an illogical series of red tape that one will acquire one's medical record, in a now dated technological format such as a fax or a CD (although admittedly all my mammogram results were emailed to me recently). For Abareshi's *Unlearn the Body*, discussed in the previous paragraph, the artist shot the video on Super 8 and then edited it so it was full of glitches and imperfections, just like the disabled body itself. The interview also discussed the continued tension in Abareshi's videos on their prosthetic medical assistive devices, and if they are in fact supports, constraints, or a mixture of both, in both a medicinal and sexual context.

In *Fetish Material* (2023), Abareshi explores how their own disabled body becomes a fetish object. This video and other recent work has seen their attention focused on disabled pornography and other fetish materials. Abareshi is interested in the tension between pleasure and pain. In this video, Abareshi is once again wearing bandages in swimsuit style, but with bright red socks, and this time they are playing with an oxygen tank which sits against a white wall on a floor covered by a large plastic sheet. They acrobatically twist and contort their body on the ground and in the air while using the oxygen tank as a support and a prop. In some scenes Abareshi has bandaged their face so that only their eyes, nose, mouth, and ears are visible, with their dyed-blonde braids cascading down their back. Abareshi's slight frame provides a powerful contrast against the oxygen tank, which they straddle, fondle, and provocatively explore with their hands, feet, arms, and legs. As the video continues, eventually Abareshi has their folded arms and folded legs taped up with bandages as well, providing more restraint for them to explore. Yellow text flashes against a blue screen, reading "the object is disabled," and intermittent images show Abareshi's body folded up and bound in plastic cellophane wrap. Abareshi's choice to use the oxygen tank as their prosthetic device this time is interesting given that this is a prosthesis that keeps us alive by literally breathing life into us.[13] Indeed, Abareshi breathes new life into the tank in a reversal of power, control, and domination.

As mentioned previously, disability performance artists define and redefine embodiment and movement. Well before Abareshi's work, there was an extraordinary proliferation of such art, beyond the iconic 1980 protest for the Americans with Disabilities Act. Through the vision and tenacity of various artistic directors, numerous dance companies have been founded on a mission to support disability dance artistry, including AXIS Dance Company, Candoco Dance Company, Dance/NYC, Kinetic Light, DanceAbility, Victoria Marks's Dancing Disability Lab at the University of California Los Angeles, and many others. Alice Sheppard is the founder and artistic director of Kinetic Light, a project-based ensemble working at the intersections of disability, dance, design, identity, and technology to create transformative art and advance the disability arts movement. Kinetic Light is a leader in the emerging form of disability dance, a field Sheppard defines as rooted in intersectional disability history, arts and culture, and work that is made by, features, and often imagines disabled people as the primary audience. While the dance field is certainly distinct from performance art within the art world, disabled dance artists nonetheless have put the moving disabled body in the spotlight, breaking barriers and taboos.

Other important individual disabled dance artists who have paved the way for artists like Abareshi include Claire Cunningham and Bill Shannon. I point out these two artists specifically because they both use their crutches to perform, which reminds me of Abareshi's own choreographic use of their crutches and other prosthetic and medical assistive devices within their moving praxis (particularly in *Unlearn the Body*). Claire Cunningham is originally from Scotland; her work is rooted in the study and use/misuse of her crutches and the exploration of the potential of her specific physicality, with a conscious rejection of traditional dance techniques (developed for nondisabled bodies). This approach runs alongside a deep interest in the lived experience of disability and its implications not only for Cunningham as a choreographer but also in terms of societal notions of knowledge, value, connection, and interdependence. Bill Shannon is a US-based artist who dances with his crutches, a practice that originated in childhood play. Since these early beginnings, Shannon has refined and expanded on a lexicon of disabled dance technique specific to his crutches. Both Shannon's techniques and his theoretical framing are referenced and adapted by other artists all over the world, and he is colloquially known as the "crutch master."

Both Cunningham and Shannon have afforded Abareshi this theoretical and choreographic framing, where the prosthesis and the medical assistive device can be wielded by the disabled body in empowering ways to articulate more complex layers of identity, relationships, sexuality, desire, masculinity or femininity, and vulnerability. In the previous section we saw how contemporary disabled artists such as Jesse Darling, Constantina Zavitsanos, Carmen Papalia, and others have developed similar approaches. Yet Abareshi's own use/misuse of their walker and crutches brings a distinct eroticism to their approach. Given this, it is instructive to compare their work with that of Lisa Bufano. Bufano became a bilateral below-the-knee and total finger and thumb amputee as a result of a life-threatening staphylococcus bacterial infection at the age of 21, and she sadly died by suicide in 2013 at the age of 40. The artist used prosthetics and props in her performance-based practice, such as strapping Queen Anne table legs to her legs and arms. She had performed all over the world and toured with AXIS Dance Company from 2006 to 2010. In an artist statement, Bufano said that she manipulated her body to explore alternative locomotion, corporeal difference, her sexual identity, and the alternative use or animation of prosthetic body parts. In a previous essay on her work, I compared Bufano's composition and choreography to the praying mantis, where she creates a magnetic tension that is dangerous and erotic, seductive and horrific all at once.[14] All these qualities, both sinister and sensual, shadow the praxis of Abareshi.

Disability performance art can be traced to figures like the Irish artist Mary Duffy, who was born without arms.[15] In her performances from the 1980s, Duffy stood nude before the audience as she spoke about her identity as a disabled woman. An excerpt of her monologue was aimed at the medical establishment: "The words you use to describe me are: 'congenital malformation.' Those big words those doctors used – they didn't have any that fitted me properly. I felt, even in the face of such opposition, that my body was the way it was supposed to be. It was right for me, as well as being whole, complete and functional."[16] During this same period, Duffy would replicate her performance, passing herself off as the Venus de Milo. With a loose shawl provocatively draped at her waist, she emphasized the tension between revealing and concealing a body that was clearly a source of great curiosity and arousal for the audience, just as such a body was in ancient times. Duffy's ingenious appropriation points to Venus's unquestioned status as an ideal in the art historical canon, and asks if this same standard of beauty is applicable to her own nearly identical body, marked by so-called disfigurement.[17] It is hard to watch this bold and gutsy performance by Duffy, both because of the confrontational nature of Duffy's nudity and her unflinching gaze toward the audience, and also because her words resonate with my own hurtful memories with the medical industry.

Here we might return to the work of Riva Lehrer, who, in a related vein, has created many self-portraits featuring candid and unflinching imagery of her nude or semi-nude body (see Figure 3.5, where the title alludes to the disabled body as terra incognita or unexplored territory).

Lehrer has been a central figure in the disability movement in Chicago since the 1980s, when she began painting her peers. Her portraits capture the tension between the need for disabled people to be visible on a more elevated platform, and their frequent depiction in public settings and in popular culture through limiting and narrow tropes.[18] Lehrer was born with spina bifida and has had numerous surgeries throughout her life. She grew up in the 1950s and 1960s when disability was even more stigmatized than it is today. Through Lehrer's revealing of her own body, she aims to

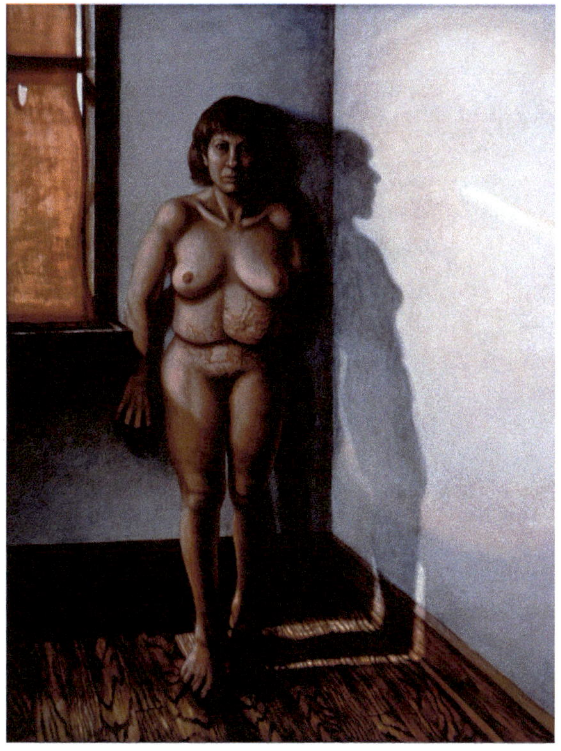

3.5 Riva Lehrer, *Corner (Terra Incognita)*, 1994. Acrylic on wood, 24 × 18 in. (61 × 46 cm) Courtesy of the artist.

Image description 3.5: A painting of a naked white woman standing in the corner of a dim room casting cool shadows on the adjoining walls. The figure has a large scar across their belly.

confront staring eyes while also showing the reality – and the normalcy – of difference.[19] The nudity displayed in work by Duffy and Lehrer aligns with imagery produced by several feminist artists of the preceding generation, such as Carolee Schneemann and Hannah Wilke, who used their nude bodies to confront the patriarchal gaze. Going far beyond Wilke and others, Lehrer's portraits advance feminist theories that challenge the male gaze from a disabled perspective, revealing its ableism.[20] Disabled artists ranging from Duffy to Lehrer can be understood as deploying bell hooks's "oppositional gaze" to empower the disabled subject, denying the viewer the pleasure of looking at a body that is stigmatized within an ableist framework.[21]

The work of these practitioners has been analyzed and theorized by numerous important disability studies and performance scholars, including Petra Kuppers, Carrie Sandahl, Rosemarie Garland-Thomson, Alice Sheppard, and Bree Hadley, among others. Kuppers is also an artist and serves as Artistic Director of the art collective Olimpias. Olimpias engages in cross-genre participatory practices, addressing and engaging with audiences directly; thus Kuppers is interested in fostering heightened awareness of complex bodily schemas within and among her participants. Directly drawing on philosopher of phenomenology Maurice Merleau-Ponty, Kuppers states that "the body of the self … is a body schema, a conglomerate and palimpsest made up of action maps and visual cues, vague sensings and acute memories."[22] Through intersubjective exchanges of bodies, Kuppers offers direct anecdotal narratives of what happens to disabled bodies when they, for example, gather underwater (in her series of *Salamander* projects, 2014–16), and she captures first-person accounts through the written word, photographs, and videos. Kuppers is especially motivated by somatic experiences that register within the interiority and exteriority of the disabled body as a type of dramatized, choreographed extension to lived experience.

Bree Hadley notes how the particular mode of disabled lived experience is portrayed by contemporary British disabled performance artists such as Katherine Araniello, Noëmi Lakmaier, and Aaron Williamson. She says,

> when people with disabilities turn to performance as a political practice, they tend to avoid … autobiographical narratives about diagnosis, crisis, overcoming and cure. Though popular on the main stage, these are, it seems, the stories others would tell about disabled people, not the preferred mode when they work as instigators of their own performances rather than interpreters of other people's well-made plays about them.[23]

Hadley is suggesting that contemporary disability performance artists, in a similar vein to the scholars and artists I have already mentioned, work toward dialogical, physical, and sensorial accounts of their lived embodied experience that avoid casting their bodies into reductive stereotypes based in the medical model of disability, where their bodies are considered "catastrophes" and removed from the public sphere. Instead, these artists emphasize the contingency of a disabled person's bodily sensation and perception, transforming meaning and capturing agency within a disabled person's own reclaimed narrative.

Scholar Rosalia Lerner builds on these ideas. She is currently working on a book entitled *Get Well Soon!: Sick Bodied Performance of Chronic Conditions*. Lerner considers how performance and dance work by twenty-first-century chronically ill artists both critiques a neoliberal ontology and enacts alternative ontologies.[24] She claims that within the neoliberal ontology, feeling unwell is deemed an "individual failing," and that the performance work of Abareshi and other artists in her study helps to reimagine sickness as a space of "political resistance and anticapitalist possibility."[25]

Another aspect of Abareshi's work that remains undertheorized and underdiscussed is how their protest work invariably folds in a rebuttal to the medical industrial complex from the perspective of a *Black* disabled woman. To provide further framing and context for Abareshi's praxis, I'd like to weave in a discussion of the history of Black performance art and its numerous threads, trajectories, and tenets. Indeed, *weaving* becomes a key word here as I introduce the work of Senga Nengudi, an African American artist who has primarily worked in sculpture and performance since the 1970s. Prompted by the birth of her son, Nengudi started to fill various shades of tan nylon pantyhose with sand to represent bodies changing shape and form. Her work has often been described as womb-like exploratory structures representing the human form. The transformation that had occurred in her own body before and after pregnancy instilled a curiosity in her about the body's ability to morph itself both physically and psychologically. Her work has been compared with that of Louise Bourgeois for its ability to capture pathos, memory, and narrative through abstractions of the hospitable and inhospitable body. Nengudi's collections of pantyhose objects, begun in 1975, came to be known as *R.S.V.P.*

Nengudi invited other artists to create performances with her pantyhose elastic sculptures; they would weave in and out of the nylon web tendrils, which were often splayed in different formations in the corners of gallery spaces. Figure 3.6 shows a performance in 1977 with Maren Hassinger, which recalls a spider in her web. Other art critics have noted that the

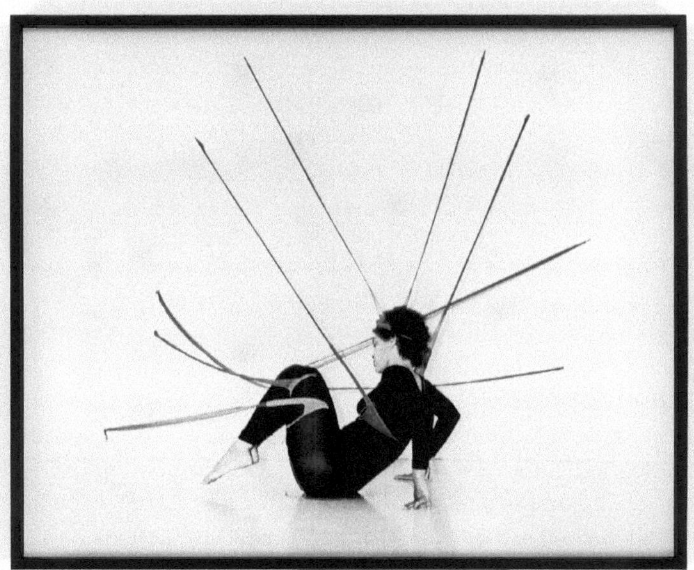

3.6 Senga Nengudi, *Performance Piece*, 1978, activated by Maren Hassinger. © Senga Nengudi, 2024. Photograph: Harmon Outlaw. Courtesy of Sprüth Magers and Thomas Erben Gallery.

Image description 3.6: A sepia tone photograph of a Black woman wearing a black long-sleeved unitard. Her torso and legs are entangled in a web of stretched nylon hosiery.

nylon would become twisted and contorted into almost impossible and painful positions, pushing beyond the capabilities of limbs and the threshold of physical possibility. Nengudi's work is important for the feminist art movement and the Black arts movement for its ability to question what it means to live in a Black woman's body. In the dancer's act of pushing the nylon skin, Nengudi has also activated for us corporal expression in the wake of Black bodily deprivation, particularly within the history of slavery.[26] Rizvana Bradley writes, "*R.S.V.P.* actively interrogates the spatio-temporal dimensions Black [and female] bodies have passed through and been barred from, illuminating figures that move through and occupy space differently."[27] She suggests that Nengudi's dancers rupture what the art historian Rosalind Krauss calls sculpture's "expanded field," because within that field the artists were white, and had unacknowledged privilege to explore normative conceptualizations of space. Nengudi's dancers thus explored alternative compositions in terms of depth, weight, scale, and physicality, showing not only how Black bodies must break free, but also how female bodies are overworked. The sand filling the nylon allowed the dancers to create new growths, bulbs, buds, and generative disfigurements of flesh that opened the door for a revised definition of bodies, in line with the work of contemporary disabled artist/performers.

Abareshi's explorations between bondage and bandage display the same malleability and flexibility that Nengudi's nylon allows. In addition to these formal material connections, both artists share a desire to demonstrate intersectional identity, corporal resistance, and the reality of unruly bodies. To my mind, Abareshi's work builds on the excellent trajectory that Nengudi has offered us, by making the disabled body a central and literal focus instead of a suggested apparition that comes and goes depending on where the grains of sand are fondled and raked. While both artists play with the tension between control and restraint, both of them ultimately maintain an emphatic agency over their own bodies as a response to the ill treatment perpetrated by a white, ableist, patriarchal system, where Black female bodies have been objectified, commodified, scrutinized, and treated with violence and degradation.

In his book *Embodied Avatars: Genealogies of Black Feminist Art and Performance*, Uri McMillan helpfully contextualizes both Nengudi's and Abareshi's work through his term "prosthetic performance." According to McMillan, the objecthood of a performance artist "acts in collaboration with inanimate props that are transformed into active agents."[28] McMillan's writing has deeper application to Abareshi's work, for he focuses on a case study where a fugitive enslaved person dons a sling and other disability-related props to pass as disabled. He is thus interested in how disability and disabled identity are implicated in prosthetic performance. McMillan importantly notes that disabled embodiment is animated through its engagement with prosthetic devices. He states: "disability here was transformed from mere bodily impairment into an elastic and *mobile* aesthetic device and a set of tactical performances."[29] Similarly, Abareshi effectively transforms their disabled body into a mobile aesthetic device that performs with strategy and political conviction. The inert prosthetic device – be it the walker, crutch, or oxygen tank – comes alive when it is engaged by disabled embodiment. To extend McMillan's thinking with my own theoretical analysis, Abareshi harnesses their disabled body's sexuality and uses it to challenge ableist assumptions, thereby contributing to the ongoing evolution of a Black feminist performance art archive. In reading Abareshi's work through the concept of hospital aesthetics, I aim to push McMillan's ideas further by bringing them to bear on the hospital, where Abareshi's treatment of their prosthetic device(s) brings disability-specific language and iconography to the cutting table.

Thinking more about performing, disability, sex, and pain

A great deal of scholarship has emerged in the past several decades on the intersection of disability and sexuality. Key scholars who have written on this subject include Robert McRuer, Anna Mollow, Margrit Shildrick, Shelley Tremain, Abby Wilkerson, Anne Finger, Tom Shakespeare, and numerous others. In the introduction to the *Routledge Handbook of Disability and Sexuality* (2021), Russell Shuttleworth, Julia Bahner, and Linda R. Mona note that early studies on disability and sexuality emerged from clinical medical practice as researchers were focused on rehabilitating the loss of sexual function, in particular of men during wartime who may have had traumatic injuries, especially spinal cord injury.[30] The editors emphasize that women and BIPOC people were completely left out of these studies. Their introduction also lays out the main critique that both Coombs and Abareshi put forward in their visual art: not only has the medical complex historically failed to provide adequate sex education for patients with acquired disabilities, but the medical framing of disabled bodies has meant their bodies have been marked as deviant, which has fostered unnecessary hardship and feelings of low self-worth in disabled subjects. The authors also note that the medical profession avoids any discussion of sexual health issues with their disabled patients. The rest of the introduction provides a historical overview of how disabled people came to reclaim their sexuality, prizing it apart and away from medical clutches in order to understand their own sexuality in a more holistic way. This included the development of a manifesto, more calls for sexual inclusion for disabled people, and discussions of how to politicize the barriers that were suppressing sexual expression.

None of the work done in the performing of disability and sex would have been possible had it not been for the pioneering practice of Bob Flanagan. In Chapter 1 I discussed Flanagan's *Pain Journal* and his *Visiting*

Hours performance and installation in relation to both Quagliozzi's and Lazard's work, but I did not touch on the sensorial aspects of his practice. In the 1980s Flanagan began both a romantic and artistic partnership with Sheree Rose, which emerged amid the Los Angeles club and art scenes. Their multimedia practice, which included performance, photography, and video, wove in aspects of bondage and discipline, sadism, and masochism (BDSM) and other erotic practices. Their work ensured a permanent place for them in the art history canon, along other prominent figures including Ron Athey, Annie Sprinkle, and Martin O'Brien. Major themes included the sexual politics in contemporary art, how pain can be utilized as an art medium, the gaze of receiving and witnessing that pain, and how art can be an erotic gesture. All three artists use aspects of endurance to highlight these themes. Flanagan paired sickness with eroticism, and according to Martin O'Brien, he even showed how passively waiting in a hospital bed could be turned into erotic suspense. For this reason, O'Brien states, Flanagan was able to "redefine the role of the patient, imagining his endurance as a worthwhile activity towards self-ownership."[31] According to O'Brien, Flanagan made the hospital room a space "imbued with pleasure."[32]

In one component of Flanagan's *Visiting Hours* installation, his body would be raised by a pulley attached to his feet and ankles. He called this "The Ascension" in reference to his own impending death and the Catholic belief that Christ rose again after death (see Figure 3.7). But "The Ascension" also confronted his audience with his participation in BDSM activity, "shattering taboos around the sick body and the nature of existence for those of us who have a chronic illness."[33] Flanagan's deviance as one who engages in BDSM and is also sick breaks mainstream understandings. This is highlighted in the sudden and unexpected moment when his body would ascend by the pulleys, lifting him high above his visiting audience, the hospital gown slipping off his body in the process to reveal his naked form. O'Brien describes how Flanagan's body looked as though it was a piece of lifeless meat hanging in the slaughterhouse.[34] Flanagan's nude body faces us, with only a cough to shatter the quiet space. The Catholic notion that "Christ will rise again" is emphatically extended to the disabled body thanks to Flanagan's work – "the disabled (penile) body will rise again" – metaphorically, politically, and physically. In many ways, this iconic performance was a proverbial BDSM slap in the face to a medical and art world that believed that disability and sex were incompatible and incommensurable.

Flanagan's interest in showing his audiences that disability and sex do indeed have a relationship with one another also reveals another element of his methodology. Flanagan's work also provides a template for how pain and anger become manifest in a portfolio of work by an artist who was told that he only had a few years to live as he was growing up. In his obituary penned for the *New York Times*, art critic Roberta Smith wrote

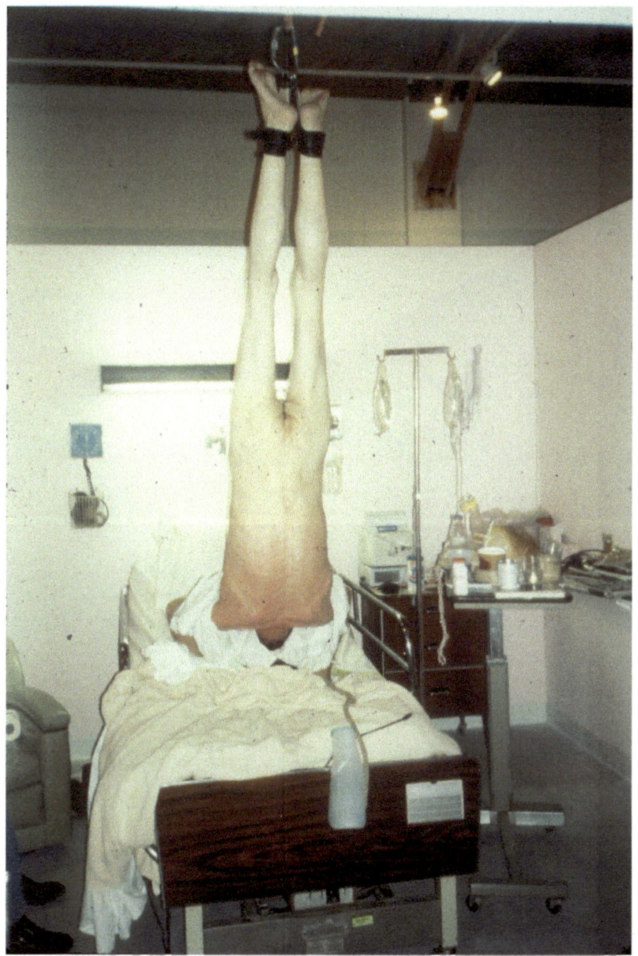

3.7 Installation view, Bob Flanagan and Sheree Rose: *Visiting Hours*, Santa Monica Museum of Art (now Institute of Contemporary Art, Los Angeles), December 4, 1992–January 17, 1993. Photograph: Sheree Rose. Image courtesy of SMMoA.

Image description 3.7: A white man is being suspended upside down nude whilst positioned above his hospital bed with crumpled white sheets. The view is of his back and buttocks. There is medical equipment surrounding the bed.

that Flanagan "attributed his longevity in part to his ability to 'fight pain with pain,' by which he meant that he took control of his suffering through the ritualized pain of sadomasochism. In time, he made his art out of his proclivity."[35] Flanagan thus channeled his physical and emotional pain into a recontextualized form of pain that not only empowered him, but that he also happened to greatly enjoy. Sadomasochism, as a sanctioned form of pain, also had the benefit of providing an activist commentary on how disabled people have sexually fulfilling lives too. Many of the artists already discussed in this book have inherited Flanagan's methodology to "fight pain with pain." Indeed, pain itself is a methodology for their work, rather than a representation, a final result, or an end game which appears in an object. This means that the artists are very much motivated by the pain and anger that they are feeling and experiencing when they encounter the medical industrial complex. This yields artwork that is bold, self-reflective, and self-aware, and arouses feelings in the audience that may include shock, surprise, shame, sadness, anger, indignation, and frustration. This approach specifically resonates with Dominic Quagliozzi and Carolyn Lazard, who were the subjects of Chapter 1, and with Robert Andy Coombs and Panteha Abareshi in this chapter.

An important development in how disabled people were able to address more fully their sexual identities came through a theoretical alignment with queer studies, otherwise known as crip–queer alliances. Since the 1970s, the disability community has found great allyship and overlap with the queer community, as both marginalized groups came to recognize that they are connected by their supposed non-normativity, which relegates them to outlier status within society at large. Disability studies had been previously criticized by Black disabled scholars for being a white discipline, and it has also been criticized for being a heteronormative discipline. Disability studies scholarship that is more intersectional has become expected and normalized. Oakland-based disability justice performance project, Sins Invalid, which Patty Berne cofounded in 2006, has been at the forefront of centering the work and the knowledge of "disabled, queer, gender nonconforming, and transgender artist-activists of color" through evenings of "art, workshops, and educational trainings."[36] Sins Invalid's performances are characterized by a vigorous energy and a provocative approach, and focus on the intersection of disability and sexuality. Disability justice as a social movement expands upon this intersection, examining ableism as it intersects with race, gender, and sexuality more broadly.[37] Berne has developed manifesto-like principles for disability justice, stressing the need for broad forms of access across marginalized groups.[38] Like the work of Flanagan, disability justice and the work of Sins Invalid have also emerged from feelings of pain, anger, and frustration at the injustices disabled people regularly experience in their daily lives. Sins Invalid also advanced early conceptions of multisensory and accessible performance by virtue of the embodied knowledges that the disabled performers brought to the stage, where they enacted the political tenets of disability justice. Disabled people of color, disabled queer people, and disabled queer people of color who initiated and set the stage for the disability justice movement – including key figures Berne, Leroy Moore, Nomy Lamm, Leah Lakshmi Piepzna-Samarasinha, and Mia Mingus – have also been vocal about intersectional conversations on gender. Sins Invalid has spotlighted these issues within disability arts and culture for decades now. Indeed, the group was founded on a mission to make space for BIPOC and LGBTQIA voices, and to recognize intersectionality within disability arts.

One of the key figures in Sins Invalid, Leah Lakshmi Piepzna-Samarasinha, who was also discussed in the Introduction, has become one of its most iconic performers for her outspoken and empowering voice. I remember watching my first Sins Invalid performance in 2009 in San Francisco at the Brava Theater when I was completing my master's degree in Visual and Critical Studies at the California College of the Arts. Piepzna-Samarasinha came onto the stage in a red lacy negligee and began a monologue about a polluted river and its disabling impact on the people who would then require medical treatment. In the performance, she asked, "what does it mean to love our bodyminds as they are, in all of their sickness and wounds and the ways they are worn down from abuse? How do we love them?" She revels in her own pleasure and sexuality, and says, "when I flare I go in my bed and I fuck myself so hard. I close all the doors and I make myself come, over and over again. Sometimes I jerk off, read library books and look at Facebook at the same time … there is no pain, just me being the slut that kept me alive."[39] I remember feeling shocked and surprised at her openness and frank revelations, but also in awe at her honesty and pride in the glory of her own imperfect body.

Another performance that remains embedded in my memory was by Maria Palacios, who is affectionately known as the "Goddess on Wheels." In the same 2009 performance of Sins Invalid, Maria came onto the stage in her wheelchair and shared the embodiment of her desire as a roaring "hunger." She says, "I mean sex with … hunger, the fire that devours you makes you kiss and makes you claw the flesh of a lover over and over because you want to hold on to the memory of that body next to yours … ."[40] In another performance at the same event, she performs "Vagina Manifesto," and asks, "Is there such a thing as a crippled vagina?"[41] Her manifesto reclaims all the ways sex, vaginas, and disabilities have been shamed, on their own and together. She celebrates the vagina, and states that her vagina is tired of being told it is dirty, and refuses to continue to be shamed and made to wear Victoria's Secret underwear to be socially acceptable. Her manifesto ends by proclaiming that vagina mounts truths and can sing reconciliation and rebirth.

All the other performances at the Brava Theater were equally powerful, and I believe that Sins Invalid were way ahead of their time. In a way, they still are. They resolutely reject the repression of disabled sexualities by the medical establishment and by the mainstream. In a chapter of Shayda Kafai's book on Sins Invalid, entitled "Crip Sex as Transformative Pleasure Universe," she shares how "crip sex helps us to create liberatory frameworks … in all their lusciousness."[42] She talks of how masturbation is pain management, and how a striptease in a wheelchair is both sexy and commonplace. Clearly, Sins Invalid's work provides a critical framework for the work of

Coombs and Abareshi; they remain the leading artists of sex and disability, and I am grateful for what they do.

A related theoretical discourse that connects to the works of Sins Invalid is pleasure activism, particularly as developed in the work of adrienne maree brown, who published *Pleasure Activism: The Politics of Feeling Good* in 2019. In this book, brown presents a politics of healing and happiness, where she draws on the Black feminist tradition through the work of Audre Lorde. In Sami Schalk's summation of the book, she says that brown "demands that our social systems contain space for rest, healing, joy, and satisfaction, particularly for those who are most impacted by oppression and most likely to have their pleasure policed, denied, and devalued."[43] Pleasure activism also contends with sex work, aging, education, fashion, and trauma, which are all areas that both Robert Andy Coombs and Panteha Abareshi are fully invested in and promote. In 2022, deaf trans artist, activist, model, and actor of color Chella Man curated an exhibition entitled *Pure Joy: 14 Disabled Visual and Performance Artists* at 1969 Gallery in Tribeca. The premise of the show was to explore how artists experience joy, and it centered ideologies of pleasure rather than pain. Man's exhibition is a manifestation of brown's pleasure activism, pairing disability with joy instead of trauma. It is notable that both Coombs and Abareshi participated in this exhibition.

Robert Andy Coombs and Panteha Abareshi perform a sensorial hospital aesthetics, using photography and video as their preferred mediums. They work within the politics of the gaze, prosthetic performance, and the Black feminist tradition, adapting and drawing from queer and trans visual culture in portraiture and body art to affront the medical industrial complex with its repressive and outdated assumptions regarding disability and sexuality. Both of them impart a bold, raw, and confrontational energy to their images that is shocking and truthful, daring and proud, and I hope that more museums and art galleries will show their work instead of censoring it. They each offer entirely new definitions of performance art, speaking to the specificities of the sensorial disabled body in ways I believe will be critical to how the genre continues to evolve in the future.

Notes

1 Jerry Saltz, "Yes, This is Me: Robert Andy Coombs Shows Us a Gorgeous Orchidology of Sexual Desire," *New York Magazine*, February 3, 2020.
2 Jeffrey Mouton Benevedes, "Shifting Identity, Emerging Self: An Interview with Robert Andy Coombs, aka CripFag," *JungJournal: Culture & Psyche* 14, no. 1 (2020): 103–23, https://doi.org/10.1080/19342039.2020.1706393
3 Saltz, "Yes, This is Me."
4 Saltz, "Yes, This is Me."
5 David J. Getsy, "How to Teach Manet's Olympia after Transgender Studies," *Art History* 45, no. 2 (2022): 342–69, https://doi.org/10.1111/1467-8365.12647

6 John Tagg, *The Burden of Representation: Essays on Photographies and Histories* (Minneapolis, MN: University of Minnesota Press, 1993).
7 Jordan Reznick, "Through the Guillotine Mirror: Claude Cahun's Theory of Trans Against the Void," *Art Journal* 81, no. 3 (Fall 2022): 53–69, https://doi.org/10.1080/00043249.2022.2110440
8 While Coombs's situation is dire, I also want to point out his privilege as a white male artist who attended a prestigious Ivy League university to complete graduate school. Furthermore, while *CripFag* is productively erotic, it also uncomfortably draws on the aesthetics of Euro-American gay pornography that is largely white, although with some exceptions.
9 Henri-Jacques Stiker, *A History of Disability* (Ann Arbor, MI: University of Michigan Press, 1999).
10 Margrit Shildrick, "Contested Pleasures: The Sociopolitical Economy of Disability and Sexuality," *Sexuality Research and Social Policy: Journal of NSRC* 4, no. 1 (March 2007): 53–66, https://doi.org/10.1525/srsp.2007.4.1.53
11 Panteha Abareshi, "Disabled, Chronically Ill, Severe Artist," *Massachusetts Review* 63, no. 4 (Winter 2022): 681–92, https://dx.doi.org/10.1353/mar.2022.0100
12 Emily Watlington interview with Panteha Abareshi, "Between Bondage and Bandage," in *Kunsthall Trondheim Podcast*, May, 2023, produced by Kunsthall Trondheim, podcast, 67:00, https://soundcloud.com/kunsthalltrondheim/18-panteha-abareshi
13 The oxygen that is stored inside a tank is compressed and is used in oxygen therapy. If someone has a lung condition or difficulty breathing, oxygen tanks help the body get the oxygen it needs to function; it comes in both gas or liquid forms.
14 Amanda Cachia, "Disabling Surrealism: Reconstituting Surrealist Tropes in Contemporary Art," in *Disability and Art History*, ed. Ann Millett-Gallant and Elizabeth Howie (New York: Routledge, 2017).
15 For more information, Rosemarie Garland-Thomson wrote an essay where she discussed the work of Mary Duffy, Carrie Sandahl, and Cheryl Wade. See Rosemarie Garland-Thomson, "Dares to Stares: Disabled Women Performance Artists & the Dynamics of Staring," in *Bodies in Commotion: Disability & Performance*, ed. Carrie Sandahl and Philip Auslander (Ann Arbor, MI: University of Michigan Press, 2005), 30–41.
16 Garland-Thomson, "Dares to Stares," 30–41.
17 The disabled art historian Ann Millett-Gallant aptly titles one of the chapters in her book "Disarming Venus," a double entendre dedicated to the work of Duffy. Here, the scholar disarms the historical and social ramifications of Venus in a close examination of Duffy's "self-objectifying act." Ann Millett-Gallant, "Disarming Venus," in *The Disabled Body in Contemporary Art* (New York: Palgrave Macmillan, 2010), 25–49.
18 Some of Lehrer's sitters have included Rosemarie Garland-Thomson, Neil Marcus, Eli Clare, Lennard Davis, Matt Fraser, Liz Carr, Tekki Lomnicki, and Susan Nussbaum.
19 Emily Watlington, "'Golem Girl': An Interview with Riva Lehrer," *Art Papers*, Winter 2018/19, www.artpapers.org/golem-girl-an-interview-with-riva-lehrer [accessed June 30, 2023].
20 Laura Mulvey, "Visual Pleasure and Narrative Cinema," *Screen* 16, no. 3 (Autumn 1975): 6–18, https://doi.org/10.1093/screen/16.3.6
21 Disability studies scholar Rosemarie Garland-Thomson has written extensively on this topic. See Rosemarie Garland-Thomson, "Feminist Disability Studies," *Signs: Journal of Women in Culture and Society* 30, no. 2 (Winter 2005): 1557–87, https://doi.org/10.1086/423352
22 Petra Kuppers, *The Scar of Visibility: Medical Performances and Contemporary Art* (Minneapolis, MN: University of Minnesota Press, 2007), 136.
23 Bree Hadley, *Disability, Public Space, Performance and Spectatorship* (New York: Palgrave Macmillan, 2014), 9–10.

24 Rosalia Lerner, "'Get Well Soon!' Sick Bodied Performance of Chronic Conditions" (PhD dissertation, UC Riverside, 2022), https://escholarship.org/uc/item/90q3435t [accessed December 5, 2024].
25 Lerner, "Get Well Soon!"
26 Rizvana Bradley, "Transferred Flesh: Reflections on Senga Nengudi's 'R.S.V.P,'" *Drama Review* 59, no. 1 (Spring 2015): 161–66.
27 Bradley, "Transferred Flesh."
28 Uri McMillan, "Passing Performances: Ellen Craft's Fugitive Selves," in *Embodied Avatars: Genealogies of Black Feminist Art and Performance* (New York: New York University Press, 2015), Kindle.
29 McMillan, "Passing Performances," Kindle.
30 Russell Shuttleworth and Linda R. Mona, eds, *The Routledge Handbook of Disability and Sexuality* (New York: Routledge, 2021).
31 Martin O'Brien, "Lie Back and Take It: BDSM, Biomedicine and the Hospital Bed in the Work of Bob Flanagan and Sheree Rose," *Body, Space and Technology* 15 (2016): http://doi.org/10.16995/bst.18
32 O'Brien, "Lie Back and Take It."
33 O'Brien, "Lie Back and Take It."
34 O'Brien, "Lie Back and Take It."
35 Roberta Smith, "Bob Flanagan, 43, Performer Who Fashioned Art From His Pain," *New York Times*, January 6, 1996, www.nytimes.com/1996/01/06/arts/bob-flanagan-43-performer-who-fashioned-art-from-his-pain.html#:~:text=Flanagan%20recalled%20that%20he%20grew,art%20out%20of%20this%20proclivity [accessed January 3, 2025].
36 Shayda Kafai, *Crip Kinship: The Disability Justice and Arts Activism of Sins Invalid* (Vancouver: Arsenal Pulp Press, 2021), Kindle.
37 Disability justice organizers include Patty Berne and Sins Invalid, Mia Mingus, Leroy Moore, Alice Wong, and the late Stacy Milbern.
38 Patty Berne, "Disability Justice – A Working Draft," Sins Invalid (blog), June 10, 2015. For more information, see https://sinsinvalid.org/10-principles-of-disability-justice/ [accessed January 19, 2025].
39 Leah Lakshmi Piepzna-Samarasinha, *Sins Invalid*, part 3, Brava Theater, San Francisco, October 2–4, 2009.
40 Maria Palacios, *Sins Invalid*, "Vagina Manifesto," Brava Theater, San Francisco, October 2–4, 2009.
41 Maria Palacios, *Sins Invalid*.
42 Kafai, *Crip Kinship*, Kindle.
43 Sami Schalk, *Black Disability Politics* (Durham, NC: Duke University Press, 2022), 152.

4

Intersectional crip networks of care

In this chapter, I examine how disabled, chronically ill, and immunocompromised women, queer, and transgender artists are formally gathering in collectives to support one another, mentally, physically, and culturally, as an alternative approach to care to that provided by the formal medical establishment. In shared spaces, such as in an art gallery or an artist's home, or online through Zoom, artists can offer mutual understanding of each other's experiences with chronic illness, disability, and the medical industrial complex, and simply be a shoulder to lean on in times of anxiety, anger, and sadness. These collectives allow artists to lift each other up, creating an environment of respect, dignity, and self-worth – a strong circle of empowerment, affirmation, and allyship. The proliferation of these support groups shows a general shift in social norms, whereby the medical field is no longer the only authoritative voice on health. This phenomenon also indicates how nonmedical health-based groups are filling a need and making up for a lack of social support networks elsewhere, particularly in sanctioned medical arenas.

Through their care-building, I argue, care collectives are practicing an art form and deepening our understanding of hospital aesthetics. Put simply, care work itself is the art. The care collectives develop access principles and practices collectively through creative methodologies. In this chapter, access is found outside the museum and gallery, and within a network of disabled folks who turn to one another for creative access solutions. Following Chapter 3's brief look at the work of Sins Invalid, this chapter also builds on notions of care work from a collaborative perspective. Sins Invalid has established that care work among disabled artists is a powerful modality for building solidarity and empowerment. In this chapter, the work generated by the diverse healthcare collectives – workshops, events, exhibitions, publications, zines, and archives – is shown to be a form of "dialogic care aesthetics." This is a new term I have coined that is inspired by the concept of dialogic aesthetics, originally developed by art historian Grant Kester.[1] My concept extends Kester's ideas, but through a disability justice lens: instead of a conversation on aesthetics, as proposed by Kester, dialogic access is a dialogue of and on care. Through these practices, disabled folks can participate in and maintain a greater hold on principles of justice and equality in art praxis and issues of access. Activist principles in healthcare become an inherent part of care-building for disability collectives and community. The collectives I examine include the Feminist Health Care Research Group (FHCRG), the Sickness Affinity Group (SAG), Power Makes Us Sick (PMS), and Black Womxn Flourish. Each of these groups aims to be intersectional in their approach, focusing on feminist, queer, and crip revisions to healthcare. Feminist, queer, and crip solidarities animate these groups, whose participants are either women, queer, transgender, or disabled, or all of the above.

Complex engagements with illness have been taken up by a plethora of artist collaboratives over the past few decades, especially the AIDS Coalition to Unleash Power (ACT UP), who have made vibrant activist contributions to the art world landscape, advocating for a range of issues during the AIDS crisis in the 1980s. The group was founded in New York City in 1987 as a political action group in response to what they perceived as the US government's lack of response to the growing number of AIDS-related deaths. The gay community was at the center of the crisis as this was the main demographic noticeably impacted by AIDS-related fatalities. Funding for patients, research, and drugs was slow to emerge from the government, a problem many perceived to be a result of antigay prejudice. ACT UP members frequently participated in nonviolent actions and protests to raise awareness about the disease and provide accurate information and access to resources. Their first march was to protest the high cost and lack of availability of HIV treatment. Collectives like ACT UP provide an important template and pathway for a younger generation of contemporary artists; this legacy allows them to feel uninhibited in sharing their intimacies, and to find solidarity in their struggles and their fraught relationships with healthcare. While this substantive history of collaborative artist groups working on issues of health provides an important background to the work being investigated in this chapter, I am mostly interested in the significant history of work by women, queer, and transgender artists wanting to take charge of their own health and their own bodies. I consider this to be the precursor to the work I examine in this chapter.

Feminist Health Care Research Group

The Feminist Health Care Research Group (FHCRG), based in Berlin, Germany, was cofounded by cultural workers, feminists, and parents Julia Bonn and Inga Zimprich in 2015. The impetus behind the group was self-empowerment with regard to one's own health from a feminist perspective.[2] The group's core activities include the publication and archiving of zines and the production of exhibitions and workshops, alongside staging oral history interviews with healthcare providers. Empowering people to make decisions about their own health and well-being is particularly important in an age when the medical industrial complex constantly tells us what is "wrong" with us. They critique the idea that we are meant to be complicit in following directions to "get better" or to fix the ailment that prevails over our vulnerable and uncontrollable disabled bodies. Instead, they encourage all of us to engage in discussions around health, puncturing the aura of the so-called medical expert. The field of healthcare is omnipresent, regulated, and expert-dominated. Personal experiences that people have with healthcare are often colored by being in a position of need and vulnerability when confronting healthcare bureaucracy. The FHCRG's workshops create space for people to reflect on their moments of exhaustion and fragility, and they invite guests into the circle to discuss "alternatives to the normative practices of the health care sector."[3] They also offer opportunities for freewriting and exchanging thoughts and ideas with other participants through bodywork and becoming attuned to one's physical needs (see Figure 4.1).

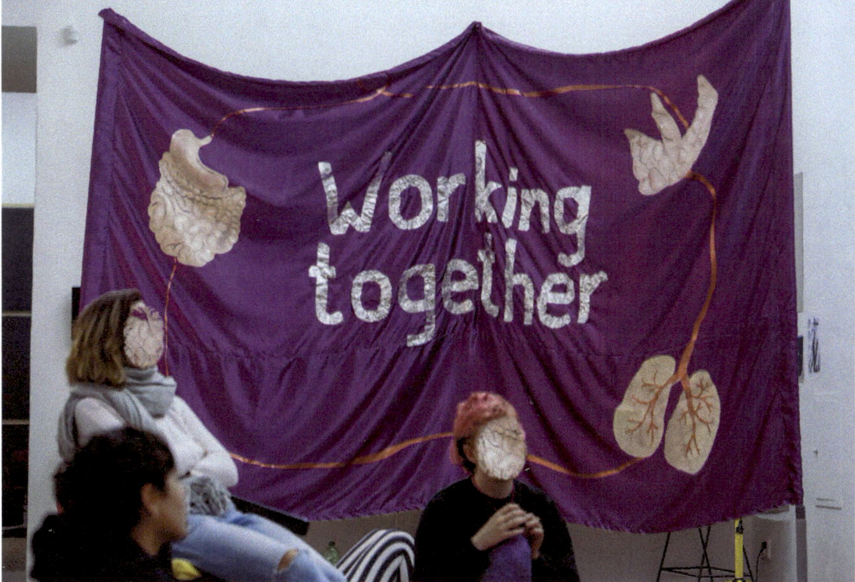

4.1 Feminist Health Care Research Group, Practices of Radical Health Care, Radikale Therapie (Radical Therapy) Workshop, Berlin, 2018. Photograph: Inga Zimprich. Image courtesy of the Feminist Health Care Research Group.

Image description 4.1: People sit in front of a large purple banner draped on a white wall. The banner reads "working together" with human organs floating around the text.

The group are inspired by the West German health movement of the 1970s and 1980s, "whose members poured their time, money, and energy into finding new models of radical mutual care."[4] The FHCRG discovered that these groups had developed new models of radical care through which they not only critiqued patriarchal power systems in conventional medicine, but also created "self-organised health centres, health magazines for squatters, vaginal self-examination classes, [and] radical and feminist therapy groups [that] overthrew both internal and external oppressive social frameworks."[5] The overarching premise of the health movement in the 1970s and 1980s, alongside the work of the FHCRG, is the notion that the state of women's healthcare is inadequate and that "casual misogyny intersects with medicine."[6] The FHCRG also brings the work from several decades ago in line with today's intersectional and queer feminisms. The research that they conduct is always based on their experience as humans confronting the medical field. These experiences are not abstract but grounded in everyday interactions.

The FHCRG's powerful collective organizing entails educating its followers regarding alternative approaches to healthcare. Creative access operates on multiple levels: the literal access being demonstrated and taught to women through the examination of their own bodies and female reproductive organs, and the creative approaches that the group take to conveying this information, alongside its own institutional documentation through exhibitions, zines, and archives. In 2020, the group participated in the Berlin Biennale, and they developed a workshop around how to support one another in moments of emotional crisis amid the pandemic. Emotional support has always been one of the main topics of the group. The questions they posed for this workshop included "What is our social, internalized, and learned understanding of emotional and mental well-being? Why is emotional crisis so stigmatized and taboo? How can we create more space as cultural workers and as friends to accommodate and support one another?" They produced a zine entitled *Being in Crises Together*, which includes a long list of resources for counseling, and features interviews with people regarding radical health initiatives.[7]

Sickness Affinity Group

The Sickness Affinity Group (SAG) is a group comprised of art workers and activists who work on the topic of sickness and disability, and/or are affected by sickness and disability themselves. SAG is also a support group that radically challenges the competitive nature of working in the art world. They share experiences and information based on the health and needs of their members, and they prioritize members' access needs. SAG was founded in 2018 by a group of artists from different parts of Europe, including the UK, Poland, and Germany, who came together because they realized that they may have been competing for the same limited funding and opportunities. They decided that they no longer wanted to compete against one another, and they started meeting once every two months in a park or in someone's house to share resources and simply check in. They supported each other in work but also in life, be it by providing a doctor recommendation or by walking a family dog. The idea was not to be a production-based group – as everyone was already overworked and underpaid – but they failed in this objective, because they eventually started inviting each other to participate in paid events, such as the Berlin Biennale in 2020.

The support group is now formalized and structured for handling work invitations and garden projects that are production-based. There is no pressure to work within the group, although there has been a shift from casual conversation toward a more structured collective. Owing to the pandemic, SAG became primarily online, with a mailing list, and while people may assume that the virtual platform is much more accessible, particularly for disabled people, one of the cofounders of SAG, Laura Lulika, notes that Zoom is not actually accessible to everyone.[8] Some low-income people may not have access to computers, and the close feeling of being in a physical space as a group is lost online. While a larger number of individuals can join an online workshop or discussion, including more international folks, it is much harder to give everyone space to communicate and share and to avoid time checks and interruptions.

Since the pandemic, there has also been a sudden influx of work invitations. On the one hand, Lulika notes, gaining paid work is positive, but they also do not want to perpetuate the ableist pressure to respond to every request, and the only people who can participate are the ones who do not have complicated access barriers.[9] These invitations are from institutions or curators who have an interest in the topic of disability and access, but sometimes they come from a shallow place, as health and illness are a "hot topic" right now. Lulika calls this trend "sexy marginalization." This type of institutional interest does not extend further into how to host and care for disabled and chronically ill folks with unique access needs.[10] This means that SAG's members find themselves performing the additional unpaid labor of explaining the basics of accessibility. Lulika believes that if a curator were genuinely interested in accessibility, then they would do the research ahead of time and learn how to manage the needs of disabled participants more carefully.[11]

The strategies that SAG uses have a logistical component; the group uses many platforms – including voicemail, email, Zoom, computers, and more – and some work better than others. There is no perfectly accessible platform, as these technologies are set up for capitalist working uses in our society, which is not what SAG supports. SAG's members are committed to finding digital accessibility that can be "softer" and more comfortable, although being in bed while chatting online is, of course, helpful. When the members get together, they have the freedom to express their access needs and to voice when things go wrong. Sometimes people do not feel comfortable with emotional check-ins in group settings, but SAG nurtures its members to discuss failure and how to move forward from challenges. SAG is also aware that they have failed to create a space that is racially inclusive, as everyone in the group is white. They are working on being critical of their whiteness through their garden project. This is also part of their ongoing work in dialogic creative access, where they address the privileges of the group, including class and economic background.

Power Makes Us Sick

Power Makes Us Sick (PMS), formed in 2017 with members based in North America and Europe, closely aligns with the objectives and impetus behind the FHCRG and SAG. The name of the collective is a double entendre, referring to the idea that power is making us sick, both literally and metaphorically. The PMS abbreviation for the collective is also clever (although its intentionality is unclear) for its reference to the stressful characteristics of women's premenstrual cycles. As stated on their website,

> Power Makes Us Sick (PMS) is a creative research project focusing on autonomous healthcare practices and networks from a feminist perspective. PMS seeks to understand the ways that our mental, physical, and social health is impacted by imbalances in and abuses of power. We understand that mobility, forced or otherwise, is an increasingly common aspect of life in the anthropocene. In this quest for placeless solidarity, we start with health. PMS is motivated to develop free tools of solidarity, resistance, and sabotage that are informed by a deep concern for planetary well-being.[12]

Power Makes Us Sick also runs workshops, meets regularly online in support gatherings, and maintains a blog in order to share resources. However, the collective's efforts have predominantly been directed toward extensive zines, which can be downloaded for free from their website. Titles include *The Accountability Model* (a tool that PMS developed to help communities take care of one another's mental, physical, and social health without so-called medical experts), *Strategies for Emotional Support*, *Emotional Support Basics*, *Building Towards an Autonomous Trans Healthcare*, and, during the pandemic, *Physically Distant, Connected by Care*. The zines focus on breathing exercises in issue 1 (winter 2017); resisting anti-sex-work legislation in issue 2 (summer 2017); and talking about death in issue 3 (summer 2018).[13] They also stand out aesthetically, featuring original line drawings that capture the collective's criticality toward power and how it dominates women.

Some of the health-based workshops PMS has led include Health Autonomy, held in London in 2018, during which it offered training on the

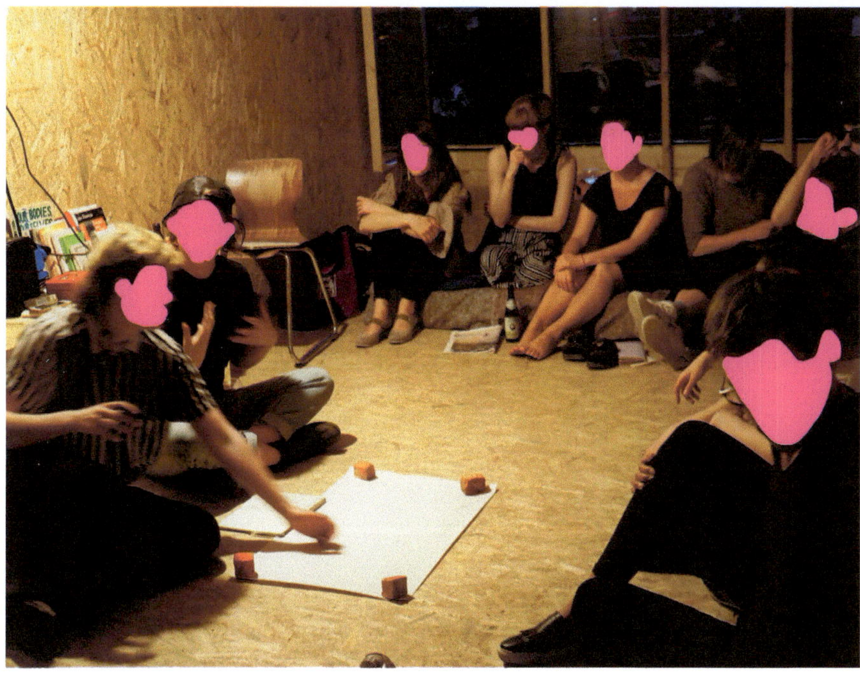

4.2 Power Makes Us Sick, Workshop in the Ständige Vertretung, 2018. Image courtesy of Power Makes Us Sick.

Image description 4.2: A group of people sit on the floor in a circle. Their faces have been obscured with bright magenta digital paint.

basics of conflict resolution and community accountability while examining examples of autonomous healthcare projects in different parts of the world, and *How Are You Feeling Today?*, also in 2018, in a temporary project space casually dubbed "The Treehouse" at the Ständige Vertretung in Berlin, where PMS facilitated a discussion on the vocabulary of sickness and illness (Figure 4.2). The session closed with a visualization exercise aimed at an aspirational idea of "health." An excerpt from this exercise can be found on the PMS website:

> Begin to imagine yourself in an environment that contributes positively to your overall sense of well-being, this can be as real or imaginary as you like. This place is bountiful and able to provide for you. Whatever you need or desire for your physical, social, and mental health is there for you to invite into the space. Free from restraints, limits, and scarcity, this environment is a vision of yourself completely taken care of. What do you see in front of you? What do you see to your right and left? What do you see above and below you? What do you hear? Are the sounds loud or soft? Near or far? How do you hold your body in this space? Are you sitting, standing, something else? Now start to move through this space? [*sic*] Walk, run, dance, whatever feels natural to you. In this real or imagined environment what aspects contribute to your

> physical health? What is making your body feel balanced and like yourself in this environment? In this environment what kind of food do you want to eat? What kind of food contributes to this feeling of balance? How do [your] lungs and heart feel? What do you notice about how your body feels as it moves through space?[14]

This visualization exercise demonstrates how the group offers its members space in which to think through more empowered and positive depictions of health on their own terms.

In 2020, PMS participated in a Zoom panel discussion with FHCRG and SAG to discuss how each collective contributes to the ongoing critical conversation on empowered anti-establishment healthcare, particularly in light of the inequities being played out during the pandemic. Clearly there is an urgent desire and need for such feminist collectives that develop creative access approaches to the health of their own bodies and their own livelihoods. This panel offered another opportunity to enlarge the circles of care even further, producing more networks of dialogic creative access that reach a truly global scale.

Black Womxn Flourish

In 2020, queer disabled designer, creative co-conspirator, and intuitive writer Denise Shanté Brown founded Black Womxn Flourish in Baltimore, Maryland. Their website states, "we're a design for wellbeing collective made up of Black Womxn Imaginaries co-dreaming and blooming new worlds for health and healing."[15] Denise Shanté's main collaborators include Precious Diamond B. (creative synthesizer and joy cultivator) and N'Deye Diakhate (intuitive design collaborator). Black Womxn Flourish uses "womxn" as an umbrella term, inclusive to femmes, transgender, and gender non-conforming people.

Black Womxn Flourish was seeded by the desire for Black womxn to self-determine their care within interpersonal relationships, communal spaces, and the healthcare system. There was a strong spiritual call to connect like-minded Black womxn and other folks from the African diaspora who were longing for more life-affirming, dignified models of care, and to enable them to lean into a nurtured space of vulnerability and learning. From these curiosities, Denise Shanté developed an emergent practice called "*Design for Wellbeing*: a shared creative process and practice of bringing experiences for whole, abundant health into existence where pleasure, healing, joy and care are possible."[16] There are a multitude of ways Design for Wellbeing showed up in the world, and one of those expressions blossomed when Denise Shanté collaborated with N'Deye on Denise Shanté's master's thesis, which she was completing at the Maryland Institute College of Art in Baltimore in 2017. Brown asked the core question, "What if there was a compassionate culture that supports the wellbeing of Black womxn?" This question led to the exploratory program, Design for the Wellbeing of Black Womxn, where members of the collective and participants "journey through an embodied and expansive curriculum to explore holistic, healing-centric practices and cultivate their creative capacity to build and implement tools for resilience, collective care, and transformation in their lives and within their communities."[17]

After prototyping the program, Denise Shanté shared a call for collaborators to create a collective that would hold, push forward, and nurture the work on a communal scale. Precious joined the collective during this visioning and building process in 2019. In July 2020, the collective was birthed and revealed to the world. Formally, Black Womxn Flourish is a design for well-being collective that centers Black creativity and dreams of well-being for those who have been historically marginalized. They draw on existing frameworks of social justice movements to collaboratively dream and design, as members of the collective and with all those who attend their community gatherings. These frameworks include emergent strategy, healing justice, disability justice, and design justice.

With Denise Shanté's training as a designer rooted in liberatory praxis, N'Deye's emergent and intuitive skills, and Precious's integrative approach to creativity and collaborative process, the collective began to talk about the ways that design should be community-led and rooted in the desires and dreams of people who are going to be impacted by anything that's created – including their care. The members of the collective realized that they had not experienced or witnessed a space where Black womxn are at the center of designing and dreaming around the things that they actually want and need, as it relates to all aspects of their well-being.

In the fall of 2020 the collective hosted three virtual workshops, with guest collaborators Teena Lewis and Aisha Shillingford, that gathered over sixty people in total. People from across the country and the world attended, and they were invited to imaginatively dream, speculate, affirm, and declare how the world needs to right itself in order for womxn, specifically Black womxn, to be held, cared for, and loved in the ways that they should be. Given that the workshops were held during the stressful first year of the pandemic, a great deal of discussion revolved around Black womxn's role as healers, and in turn, what it means to receive healing or to be a recipient of healing. Oftentimes Black womxn didn't have the luxury of working at home during the pandemic. Many were still on the front lines, going into either the office or the hospital to be the caretakers. During the gatherings, participants moved through a generative journey of somatic exploration and guided visualizations rooted in Black Imagination, collective collaging, affirmation writing, and the creation of artifacts from a Black womxn's flourishing future from the chosen years of 2025 to 9262. The following questions were used as a basis for discussion in the workshops:

What is our flourishing future?
What do we need to affirm and declare to fully experience a flourishing future in which we are healing, joyful and well?
How would our lives, communities and worlds be transformed by a flourishing future designed by Black womxn?

What was imagined and conjured through the collaborative workshops was their manifesto, *Dreaming Flourishing Futures: A Black Womxn's Manifesto for Designing the Worlds we must Have to be Well*, which can be purchased from the Black Womxn Flourish website. The manifesto takes the explorer on a journey of reflection, visioning, imagination, meditation, time travel, and self-discovery. It was a labor of love made possible with the additional support of "manifesto creation crew organizers" Aki Younge, Alexandra Antoine, and Nechari Riley. This luminous collection includes an introductory statement capturing the Black Womxn Flourish two-year co-creation and design journey; "breath pages" that offer soft landings and moments of visual contemplation (see Figure 4.3); thematic summaries that open the doors to collective imaginative planes; affirmations and declarations from the gathering participants; recipes, rituals, and meditations associated with

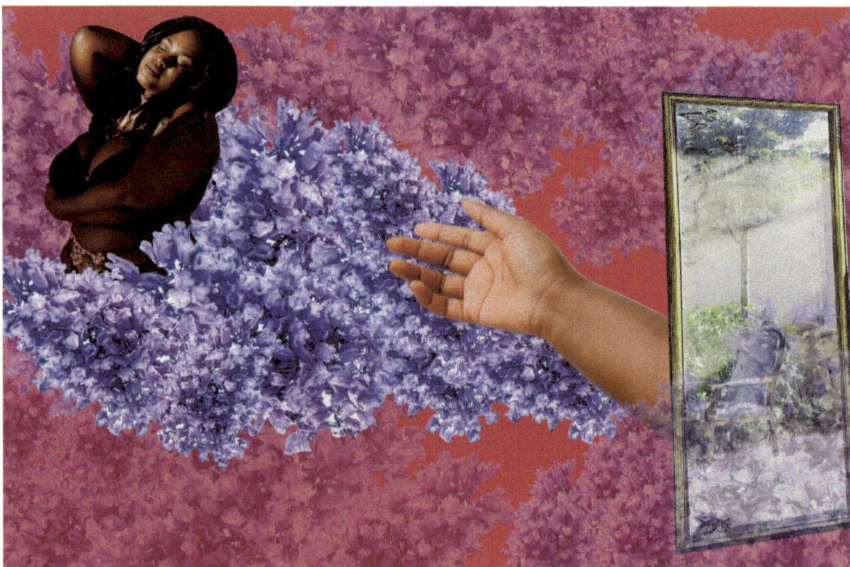

4.3 One of the "breath pages" that offer soft landings and visual contemplation from *Dreaming Flourishing Futures: A Black Womxn's Manifesto for Designing the Worlds We Must Have to Be Well*, 2020. Designed by Precious Diamond B., Creative Synthesizer and Joy Cultivator for the Black Womxn Flourish Collective.

Image description 4.3: A digital collage depicting a Black woman luxuriating in a cloud of lavendar blooms. An outstretched arm with light brown skin appears from behind a framed image.

various themes of the workshops, and highlight pages as a reminder of Black womxn's creative power, aliveness, and sacredness. The manifesto also offers interactive pages that invite the reader to co-dream and design in the spaces of the book. At the time of writing, Black Womxn Flourish are in a period of transformation, where they are individually tending to themselves, their nourishment, and joy.[18]

A brief history of collective care and empowerment

Of particular importance in framing the work discussed in this chapter is the work of the first known women's health collectives, which formed in the 1960s and 1970s alongside the second wave feminist art movement as a means for women to take more control over their own bodies and their own healthcare. While disability perspectives may not have been explicitly represented in these groups, the issues that these women addressed would nonetheless resonate with other minority groups of the time, and in the future. Some of these issues included the experience of being dismissed by the medical establishment, particularly by white male doctors who refused to share knowledge or kept medical information inaccessible, and a general restriction to healthcare. This asymmetrical power dynamic is what the women's health collective aimed to dismantle so that women could better understand their own health and medical needs. A group of women in Boston who were a prominent part of the women's liberation movement in Boston formed the Boston Women's Health Book Collective (BWHBC), which turned into a course and a book published by New England Free Press in 1971 entitled *Our Bodies, Ourselves*. The goal of both the course and the book was to fight patriarchy and the "historic oppression and self-alienation perpetuated by the medical establishment."[19] The book was developed as a critical resource, providing medical knowledge to help women navigate their own health. The book has sold millions of copies all over the world, and has been translated into more than twenty-five languages. Amber Jamilla Musser states: "by providing women with knowledge, it strove to dismantle the medical establishment from the inside out, thereby repossessing health and making it something individuals could attain from communal knowledge without interference from the medical establishment."[20] In Figure 4.4, two original members of the collective, Norma Swenson and Betsy Cole, chat at their exhibition booth to promote the various activities of the collective in 1980. The collective has also distributed information about women's health through websites, blogs, and other related publications, and hundreds of people have contributed to the wealth of knowledge shared across each of these platforms, including staff, advisory board members, board members, founders, and consultants.

The work of the Boston Women's Health Book Collective remains deeply influential for many artists, activists, and health and care practitioners today. Contemporary British artist Olivia Plender, who is based in both

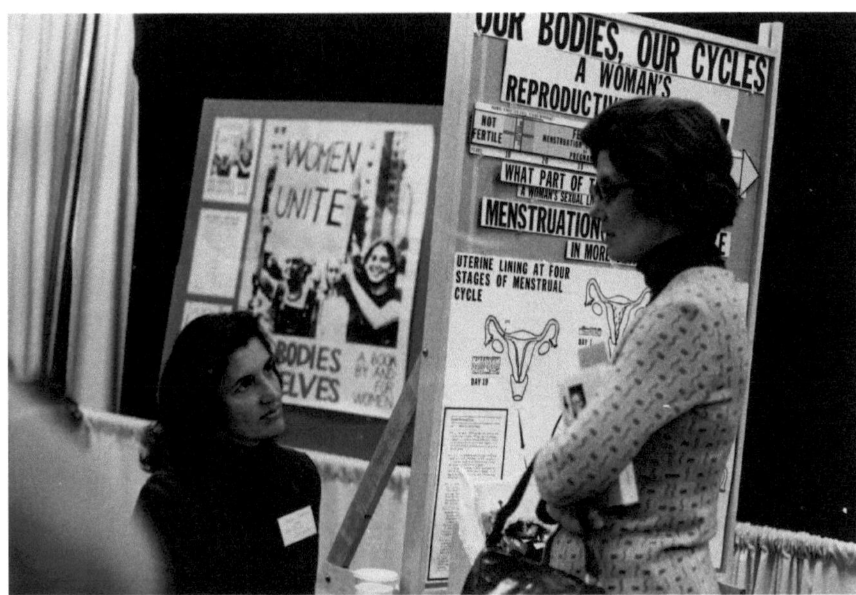

4.4 Norma Swenson and Betsy Cole at exhibit booth for "Our Bodies, Ourselves," *c.*1980. Gelatin silver, 5 × 4in. (13 × 10cm) Records of the Boston Women's Health Book Collective, MC503-PD.5-4. Courtesy of Schlesinger Library, Harvard Radcliffe Institute.

Image description 4.4: A black and white photo of two women talking in front of women's reproductive rights posters.

London and Stockholm, produced drawings inspired by the collective. Her projects generally start with research into the histories of social movements, and she is interested in the relationships between gender, power, and authority. In her series of drawings and printed posters, *Our Bodies are not the Problem, the Problem is Power* (2021), Plender depicts materials from the archives of the collective housed at the Glasgow Women's Library in Scotland, including pamphlets and zines which challenge health inequalities and ableist systems of care (Figures 4.5 and 4.6). These materials also show how communities have developed alternatives for educating themselves about their bodies and health, countering deficiencies in mainstream provision. Plender states: "across all these components, I highlight the relationship between ill health and structures of inequality, including racism, sexism and transphobia."[21] The posters were developed for a group exhibition entitled *Life Support: Forms of Care in Art and Activism* held at the Glasgow Women's Library, and were just one component of a larger installation that Plender developed which consisted of her redesign of a community room to make it more welcoming and accommodating for all kinds of bodies. She domesticated the space by introducing new carpets, comfortable furniture like beanbags, and dim lighting. She also changed the color of

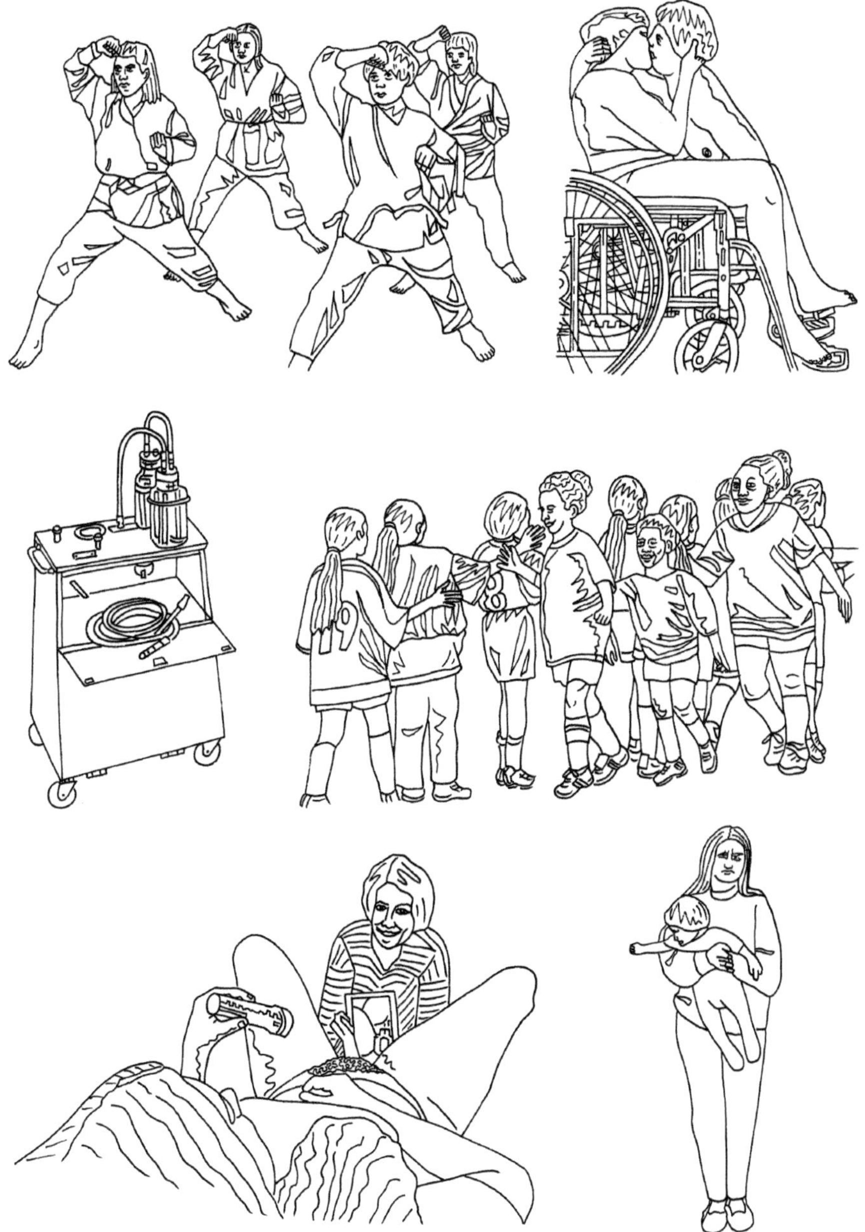

4.5, 4.6 Olivia Plender, *Our Bodies Are Not the Problem, the Problem is Power*, 2021. Printed poster, 23.4 × 33.1in. (59.5 × 84cm). Courtesy of the artist.

Image description 4.5, 4.6: Twelve contour line drawings depicting people in the midst of various activities such as kissing, practicing karate, visiting the doctor, reading braille, and practicing prenatal yoga.

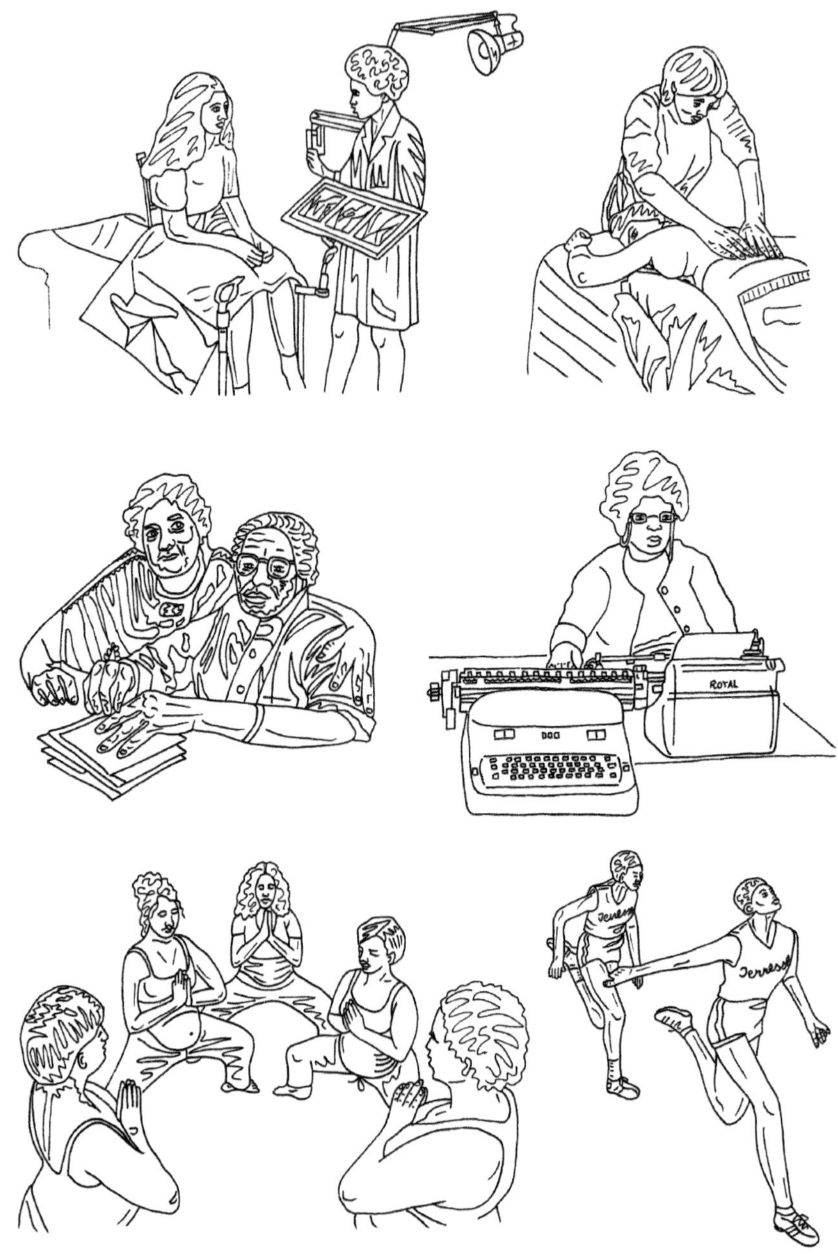

4.5, 4.6 Continued

the walls and ceiling to a calming lavender. Plender realized that women needed a relaxing environment in which to recuperate from the challenges of everyday life and from dealing with a medical establishment that consistently failed to take women's health concerns seriously. Plender's design aligns with the objectives of the women's collectives discussed in the previous sections, including women's empowerment of design, health, and their bodies, as well as prioritizing self-care. I enjoyed learning of Plender's work as another iteration of the Boston Women's Health Book Collective, but also because Plender is literally illustrating their work in a visual format, and thus sharing their history and their knowledge with new generations of communities in need of these resources.

In addition to the formal coalitions developed through the healthcare collectives I have discussed, other contemporary disabled artists have also been deeply committed to the topic of care through individual practices. I believe the genesis of these ideas around collectivity and care as art praxis arose through the foundational work of artist Park McArthur, whose own personal collective of care workers-cum-performers became an essential part of her art practice.[22] In the video *It's Sorta Like a Big Hug* (2012), McArthur recorded the routine of her care workers as a type of performance: a coterie of people would come to her New York apartment for scheduled visits in order to help McArthur move from her wheelchair into her bed at night, and return in the morning to assist her with moving from the bed back into the wheelchair, or to use the toilet or the shower, and so on. McArthur's compelling work portrays an intimacy among bodies that had rarely been considered previously as anything but laborious care work. Through the artist's clever reframing, viewers are forced to recognize and reckon with the act of collective care and collective access as one to be valued, uplifted, and shared.

In tandem with the video, in 2011 McArthur collaborated with Constantina Zavitsanos to codevelop a series of text-based idiosyncratic scores, which explore the intimacies of care and collaboration around meeting specific access needs for someone who navigates the world in a wheelchair (see Figure 4.7). The scores resemble and riff on the Fluxus strategy for drawing attention to everyday actions. These scores were an outcome of the care collective that McArthur established, made up of ten people who engaged in a care routine for the artist as she navigated transfers from her wheelchair to the shower, changing into pajamas, and getting into bed at night. Other routines that the artists have recorded include making dinner, drinking, talking, reading, massaging limbs, drawing, videotaping, and sharing stories. The scores aim to lift up the value of care work, which has historically been ignored and diminished, and through which disabled people have frequently been subjected to violence and assault. The artists aim to explore convivial forms of care work that do not depend on an exchange under a capitalist regime, instead pointing to care as an event. Their scores

SCORE FOR BACKING UP

Think about your first lift with your partner.

Know that your partner has done this one million times more than you and that in twelve point font, a list of names of people that have done these lifts with her is 38 inches long when printed and leaves a 14 inch block of space for all the names that will come after you.

Realize you don't remember the occasion of your first time, despite never having done this before.

Realize that she probably does remember.

Consider this discrepancy.

Know that now feels like the first time precisely because the first time felt like you've done this forever.

Pull the manual chair down the ramp backwards.

4.7 Park McArthur and Constantina Zavitsanos, *Score for Backing Up*, 2013. Text in vinyl: scores for acts of care with two or more, dimensions variable. Courtesy of the artists.

Image description 4.7: An event score titled "Score for Backing Up" reads as follows: Think about your first lift with your partner. Know that your partner has done this one million times more than you and that in twelve point font, a list of names of people that have done these lifts with her is 38 inches long when printed and leaves a 14 inch block of space for all the names that will come after you. Realize you don't remember the occasion of your first time, despite never having done this before. Realize that she probably does remember. Consider this descrepancy. Know that now feels like the first time precisely because the first time felt like you've done this forever. Pull the manual chair down the ramp backwards.

take various forms, and have been exhibited at The Schinkel Pavillon in Berlin, at Gebert Stiftung für Kulture in Rapperswil-Jona, Switzerland, and at the Brooklyn Museum in New York. McArthur and Zavitsanos's work is also responsive to central tenets within the academic field of disability studies, particularly its critique of the notion of an independent self, and gestures to thinkers such as Marta Russell, Eva Feder Kittay, and Rosemarie Garland-Thomson.

McArthur and Zavitsanos were also part of the New York City-based healing and arts care collective Canaries, which was founded in 2016, and included core members Jesse Cohen, Catherine Czacki, Taraneh Fazeli, Citron Kelly, Carolyn Lazard, Bonnie Swencionis, and Rebecca Watson Horn. Canaries was "a network of women-identified, femme-presenting, and gender non-conforming people living and working with autoimmune conditions and other chronic illnesses."[23] The group's name, Canaries, was inspired by the idiom "canaries in the coal mine," which references the nineteenth-century practice of using canaries to indicate potential hazards and adverse conditions in the coal mine and in the environment. Like the other groups discussed in this chapter, Canaries held monthly support meetings, maintained a listserv with many members, and would come together to exchange stories and strategies for coping with their disabilities and illnesses.

Canaries and McArthur's ideas have had a profound impact on current generations of disabled artists, who have been emboldened to share their personal and collective experiences of chronic illness and their encounters with ableism in the medical industry over the years, both on social media and in art praxis. Each hospital visit, therapy appointment, or treatment has been documented and discussed through the lens of a personal journey by disabled and chronically ill artists, then shared with others going through similar experiences (most often on social media or blogs), offering a form of dialogic creative access. Eventually, more formal collectives have developed organically, allowing this work to be documented, archived, and formalized through regular meetings, online encounters, and exchanges of conviviality and care.[24]

An important critique that Musser makes in her article about the Boston Women's Health Book Collective is that while the collective treated access to health as an inherently political move, there is an assumption that the subjectivity of the group's membership is white, straight, and middle class. There was therefore an omission of lesbian sexuality, racialized groups, lower socioeconomic classes, and indeed disability, as mentioned at the outset of this section. Some of the collectives discussed in this chapter have also acknowledged the absence of representation of other minorities, which they hope to rectify in the future. However, while noting these absences in collectives such as SAG and PMS, other minorities have also created space for themselves, for instance Black Womxn Flourish. Historically,

Black women have also made space for themselves to gather and discuss vital issues of health, too. Sami Schalk uses the National Black Women's Health Project (NBWHP) as one of her central case studies in *Black Disability Politics*. Now known as the Black Women's Health Imperative, the organization outlines their mission on their website:

> BWHI is the first and only national non-profit solely dedicated to achieving health equity for Black women globally. Founded in 1983 by Byllye Y. Avery as the National Black Women's Health Project at a conference on the campus of Spelman College, BWHI has evolved into a nationally recognized organization leading health policy, education, research, knowledge and leadership development and communications designed to improve the health outcomes of Black women.[25]

In her book, Schalk argues that the National Black Women's Health Project played a critical role in Black feminist health activism, and that they "engaged in a multifaceted, comprehensive, intersectional, and explicitly political approach to health that built on the legacies of previous health activism in feminist, civil rights, and other progressive movements."[26] Schalk argues that the NBWHP were enacting a health activism in a specifically Black feminist form, where to be well was to be empowered.

A Black artist whose socially engaged art practice intersects with Black Women's Health in a contemporary context is Simone Leigh. In two lauded works, *Free People's Medical Clinic* (2014) and *The Waiting Room* (2016), Leigh addressed health and self-determination, drawing from a lineage of radical health activism encompassing the Black Panthers' Free Clinics and The United Order of Tents. The Black Panther Party was a Marxist organization founded by college students Bobby Seale and Huey P. Newton in 1966 in Oakland, California. They had chapters across many major American cities and internationally. While the initial impetus for the party was to decry police violence against Black citizens, the party also initiated many important social advocacy programs to serve underrepresented populations. The United Order of Tents was an organization of African American churchwomen who cared for the sick and elderly and helped those in need bury their dead. They were founded in Norfolk, Virginia in 1867 by Annetta M. Lane and Harriet R. Taylor. Influenced by the many social service and community programs that both these organizations implemented for members of the public, Leigh wanted to offer "care sessions" that ranged from "lessons in Caribbean medicine to free HIV screenings."[27] Leigh's projects were "devoted to promoting healing and agency among women of color."[28]

Free People's Medical Clinic was held in 2014 at the Stuyvesant Mansion in Brooklyn as part of an event hosted by Creative Time. The site of Leigh's health workshops for Black women was significant in that it was built in 1914 and owned by the family of Dr. Josephine English. English was the first African American woman to have an OB/GYN practice in New York,

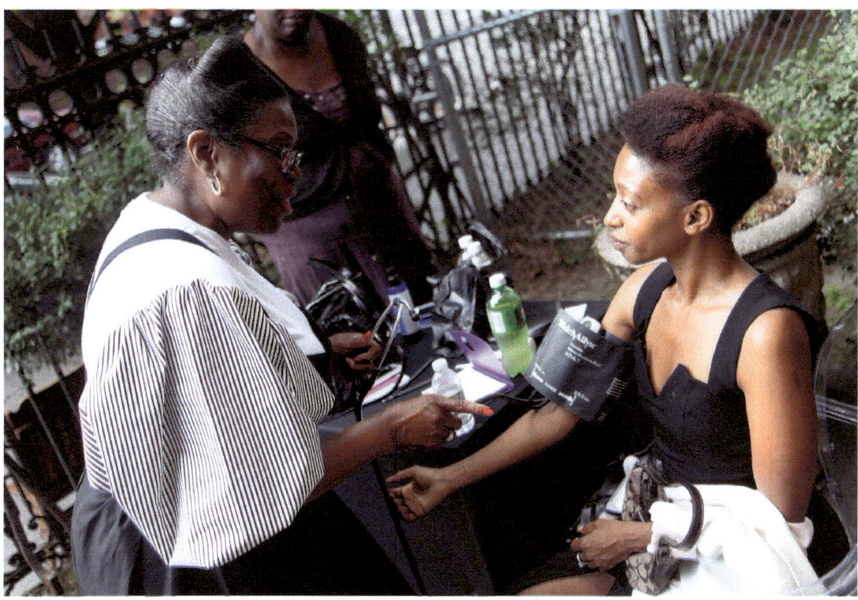

4.8 Simone Leigh, *Free People's Medical Clinic; Funk, God, Jazz, and Medicine: Black Radical Brooklyn*, 2014. Photograph: Shulamit Seidler-Feller. Courtesy of Creative Time.

Image description 4.8: A Black woman sits getting her blood pressure measured while listening to another Black woman who speaks animatedly.

and was a prominent member of the community as both a supporter of the arts and a doctor, among other professional titles. At the entrance to the mansion were site attendants taking visitors' blood pressure (see Figure 4.8). Women dressed in nineteenth-century period costumes would welcome visitors once they had entered through the mansion front doors, and provided information about the clinic's scheduled classes and performances. Some of the classes included ancient song, doula services, Black folk dance, massage therapy, acupuncture, Afro-centering pilates, and yoga.

Leigh's next event was *The Waiting Room*, held at the New Museum in New York in 2018. *The Waiting Room* had a particularly tragic premise, as it was based on the story of a Jamaican woman, Esmin Elizabeth Green, who died in 2008 at the age of 49 after waiting twenty-four hours in an emergency waiting room without being seen. For this reason, Leigh made the waiting room at the mansion in *Free People's Medical Clinic* one of the most dynamic spaces, where yoga and dancing helped cut through the opaque quality of what happens behind closed doors in the doctor's office, and to endow the waiting room – and thus those who wait in it for prolonged periods – with more power, care, and agency. Similar to *Free People's Medical Clinic*, visitors were able to attend an array of workshops and programs focused on caregiving and health. It is notable that Leigh's series of events were only open and available to those who were "in the know" as part of Leigh's circle of friends and acquaintances. Giulia Smith states that "secrecy and separatism are Leigh's cardinal tactics, reflecting not only the chronic erasure and deferral of Black subjects, but also their capacity to self-organize and go underground."[29] Helen Molesworth wrote that when she visited Leigh's *The Waiting Room*, all she witnessed was an empty room with a display cabinet filled with glass jars stuffed with herbal recipes.[30] Experiencing this lackluster space and raising questions about the specific nature of the installation and its socially engaged aspects henceforth kicked off a period of reciprocal waiting for the white visitor that was as anxiety-filled as being in a waiting room in a medical setting. An antagonistic turn to health, waiting, and putting on hold was thus very much the point of Leigh's work, where turning the tables (or the waiting room chair as the case may be) on the white person meant turning the tables of equal access.

It is important to underscore that Leigh's interventions were intersectional because she incorporated Black, queer, and disabled individuals into her events. As Schalk has articulated, a history of Black intervention (such as the Black Panther Party or the National Black Women's Health Project) incorporates a disability history, but within Black activist communities "disability" shows up in specific and different ways, such as through medical neglect, or lack of access to resources. As mentioned in the Introduction, sometimes disability activism is harder to recognize in Black communities because the language of disability may not necessarily be used, but Schalk argues powerfully that disability activism is nonetheless being practiced. Based on Schalk's theorizing, perhaps I could venture that Leigh's work falls into this category, where Blackness comes first, and disability politics is a quieter interlocutor, but an interlocutor nonetheless.

This brings me to a question that has likely already gone through the reader's mind as they have read this book – aren't all patients disabled, if disability is now much more expansively defined and encompasses all illness and a myriad of health conditions? The answer to this question lies in the intersectional identity of the patient. As I have already remarked numerous times throughout the book, the intersectional identity of the disabled patient is what dictates the type of treatment they get – hence the difference between Dominic Quagliozzi's treatment in hospital as a white cis man, compared with the work about medical racism by Carolyn Lazard, as discussed in Chapter 1.

The last but not least important manifestation of collective care and empowerment comes in the form of a doula. A doula is conventionally understood as a woman who guides and supports another woman through the final stages of pregnancy and childbirth, who can be present both inside and outside hospital settings. A doula does not necessarily have medical training, unlike a midwife; the doula is more interested in providing emotional support, comfort, and care through this major life transition. In the past few years, the term doula has been adopted by the disability community in various ways, in recognition of the formal caring qualifications that make up the doula role. Queer Korean American disability justice activist Stacey Park Milbern developed the terms “crip doula” or “disability doula” to signify a doula who specifically helps an individual to transition into becoming disabled, especially for those who have newly acquired disabilities and are trying to navigate a world that wasn’t made for disabled people. A crip doula has intimate embodied knowledge, resources, tricks, and skills regarding disability as they are disabled themselves and can share their lived experiences with others. The associations that a crip doula has with a traditional doula are symbolic, in that both are involved in “birthing practices” in different contexts. Milbern has noted that a crip doula is able to help with rebirthing a person through disability. She states: “this looks like a lot of things – maybe learning how to get medicine, drive a wheelchair, hire attendants, change a diet, date, have sex, make requests, code switch, live with an intellectual disability, go off meds, etc. etc.”[31] This type of crip mentorship and crip doulaship is often invisible, but activists such as Milbern, Sami Schalk, and Leah Lakshmi Piepzna-Samarasinha have written and talked about this topic at great length in the past few years, so there is now more widespread recognition of the importance of this work. Typically the work of a disability doula is practiced within a community of disability friends, which is why I perceive this as a socially engaged art practice alongside the other work discussed in this chapter. Piepzna-Samarasinha wrote that “crip doulaing is both an interpersonal dynamic and one that creates new disability justice space.”[32] Thus, alongside all the collective/collaborative making work in this chapter, crip doulaing is key to providing advocacy, and another component to the politics that stems from hospital aesthetics.

Disability doula work has much in common with HIV doula caregiving. What Would An HIV Doula Do? is a collective of artists, academics, chaplains, doulas, healthcare practitioners, nurses, filmmakers, AIDS service organization employees, dancers, community educators, and more from across the HIV spectrum. They have joined together to collectively respond to the ongoing AIDS crisis, and their goal is to offer support to individuals with HIV within a community of people who also have HIV. In a statement on their website, they write, “We know that since no one gets HIV alone, no one should have to live with HIV alone. We doula ourselves, each other, institutions and culture. Foundational to our process is asking questions.”[33] The collective understands that individuals with HIV need support around testing, diagnosis, and treatment, and navigating what can be a toxic culture of stigma and criminalization of HIV. Like the other collectives featured in this chapter thus far, What Would An HIV Doula Do? has developed various public engagement programs hosted by museums, and has received press across a number of media outlets and social media platforms. They have also produced digital zines, such as *Harm Reduction is a Not a Metaphor: Living in the 21st century with Drugs, Intimacy, and Activism*, developed in collaboration with MoMA PS1 in their Homeroom gallery. Homeroom is a new program that seeks to amplify the work of collaborative groups such as those I have discussed in this chapter. The collaboratives are offered this space at MoMA PS1 in which to work, to recall and revive the history of the PS1 building, which was founded as the first school in Long Island City in 1976. I find it interesting that museums and contemporary art spaces are responding to the demands and needs of socially engaged art practices by implementing new permanent spaces in which this work can be held. Overall, socially engaged art practices and collectives that are forming around health and access needs reinforce the argument that I made at the outset of this chapter: that the proliferation of these support groups shows a general shift in social norms, where the medical field no longer has the only authoritative voice on health. The work of these groups indicates how nonmedical health-based groups are making up for a lack in social support networks elsewhere, particularly within sanctioned medical arenas.

Theoretical frameworks on collectivity and care

Thinking on the topic of care has proliferated across the humanities, particularly in disability studies, gender and sexuality studies, communication studies, ethnic studies, art history and visual culture, philosophy, and the medical humanities. I want to give the reader a sense of the broad range of approaches to and interpretations of caring, both because we are living in the aftermath of COVID-19, a moment when this topic is even more relevant and timely than ever before, and because this is a critical concept that ultimately has resonance across all of the chapters. The lens of collective care will further elucidate the concept of "hospital aesthetics."

As I mentioned at the start of this chapter, my term "dialogic care aesthetics" is greatly informed by the groundbreaking work of art historian Grant Kester, who developed the term "dialogic aesthetics" over a decade ago as a way to frame the practices of socially engaged artists who were creating new work based on their direct conversations with their community.[34] The conversations, in fact, were the art; artists involved in these practices moved away from the tradition of making and producing objects entirely. Kester, along with a cohort of other prominent art historians and cultural producers, including Claire Bishop, Shannon Jackson, Nicolas Bourriaud, and others, fashioned an entirely new art movement – socially engaged art practice – based on these important propositions.[35] While a few disabled socially engaged artists have emerged in the past decade, most prominently nonvisual learner Carmen Papalia in Vancouver, the question of how the disability community participated in the movement has been difficult to assess up until this point. As the various disability justice care collectives have begun to emerge and engage with each other, it has become clear to me that their work contributes to the landscape of dialogic aesthetics, albeit through a framework of care – hence my coinage, dialogic care aesthetics. It is encouraging to witness disability's representation and voice in the socially engaged art movement, as it had been largely absent until COVID-19 hit. Not only is the voice of disability important to add to this critical new genre and movement in contemporary art history, I argue that disabled artists have also become the (initially unintentional) leaders in addressing the complexities of care across all genres and mediums of contemporary art.

In the previous section, I mentioned the impact that disability studies scholars such as Eva Feder Kittay have had on contemporary disabled artists like Park McArthur, Constantina Zavitsanos, and Carolyn Lazard, among others. Emeritus professor of feminist philosophy, feminist ethics, social and political theory and disability studies, Kittay has long theorized on the issue of care, examining how care is structured in society as a matter of social justice. She has analyzed in particular the relationship between care and labor, the role of women, and socioeconomic status. Kittay's daughter Sesha has cerebral palsy and is intellectually disabled, and Kittay has written from her lived experience as Sesha's caregiver. Kittay is considered to be a pioneer in writing about an ethics of care based on interpersonal relationships which are responsive to the specific needs of the caree, and about the nuanced relationships of dependence and interdependence in the disability community. Kittay's concepts of care are not designed based on any so-called universal principles, which are often rendered from an able-bodied perspective; instead, Kittay offers a deeply felt and deeply knowing experience of careship where the carer and the caree are partners and collaborators. Kittay's books include *Learning From My Daughter: The Value and Care of Disabled Minds* (2019) and *Love's Labor: Essays on Women, Equality, and Dependency* (2nd edition, 2020), among other publications.[36]

Following Kittay's groundbreaking and foundational work, I want to explore other recent and important scholarship that has contributed to the evolving rhetoric on networks of care and kinship in the aftermath of COVID-19. For example, Akemi Nishida's book, *Just Care: Messy Entanglements of Disability, Dependency, and Desire* (2022), examines what Nishida calls care injustice.[37] Nishida argues that care has become a business opportunity and has been wielded as another mechanism through which to control vulnerable citizens. She provides detailed case studies on people who must negotiate complex care situations as both caregivers and receivers, dialoguing with numerous artists discussed in this book, such as Park McArthur and Constantina Zavitsanos. Nishida gives great detail on the activism of numerous members of the disability community, and highlights how bed activism, which she defines as resistance from the bed, is helping to redefine care as we know it. One very powerful scholarly move that Nishida makes in the book is to deploy the sociopolitical theory of necropolitics, originally developed by Achille Mbembe, in conjunction with care, calling this concept a "necropolitics of care." Mbembe used necropolitics to define how social and political power is used to determine whose life is worth living. In Nishida's construction, *necropolitical care* is contrasted with *biopolitical care*. The difference between the two terms is that within the scholarship of biopolitical care, disabled people are kept alive "at the expense of the weathering care worker population" whereas in necropolitical care, both the workers and the disabled patients are victims of a larger corrupt system.[38] In Nishida's words, both workers and patients "experience constant debilitation in the shadow of a flourishing healthcare assemblage."[39] Nishida's scholarship shows us that both disabled patients and care workers are equally caught in the jaws of the industrial complex and the biomedical complex, rendering the act of turning to each other within self-sustaining care collectives even more important.

In Marty Fink's *Forget Burial: HIV Kinship, Disability, and Queer/Trans Narratives of Care* (2021), he argues that the archival narratives of HIV caregiving from the 1980s and 1990s provide a revelatory model of disability kinship "that supports ongoing sexual and gender self-determination into the present."[40] For Fink, kinship – generally defined as a web of social relationships that form an important part of the lives of humans across societies – is therefore invaluable for providing support in self-proclaiming one's identity and empowerment. Fink shows us that there are important historical models for this type of kinship based in the HIV community. Although certainly not the first to do this, Fink also does important work by showing how those diagnosed and living with HIV are disabled as well. Although bridging HIV with disability is not universally accepted by all those who belong in the HIV community, Fink nonetheless does their own work in building kinship and demonstrating that there is strength and safety in numbers. Another interesting point that Fink makes is how caregiving within the HIV community needs to be recognized as important work too, as historically it has received scant attention owing to its so-called "less revolutionary" nature compared with the HIV street protest.[41] This is another important addition to the work being done by artists like Park McArthur and scholars like Eva Feder Kittay, who have brought attention to the labor of care workers as they engage with disabled individuals. Additionally, Fink shows that the HIV archives also reveal epistemic racism and colonialism, and that access to institutional care has been blocked in myriad ways under our capitalist system.

Lastly, in *Medical Entanglements: Rethinking Feminist Debates About Healthcare* (2020), Kristina Gupta analyzes a glaring contradiction within the biomedical industrial complex that many other scholars in disability studies and other humanistic disciplines have wrestled with.[42] Namely, that the mainstream medical industrial complex will always simultaneously reinforce social inequality while alleviating patient suffering. Gupta examines the political/ethical and policy/practical implications of this contradiction. Like the other scholars mentioned here, Gupta uses intersectional feminist, queer, and crip theory to build her analyses of case studies in gender-affirming surgery, pharmaceutical treatments for sexual dissatisfaction, and weight loss interventions. She ultimately argues that every individual will have to decide for themselves the best path for their healing and wellness, whether it be through allopathic or alternative treatment plans. At the same time, we each have a responsibility to dismantle systemic oppression in mainstream medicine, so that we can all gain equal access to it, if that is indeed the most desirable pathway. I appreciate Gupta's work for its realistic and frank observations, and for sharing how a combination of allopathic and alternative medical interventions and rituals is likely a good path to follow for anyone who desires to take the best of both.

As with the many arts-based collectives who are focused on various forms of care activism, it is impossible to capture all the excellent scholarship taking place on this topic, but this section is intended to provide a small window into some of the many excellent ideas being shared by scholars and important thinkers today.

The right to rest and conveyers of power

In the second half of this chapter, I am shifting gears a bit. While the work I'm about to discuss continues to develop the concept of hospital aesthetics, it moves away from art objects or socially engaged art that is primarily medical, such as X-rays, hospital gowns, or prostheses. Instead, Finnegan Shannon's latest installation casts hospital aesthetics in a more understated way, where care is being shown to disabled, sick, and immunocompromised bodies through rest, as designed by a cadre of artists and their friends within the disability community. Shannon's work fits into this chapter because the artist is developing a socially engaged work in collaboration with others as an iteration of an intersectional crip network of care. The central thesis behind this work is that disabled visitors need to be taken care of in the gallery, and they need rest, just as much as they need care and rest in other settings – the hospital, or the care collective. The point of connection, then, between Shannon's work and that of the collectives discussed in the previous section is the desire to care for one another, both inside and outside of hospital settings. In Shannon's case, I am particularly taken by how they are enacting a direct intervention in caring for weary bodies in the museum, changing its culture and its spatial politics in exciting and dynamic ways. More than any other work in the book so far, this work speaks to what a caring museum intervention might look and feel like in a museum.

Seating has been a critical part of Shannon's practice for the past five years. Their institutional critique centers the absence of benches in museum and gallery spaces. Galleries usually accommodate for standing only. But for Shannon, there can never be enough benches; having many benches throughout the wayfinding experience of an exhibition is helpful to them, and gives them many opportunities to rest. But the artist's intervention in making their own benches, a skill which they have learned over time by working with various furniture fabricators, makes visible this absence. Their blue benches (a color which intentionally mimics the color of the ADA accessible sign of a person in a wheelchair) are always loudly splashed across the upright back and flat seated area with white slogans in their whimsical signature font, such as "Museum visits are hard on my body, rest here if you agree," or "I'd rather be sitting, sit if you agree," or "I focus better seated, sit if you agree" – or their most famous slogan, "This exhibition has asked me to stand for too long, sit if you agree." The choice of words, along with the color and even design of the bench, which does not mimic a conventional museum bench but a rather quirkier iteration, makes clear that this work is activist in its orientation. These are not benches that people may easily gloss over and mistake for common furniture. As Shannon worked with furniture fabricators on the design of the benches, they consulted the Smithsonian Guidelines for Accessible Exhibition Design to ensure the benches were of the right proportions. They also took care to ensure the benches were sturdy and could accommodate a range of body weights. Shannon's benches are always accompanied by labels that explicitly invite museum visitors to sit on them, urging visitors to break with the familiar norm of not touching artwork.

In 2023, Shannon developed a large-scale solo work entitled *Don't Mind if I Do* for the Museum of Contemporary Art (moCa) in Cleveland which opened in summer of that year. This project includes a full-scale reconstituted conveyer belt (see Figure 4.9) which was partially sourced and funded by the Ford Foundation in New York City, and is toured across the country throughout 2024–25. Curated by moCa curator Lauren Leving, this show featured artwork that became mobile and traveled to the visitor, instead of the visitor walking over to see the typically stationary art. This revised flow of movement resists historic and ableist structures of museum engagement that suggest specific methods of movement and mobility are necessary to experience the work on display. All the items on the conveyer belt could be picked up and touched, and the items themselves were supplied by a collective of disabled artist friends whom Shannon is in disability arts community with. Some of the objects include 3D scans of small sculptures by Emilie Gossiaux, pom-poms by Felicia Griffin, and tools for interpersonal interaction by Jeff Kasper. Other artists who were involved

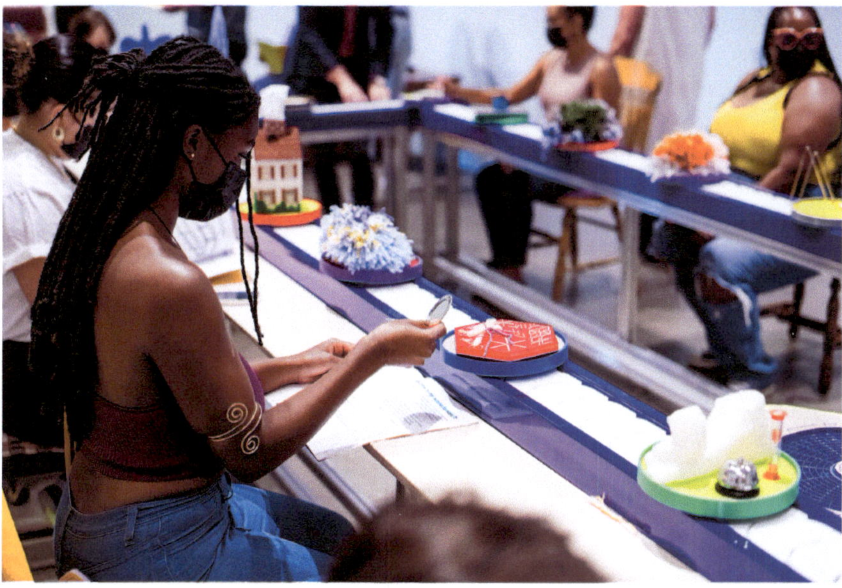

4.9 Finnegan Shannon, installation of *Don't Mind If I Do*, Museum of Contemporary Art, Cleveland, 2023–2024. Photograph: Mckinley Wiley. Courtesy of the artist and the Museum of Contemporary Art, Cleveland.

Image description 4.9: An installation where a few people sit around a conveyor belt that circulates small works of art to the seated viewers. The conveyor belt is placed in the center of the exhibition.

included Lukaza Branfman-Verissimo, Pelenakeke Brown, Rebirth Garments, and Joselia Rebekah Hughes. Audience members became participants in this experimental project, as Shannon encouraged visitors to handle artworks as a mode of haptic activism.

The conveyer belt is 25 feet long and was organized in a circular shape which sat inside a wooden table structure built on-site. The mechanism weighs approximately 300 pounds, and the conveyer belt was built in sections similar to a kid's train set. For future iterations, it can be scaled according to the size of the gallery. As part of the installation, the artist purchased comfortable chairs and benches from Craigslist, which were placed evenly around the conveyer belt so that visitors can take a seat and engage with the full sensorial qualities of the art while seated comfortably at the table. Shannon has cited inspiration from conveyer belt sushi or sushi train eating, where the food comes to the diner by way of a mechanical system while they are seated at a bar, and they can pick up and choose what they want to eat and enjoy at a whim. The title of the work, *Don't Mind if I Do*, is a playful acceptance of this invitation – similar to the casual remark one murmurs as one grabs a spicy tuna roll passing by. The exhibition is also intentionally situated outside the conventional scope of museum exhibitions, as *Don't Mind if I Do* fosters visual and tactile encounters with artwork that support experiential learning. Shannon desires a more comfortable viewing experience for their audiences that involves seating but also spaces where the art is within reach, making possible an enhanced viewing experience.

When I started to think about Shannon's brilliant new work, I was struck by how the history of the conveyer belt and its relationship with disabled bodies might open up an interesting tension within the artist's intervention. While, in the context of Shannon's new project, the conveyer belt works for the needs of disabled body-minds effectively, radically, and in a way that fosters agency, there was a time in the not-so-distant past when the conveyer belt had a more fraught relationship with disabled individuals. In *No Right to Be Idle*, the historian Sarah F. Rose traces a history of disability in the workplace, specifically within capitalist infrastructures that relied on an able-bodied and healthy body that could speedily execute tasks for the good of a sustainable, thriving economy.[43] How, then, did disability (mis)fit into this polished and seamless system of labor? Henry Ford's car factories in Detroit, Michigan became the first in the world, in 1913, to introduce conveyers and a moving assembly line so that the laborers' actions could be reduced to simple repetitive tasks for the more efficient production of objects. In this new system of mechanization, disabled people had a place. Prior to Henry Ford and his auto empire, disabled workers found it challenging to find employment as they were seen as unfit and unproductive compared to fully able-bodied employees. As Rose states, "Henry Ford, however, challenged the simple equation of disabled people with inefficiency, demonstrating that workers with a broad array of disabilities could in fact be productive in the increasingly mechanized economy of the twentieth century."[44] Henry Ford stood apart from his fellow capitalist entrepreneurs who failed to employ disabled workers, and Ford believed that the wonders of mechanization helped to make disabled workers more employable, not less.

From the outset, it would seem as though disabled individuals had an amicable relationship with factories and their brand of scientific management of workers' bodies, but these bodies – disabled or otherwise – were still treated as machine-link cogs which interlocked on assembly lines. Although the assembly line was more efficient, the workers themselves were still suspicious of it, and the conveyer gave Ford even more control over the bodies of his workers.[45] Stephen Phillips also notes that "Fordist practice ... attempted to mold the body to the specialized demands of an efficient technological, mechanized workplace."[46] The European architect, artist, and designer Frederick Kiesler suggested that needs are not static and should evolve in the ways that bodily needs evolve, and thus architecture should be organic and consist of a living machine that "modulate[s] to one's motion in time as a consequence of one's societal and bodily habits."[47] In Kiesler's notion of mechanization, there is a mutually beneficial relationship between man and technology, in contrast with Ford's technology, which put profit first. Kiesler did not want bodies to strain within an environment of fixed and repetitive actions such as was typical in the Ford factory; rather, he wanted architecture to shift the strain from the human to their tools. For Kiesler, technology engaging bodies in such harmony was a way to ensure that the environment was balanced and provided a good tension between comfort and discomfort. Shannon's conveyer belt, then, might be seen as operating under Kiesler's good design principles, while empowering disabled bodies through the reconstitution of a device that has historically presented hardship for all kinds of bodies under laboring conditions. While the conveyer belt has presented many advantages to our contemporary society in various environments and contexts, from shopping malls to airports or sushi trains, Shannon's installation turns the table on the spectatorship experience, so that it becomes one of leisure, idleness, and radical activism for disabled bodies, where we (re)claim the right to rest.

Finnegan's furniture design shows a clear connection to Kiesler's through its sympathetic and humanist approach to bodies of different shapes and sizes, and bodies that are in need of comfort and care. Kiesler had collaborated with a number of cabinetmakers to create his custom furniture, consisting of instruments and rockers that were very popular with gallery visitors, who sometimes wanted to purchase them (alas, they weren't for sale). The seating that Kiesler was executing in the 1940s was organic in shape and evocative of curving or falling waves, meant to encase the curves of the human body with ease.[48] Kiesler included these seating designs as part of Peggy Guggenheim's Art of this Century gallery on 57th Street. While the seating was inspired by surrealism, Kiesler also showed an interest in the comfort of the gallery visitor through his highly attuned design and its ability to merge object with subject. Shannon's conveyer belt installation extends from a similar interest. In addition to being a powerful and distinctive example of hospital aesthetics, Shannon's work also provides a schemata for how micro-architectures – or to use Arseli Dokumaci's phrase, "activist affordances" – can be rendered in the art gallery so that the museum might become a more accessible and habitable place, or an affordance, for a disabled body.[49]

It would be interesting to imagine what the conveyer work might look and feel like in the hospital setting, and how it could bring a greater degree of medical attention to patients. At this time, conveyer belts in hospital settings are not necessarily conducive to a more humane and personalized approach, a reality examined in work by Dominic Quagliozzi. Quagliozzi adds another dimension to the question of disabled movement by examining the life cycle of the tissue paper in a doctor's office. Quagliozzi became interested in the fragility of this tissue paper, which is used as a type of protective covering for the patient examination bench. Quagliozzi uses it as a way to reference the movement of bodies that come into and out of the doctor's office. The tissue paper bears the traces of those bodies as the doctors and nurses unfurl it in a continuous and mechanical looping fashion; it captures the crinkled outlines of bodies as they lie prone on its crunchy surface. Most potently, the paper records the physical and psychological experiences that patients are having in that moment in time, portraying the residue of their presence in their absence. The paper is clearly a fragile medium to deploy, but in synthesis with its delicate materiality is the paradoxical weight it literally carries – fragile minds of disabled, ill, and immunocompromised bodies. Further, at the end of each patient visit, the nurse comes and rips the paper off the bench and throws it in the trash, and she proceeds to pull down a fresh section of paper from the roll to lay over the bench again, ready for the next patient. The implication of this movement is that people are made disposable just like the paper (for example, through medical experimentation or death), but also that the medical industrial complex moves through disabled bodies speedily and with a depersonalized bedside manner. While people and paper are expendable in this world (a world that disability has long held with ambivalent, if not hostile, regard), Quagliozzi reconstitutes the paper as serious material for mark-making. He is interested in the idea that once the tissue paper has been recontextualized into works of art, thanks to his efforts, the museum world's job is to take care of it and protect its longevity. Quagliozzi first displayed these drawings in a group exhibition at the Rhode Island School of Design in 2022, and he requested that the drawings be hung loosely with magnetic pins so that the drawings would be able to flutter and flit in response to the wind generated by bodies moving through the gallery space. Quagliozzi thus ensured that the tissue paper once again became a living record of bodies rotating through a specific environment. The fluttering evinces fragility once again, but in this context it becomes a beautiful denotation of the fleeting quality of life itself.

On being even more caring

The four intersectional feminist, queer healthcare collectives discussed in this chapter all apply dialogic care aesthetic approaches to self-empowered healthcare work for the disabled community through publishing, workshops, and activist care-building. All four demonstrate the growing need for disabled communities to turn to one another for mutual aid and support in the absence of a reliable medical industrial complex – support that is not sexist, ableist, racist, or classist. Stories that members of these collectives share center on society's apparent lack of attention to access. Therefore, a dialogical care aesthetics within networks of care builds powerful bonds of friendship and support. The exigent work of these collectives is important and offers a much-needed alternative, and a radical critique of the hypocrisy and assumed superior knowledge of the healthcare system. Feminist, queer, and trans crip perspectives on health have offered an insight into our own bodies and our own medical scripts and narratives, complete with vaginal self-exams. Nonetheless, the compelling, remarkable work of the FHCRG, SAG, PMS, Black Womxn Flourish, and many other groups with similar missions offers space for reflection, counsel, and new direction amid the reality of disability and the malaise of everyday life.

The care and rest work of Finnegan Shannon and their conveyer belt intervention in the museum is another iteration of a cadre of artists working together to transform how the body – the disabled body specifically – is treated in public space. Shannon's work also shows how museums can change spatial and viewing positionalities though innovative exhibition design practices that offer care and comfort, instead of discomfort and exhaustion, similar to the work of Frederick Kiesler in seating design. In their artistic practice, Shannon is committed to working with other disabled artists as part of a community, where they collaborate to provide allyship and strength – or care – in numbers, especially when positioned within ableist museum cultures that are difficult to transform and shift. The next chapter continues this discussion of how architecture, design, space, disability, and health intersect, focusing on the work of contemporary disabled artist Lauryn Youden, who appropriates and critiques the furniture of another historical design figure, Le Corbusier, and connects it to the ableism pervasive in medicine.

Notes

1 See Grant Kester, *Conversation Pieces: Community and Communication in Modern Art* (Berkeley, CA: University of California Berkeley Press, 2004); and Grant Kester, *The One and the Many: Contemporary Collaborative Art in a Global Context* (Durham, NC: Duke University Press, 2011).
2 Julia Bonn, Inga Zimprich, and Chloe Stead, "The Feminist Health Care Research Group Fights Art-World Exploitation," *Frieze*, April 19, 2021, www.frieze.com/article/feminist-health-care-research-group-fights-art-world-exploitation [accessed December 5, 2024].
3 Inga Zimprich and Julia Bonn, *Practices of Radical Health Care: Materials of the Health Movement of the Seventies and Eighties* (Berlin: Self-published by Feminist Health Care Research Group, 2019), 2.
4 Zimprich and Bonn, *Practices of Radical Health Care*, 2.
5 Zimprich and Bonn, *Practices of Radical Health Care*, 3.
6 Caren Beilin and Feminist Health Care Research Group, "Medicine & Misogyny," *Art in America*, October 8, 2021, www.artnews.com/art-in-america/interviews/feminist-health-care-research-group-caren-beilin-1234606473 [accessed December 5, 2024].
7 Feminist Health Care Research Group, *Being in Crises Together*, www.think-tank.nl/health/zines.html [accessed December 1, 2021].
8 "Art, Health, and Accessibility: A Conversation with Laura Lulika of the Sickness Affinity Group," podcast, 44:59, October 26, 2021, in *Critical Diversity Podcast*, produced by Critical Diversity AG, Berlin University of the Arts, https://anchor.fm/

critical-diversity/episodes/Art—Health—and-Accessibility-A-Conversation-With-Laura-Lulika-of-the-Sickness-Affinity-Group-e19a8p6 [accessed December 5, 2024].

9 "Art, Health, and Accessibility."

10 "Art, Health, and Accessibility."

11 "Art, Health, and Accessibility."

12 "About Us," Power Makes Us Sick, https://powermakesussick.noblogs.org/about-us/ [accessed January 19, 2025].

13 *Power Makes Us Sick*, issue 1 (winter 2017) includes topics such as breathing exercises, discussion of unsafe spaces, Greek solidarity clinics, harm reduction and needle exchange programs, and autonomous health projects in New York City and Standing Rock; *Power Makes Us Sick*, issue 2 (summer 2017) includes topics such as witches, resisting anti-sex work legislation, sex workers' organizing, DIY abortions, pressure point exercises, probiotics, the Prostitutes War Group, and more; *Power Makes Us Sick*, issue 3 (summer 2018) includes topics such as healers, becoming undiagnosable, talking about death, accountability in practice, the Olympia blockade, street medic skills, illegalist herbalism, Mutual Aid Disaster Relief, poetry and art; other zines include *Introduction to the Accountability Model* (2018); *Strategies for Emotional Support* (poster); *Emotional Support Basics*; *Building Towards an Autonomous Trans Healthcare* (fall 2018); *Physically Distant, Connected by Care* (spring 2020). All issues and posters can be accessed from https://powermakesussick.noblogs.org/zines-and-resources/ [accessed January 19, 2025].

14 "'Power Makes Us Sick,' Most of us are not doctors and some of us can't go to the doctor, but everything that is living will at some point fall ill. Although we prefer to thrive amongst the well, illness rests like the other side of the coin. And in another way, we are all sick under late capitalism or, we are all sick when alienated from our activity, from the places where we rest, from one another. We are all crazy when someone or something else has the ability to diagnose us against our will. When the air we breathe is toxic, we all suffer indeterminately. As we learn to take care of one another's health the state can't but fail, or at least we would no longer be bothered if it did. In May PMS led a workshop called How Are You Feeling Today? We facilitated a playful discussion to dissect the vocabulary of sickness and illness. We closed with a visualization exercise towards an aspirational idea of 'health.'" Tumblr post, https://powermakesussick.tumblr.com/post/175046750302/workshop-in-the-st%C3%A4ndige-vertretung-we-call-it [accessed December 1, 2021].

15 Black Womxn Flourish website, www.blackwomxnflourish.co [accessed April 10, 2024].

16 Black Womxn Flourish website.

17 Black Womxn Flourish website.

18 Black Womxn Flourish (@blackwomxnflourish), "Our Collective Update: We're Entering an Extended Period of Trans Formation," Instagram post, March 15, 2023, www.instagram.com/p/Cp0gSPbuLq9 [accessed January 6, 2025].

19 Amber Jamilla Musser, "From Our Body to Yourselves: The Boston Women's Health Book Collective and Changing Notions of Subjectivity, 1969–1973," *Women's Studies Quarterly* 25, no. 1/2 (Spring/Summer 2007): 93–109, www.jstor.org/stable/27649656

20 Musser, "From Our Body."

21 Olivia Plender, *Our Bodies Are Not the Problem, the Problem is Power* [installation, Glasgow Women's Library], https://oliviaplender.org/many-maids-make-much-noise/installation-life-support–forms-of-care-in-art [accessed April 10, 2024].

22 Park McArthur and Constantina Zavitsanos, "Ode to 1 & Under," *Arika*, https://arika.org.uk/ode-1-under/ [accessed January 19, 2025].

23 "Refuge in the Means," Recess Art website, www.recessart.org/projects/50-refuge-in-the-means [accessed April 11, 2024].

24 Park McArthur and Constantina Zavitsanos, "Other Forms of Conviviality: The Best and Least of Which is Our Daily Care and the Host of Which is Our Collaborative

Work," *Women & Performance: A Journal of Feminist Theory* 23, no. 1 (2013): 126–32. https://doi.org/10.1080/0740770X.2013.827376

25 Black Women's Health Imperative, https://bwhi.org [accessed April 10, 2024].

26 Sami Schalk, *Black Disability Politics* (Durham, NC: Duke University Press, 2022), 82.

27 Guila Smith, "Health v Wealth," *Art Monthly*, July–August 2018, www.artmonthly.co.uk/magazine/site/article/health-v-wealth-by-giulia-smith-jul-aug-2018 [accessed December 5, 2024].

28 Smith, "Health v Wealth."

29 Smith, "Health v Wealth."

30 Helen Molesworth, "Art is Medicine: Helen Molesworth on the Work of Simone Leigh," *Artforum*, March 2018.

31 Leah Lakshmi Piepzna-Samarasinha, *Care Work: Dreaming Disability Justice* (Vancouver: Arsenal Pulp Press, 2018), Kindle.

32 Piepzna-Samarasinha, *Care Work*, Kindle.

33 "What Would a HIV Doula Do?," *HIV Doula Work*, https://hivdoula.work [accessed April 15, 2024].

34 See Kester, *Conversation Pieces*; and Kester, *One and the Many*.

35 For a brief selection of readings on socially engaged art practice, see Claire Bishop, *Artificial Hells: Participatory Art and the Politics of Spectatorship* (London: Verso, 2012); Shannon Jackson, *Social Works: Performing Art, Supporting Publics* (New York: Routledge, 2011); and Nicolas Bourriaud, *Relational Aesthetics* (Dijon: Les presses du reel, 1998).

36 Eva Feder Kittay, *Love's Labor: Essays on Women, Equality and Dependency*, 2nd ed. (New York: Routledge, 2020); Eva Feder Kittay, *Learning from My Daughter: The Value and Care of Disabled Minds* (Oxford: Oxford University Press, 2019).

37 Akemi Nishida, *Just Care: Messy Entanglements of Disability, Dependency, and Desire* (Philadelphia, PA: Temple University Press, 2022).

38 Nishida, *Just Care*, 79.

39 Nishida, *Just Care*, 79.

40 Marty Fink, *Forget Burial: HIV Kinship, Disability, and Queer/Trans Narratives of Care* (New Brunswick, NJ: Rutgers University Press, 2020), 2.

41 Fink, *Forget Burial*, 4.

42 Kristina Gupta, *Medical Entanglements: Rethinking Feminist Debates About Healthcare* (New Brunswick, NJ: Rutgers University Press, 2020).

43 Sarah F. Rose, *No Right to be Idle* (Chapel Hill, NC: University of North Carolina Press, 2017), Kindle.

44 Rose, *No Right*, 112.

45 Kat Eschner, "In 1913, Henry Ford Introduced the Assembly Line: His Workers Hated it," *Smithsonian Magazine*, December 1, 2016, www.smithsonianmag.com/smart-news/one-hundred-and-three-years-ago-today-henry-ford-introduced-assembly-line-his-workers-hated-it-180961267 [accessed December 5, 2024].

46 Stephen J. Phillips, *Elastic Architecture: Frederick Kiesler and Design Research in the First Age of Robotic Culture* (Cambridge, MA and London: MIT Press, 2017), 104.

47 Phillips, *Elastic Architecture*, 104.

48 Don Quaintance, "Modern Art in a Modern Setting: Frederick Kiesler's Design of Art of This Century," in *Peggy Guggenheim and Frederick Kiesler: The Story of Art of This Century*, ed. Susan Davidson and Philip Rylands (New York: Guggenheim Museum Publications, 2004), 207–73.

49 Arseli Dokumaci, *Activist Affordances: How Disabled People Improvise More Habitable Worlds* (Durham, NC: Duke University Press, 2023).

5

Alt medicine

A black BDSM (bondage and discipline, dominance and submission, and sadism and masochism) rope and noose is suspended from the ceiling inside a dazzling white cube gallery space. Hanging and tilting at the end of the noose is a small round fitness trampoline, of a size that would be suitable for toddlers to jump on. Equipped with short chrome-finished steel legs, the black polypropylene canvas surface of the trampoline is stretched by coiled steel springs. On the surface is a collage of additional objects tethered with black thread, including a crystal glass vibrator, a used prescription pill bottle, a half-used blister pack of red pills, a pink and red queer anime illustration of a girl lying on a bed, a pair of silver medical scissors, theoretical texts, including the 2021 book *Ill Feelings* by Alice Hattrick, and other small packets, charms, and bottles.[1] The circumference of the trampoline is lined with black cowboy/girl tassels, thin threads capped off with yellow beads, and additional tendrils from the noose. The title of the work is *But Have You Tried Yoga?* (2023) by Lauryn Youden (Figure 5.1). Youden has fibromyalgia, chronic pain, and a host of other disabilities. When she first approached doctors to help determine the cause of her pain and other ailments, the doctors were dismissive and lacked empathy and understanding. One of their responses was, "but have you tried yoga?" Youden's appropriation of this question "mocks the illusion of wellness-culture cures and nods to the appropriation (and bastardization) of Eastern treatments and practices in the West."[2] In Youden's powerful act of suspending the trampoline from the noose, she blends exercise, fitness, and yoga into a political assemblage. Is the artist mocking the doctor's feedback by hanging it up so that it translates into a precarious life? Or is the act of precarity a moment of honesty on Youden's part, in which the reality of vulnerable bodies is reinforced? Either way, I argue that this work is another iteration of hospital aesthetics,

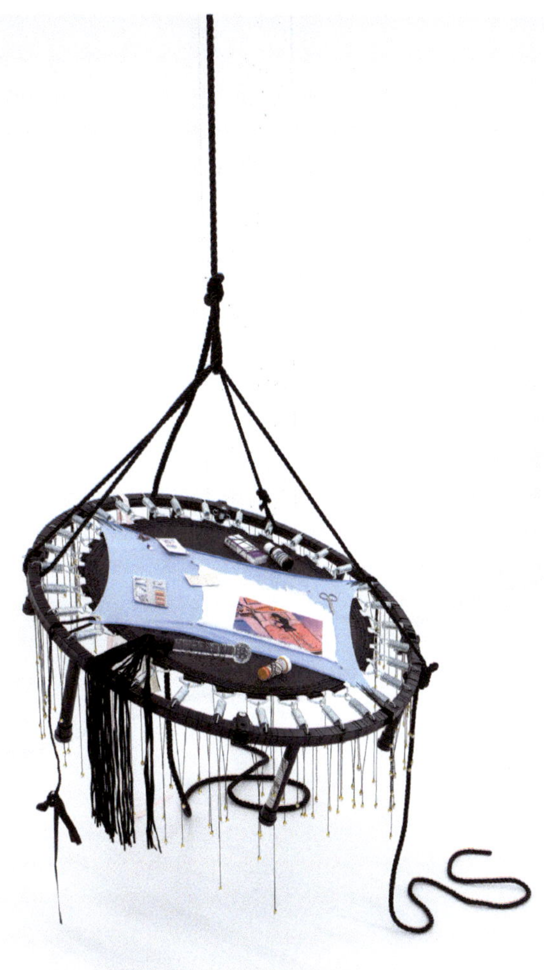

5.1 Lauryn Youden, *But Have You Tried Yoga?*, 2023. Kinetic sports fitness trampoline, various materials, 35.8 × 35.8 × 185in. (91 × 91 × 470cm). Courtesy of the artist.

Image description 5.1: A trampoline suspended a couple of feet off the ground, held up by thick black rope. A bolt of fabric is stretched on top of the trampoline featuring an anime character lying face down on their bed. Several objects are placed on top of the trampoline, including various medicine bottles, a playing card, and flogger.

one that embraces the still-present tension between the medical industrial complex, biopharmaceutical industries, and alternative medical practices and rituals. In this chapter, the artists I examine appropriate aesthetics from hospitals and bring them into domestic spaces, showing how design principles intended to promote wellness can be found in unexpected places, in both historical and contemporary contexts.

In this final chapter, I return once again to a quieter form of hospital aesthetics, but now I show how contemporary disabled artists are finding solutions for the application and ingestion of literal and metaphorical medicine itself in comical and empowering ways. I examine how these artists lean into alternative medicine and therapies for self-medication, pain management, and more. Such therapies might include massage, acupuncture, t'ai chi, and medical marijuana. While it is true that alternative medicine can also be defined as integrative or complementary medicine in line with more mainstream treatments for ailing health, in this case I argue that disabled artists are using alternative medicines as a political means to refute mainstream attitudes toward disabled body-minds. This chapter includes longer discussions of work by Lauryn Youden and Sharona Franklin, with a brief examination of pieces by Carmen Papalia and Maryam Jafri. The title of the chapter, "Alt medicine," references the term "alternative medicine." Alternative medicine is commonly not accepted within mainstream Western medical settings, as it might incorporate more ancient traditions from Eastern cultures, such as acupuncture, Reiki, chiropractic manipulation, herbal medicine, and yoga. Standard medical practices, otherwise known as allopathic approaches, tend to focus on the disease and how it can be eradicated; alternative medicine focuses on the entire body. While allopathic and alternative medicine have often been at odds with one another, as there have been varying levels of success with each approach, today many people use a combination of these approaches to treat their bodies through periods of both wellness and unwellness. In this chapter, the artists turn toward alternative medical practices to empower themselves against the overwhelming force of the biopharmaceutical industry, based on their lived experiences as disabled individuals. The other intention behind my abbreviation of "alternative medicine" in the title of this chapter was to connect it with the term "alt text." The "alt" in alt text is also an abbreviation for "alternative." Alt text is a practice whereby images are described for people who are blind or have low vision, to help them understand the content of an image. Alt text makes images more accessible. Given how the practice of "alt text" empowers disabled people, it made sense to suggest that "alt medicine" is a way of making medicine more accessible for disabled people, based on the work discussed in this chapter.

As in the previous chapters of the book, I will focus on work by two main artists, while also making mention of other artists whose work further contributes to this important topic. I also incorporate historical, artistic, and theoretical materials from the fields of design, architecture, biocitizenship, pharma art, bio art, and the medical humanities to help contextualize the work by Youden, Franklin, and others. While Chapter 4 showed how artists are working together in collectives to hold each other up within powerful networks of labor and love, in this chapter, care work is found within the object again, be it through a suspended medical chime, a jelly cake, a joint, a vibrator, or a quilt. Indulgence becomes an active ingredient in the pleasure of healing and taking care of oneself. I continue to thicken my concept of hospital aesthetics in this chapter, showing how idiosyncratic ritualistic practices can be used to ground and heal bodies who have experienced trauma and pain. By noting intersections among the artists' methodologies and interests across the five chapters, the reader will understand how hospital aesthetics is a vital and impactful phenomenon and field that will continue to resonate into the future.

Venus in Scorpio: a personal astrology chart

Lauryn Youden is an artist from Vancouver, Canada, who currently lives in Berlin, Germany. Youden's research-based art practice revolves around performance, installation, poetry, and curating. Her research focuses on her chronic illness and the treatments she takes. Youden is invested in alternative healing practices, defined as everything outside of the pharmaceutical–medical industrial complex. She is part of the Sickness Affinity Group, who were discussed in Chapter 4, and she has acquired much of her knowledge about medication through her experiences as a regular participant in the group. Youden's investment in these topics is also connected to her own family's personal history of mental illness. Her grandmother was severely mentally ill and died by suicide before Youden was born. As a result of the familial trauma that ensued from this life-changing event, Youden found herself dealing with her chronic illnesses independently and seeking support outside of her family.

Youden's series *Venus in Scorpio* (2023) consists of six large sculptures suspended from the gallery ceiling (see Figure 5.2). The trampoline work I described at the beginning of the chapter, *But Have You Tried Yoga?*, is one of the sculptures in the series. The series was sparked when Youden started looking for new furniture on Craigslist.[3] She noticed there were many replicas of Le Corbusier furniture in Berlin, and she came to learn that, historically, the industry of Le Corbusier furniture was indeed rooted in her home city. Le Corbusier was a French-Swiss architect, designer, writer, and urban planner, and is regarded as a pioneer of modern architecture. He was active across five decades, from approximately 1900 to 1960, and designed in Europe, North and South America, and Asia. Today, this furniture style has become archetypal, and having a Le Corbusier piece in one's home in West Berlin is considered a status symbol. As Youden studied the Le

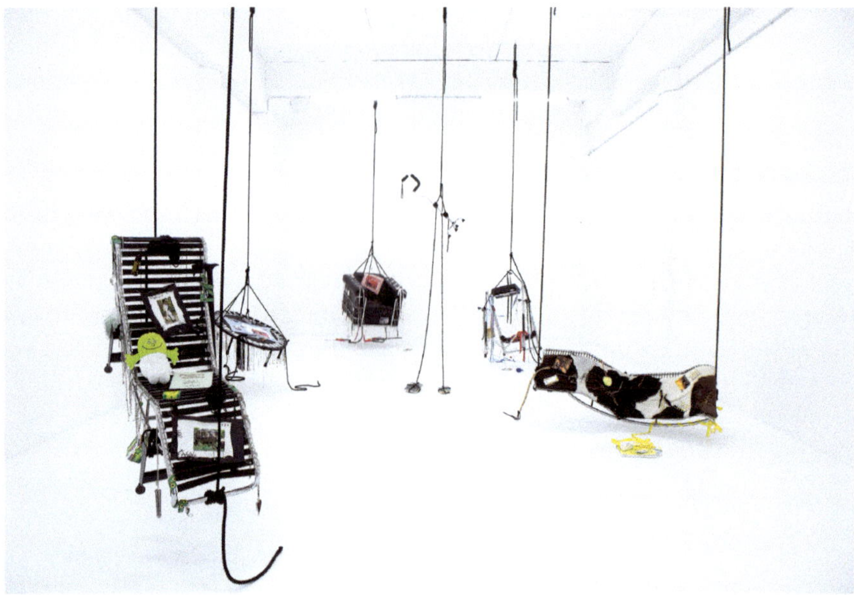

5.2 Lauryn Youden, *Venus in Scorpio*, 2023. Exhibition view, Open Forum, Berlin. Courtesy of the artist.

Image description 5.2: A stark white gallery space displaying large objects suspended in the air with the use of thick black ropes. Objects include pool chairs, a trampoline, a cane, a walker, and a lounge chair. The floating objects all have other objects and images embedded or balanced on top of them.

Corbusier furniture on Craigslist, she noticed that physically and aesthetically it resembled some of her medical devices. Common characteristics of the furniture include black leather and tubular steel, which, combined, make for a clinical look and feel.

When Youden read the book *X-Ray Architecture* by architectural historian Beatriz Colomina, she found that modernist architecture was greatly impacted by the X-ray, tuberculosis, and medical imaging technologies, which were developed around the same time.[4] Le Corbusier's furniture was responsive to these developments, and he tried to design furniture that would encourage wellness and deter serious illness. Owing to his obsession with health, he felt that the "ailing city and its sick inhabitants could only be cured through complete reconstruction."[5] Youden realized that Le Corbusier's approach to building the home and the city was to become a quasi-doctor-architect, designing architecture intended to mitigate the possibility of people getting sick with tuberculosis. While Le Corbusier's approach may seem strange based on our contemporary understanding of tuberculosis as something treated with an injection, during the period when Le Corbusier was working, tuberculosis was a mystery and people were trying to come up with strategies for reducing the risk of becoming infected. At the time, people thought that tuberculosis was caused by the environment and "incubated by the murky, festering dampness of industrial cities."[6] Patients with respiratory illness were urged to choose environments where they had access to fresh, well-ventilated air and sparse surfaces that were "guaranteed minimal dust accumulation."[7] Le Corbusier's blueprints reflected this imperative, aiming to foster better bodily health through features such as flats with individual garden terraces; running tracks on the roof of apartment blocks that occupants could use to exercise in the fresh air; and sun parlors that allowed exposure to sunlight, which studies at the time found effective in combatting tuberculosis.[8] Colomina writes:

> Modern Architecture, launched in the 1920s by an international group of avant-garde architects, has usually been understood in terms of functional efficiency, new materials (glass, iron, reinforced concrete), new technologies of construction, and the machine aesthetic ... In contrast to how modern architecture was actually shaped by the dominant medical obsession of its time – tuberculosis and the technology that became associated with it, X-Rays ... we are still living in the architecture shaped by [tuberculosis] ... Modern architecture remains the default everyday environment, the norm produced by vast industrial systems, rather than the transgressive work of an avant-garde inspired by a specific disease. Modernity was driven by illness. The engine of modern architecture was not a heroic, shiny functional machine suspended outside daily life in a protective cocoon of new technologies and geometries. It is the difficulty of each breath and therefore the treasure of each breath: the melancholy of modernity.[9]

Youden shows us that, like Le Corbusier's architecture, his furniture was also designed with health and wellness in mind. Le Corbusier drew directly from medical devices to inspire his chairs, lounges, and chaises, where black leather and tubular silver steel reign as part of his aesthetics of modernist design. Compare Le Corbusier's LC2 armchair and LC4 lounges with Youden's MU Quad Cane Walking Stick or the Invertrac inversion table traction unit. The Invertrac inversion table traction unit is used to relieve pinching and pressure on the nerves in the spinal column, which causes lower back pain, by flipping a person upside down to increase circulation, and to decrease stress and tension. Le Corbusier was attracted to the aesthetics of these medical devices because it was clean, sterile, and minimal, and was able to blend into the decor of the home owing to its inconspicuous nature. Youden also found it quite interesting that despite the obvious aesthetic consonance between medical devices and Le Corbusier's furniture, Le Corbusier's luxury chairs were vastly more expensive. Le Corbusier was, in fact, not the only designer who drew inspiration from medical devices for their architecture and furniture design. Youden mentions that Herman Miller, an American home furnishings company, was also inspired by medical furniture, as were the industrial designers Charles and

Ray Eames. The histories of medical design and mainstream furniture are thus more intertwined than most people know.

Le Corbusier's architecture was also riddled with controversy, given his ties with eugenics and antisemitism. He based his architectural measurements of the so-called average person on the physical body of a white 6-foot cis man. These measurements were clearly limiting and didn't account for the full diversity of bodies in society, particularly the disabled body. Yet modernist architecture was formed with these narrow perspectives in mind, alienating a large part of the population. Additionally, while it may have seemed as though Le Corbusier was interested in keeping people healthy in the buildings he designed, the sanatoriums that he designed in Europe at this time were actually used as places where modernist architects could test out theories on design, health, and wellness. This suggests that the good intentions behind the construction of sanatoriums were less important than what they could offer for even greater and more ambitious projects later down the line. Adding to this, sanatoriums were not exactly places for the average person; they catered to rich people who could afford the facilities to get self-care and rest. Ultimately, Le Corbusier's ideal of designing architecture that was healthy and accessible to all was riddled with problems and challenges that cut across – and impacted – class, ability, gender, and race. In the ten years that I have been thinking about access, disability, and contemporary art, I have always been a critic of Le Corbusier, pointing out how his architectural measurement for the so-called average height of a 6-foot man is deeply problematic and limiting, particularly from my perspective as a disabled art historian who has a rare form of dwarfism. Youden understands these problems and tensions inherent within Le Corbusier's work and folds this awareness into her use of his furniture in her *Venus in Scorpio* installation.

Youden's approach to using secondhand Le Corbusier furniture sourced from Craigslist was to suspend everything from the ceiling. Within the *Venus in Scorpio* installation, Youden has included a strung-up LC2 armchair entitled *Hot Topic Esoteric Bimbo* (2023); two LC4 lounges, one covered with a cowhide rug and entitled *Bitch I'm a Cow* (2023), the other entitled *ACAB ("Mary Kate" Olsen)* (2023); *The Fear of Disease* (2023), a MU Quad Cane Walking Stick attached to Colomina's *X-Ray Architecture* book and Susan Sontag's *Illness as Metaphor* text; and lastly *Beautiful … This is the Skin of a Killer Bella* (2023), which is the Invertrac inversion table traction unit. All contain elements of black leather and tubular silver steel except for the reclining lounge covered in a cowhide rug. In treating the furniture in this way, Youden is engaged in an act of protest, which has both serious and humorous implications. For starters, Youden has noted that when Le Corbusier started to develop these pieces of furniture, he was in conversation with a French doctor who was known to be a fascist and eugenicist. In that period, the concept of the athlete was still quite new, as was the concept of exercise. But athleticism and exercise were already constructed in very ableist ways, a framework that stubbornly persists today. When Youden was first diagnosed with fibromyalgia, which is a chronic disorder that causes pain and tenderness throughout the body, as well as fatigue, her doctor wanted her to try yoga as a remedy. The doctor told her to jump on the trampoline three times a day for fifteen minutes per session; this was impossible for the artist, as she could barely walk at the time. The doctor was offering a very ableist remedy, which also came over as dismissive and ill-informed.

Youden's noose and rope also have serious and sinister associations, and the *Venus in Scorpio* installation is powerfully influenced by Youden's grandmother's suicide. Youden feels there is still not enough discussion around mental health and disabilities that might include schizophrenia and bipolar disorder. Mental health often feels relegated to the sidelines, or like an elephant in the room that even the disability community are reluctant to discuss. Youden was also conscious of the noose's associations with slavery and the lynching of Black people in US history. The imagery she draws on, then, simultaneously evokes grief and an egregious historical act, and is thus imbued with contrasting feelings of vulnerability and violence. To start, Youden wanted to emasculate the furniture, as these are objects that are typically found in men's offices or rich bachelor pads, symbolizing power, authority, and control. Given that this furniture confronted her on a daily basis as part of her life in Berlin, Youden wanted to confront its toxic masculinity and its ableist, eugenicist history. By hanging the objects, Youden literally ungrounds them from this masculinist zone, floating them, and rendering them fragile and free. The floating aspect of the furniture also creates a sense of uneasiness because the objects can now move and sway in space depending on body movements and the rush of wind flowing in and around their forms. Youden states of this aspect of the work, "they do move in-person. They spin and they ... are floppy. So, it really brought a lot more life into these ... very dead masculine pieces, as well. I think something that happened ... through the process is that ... they became more relatable to bodies rather than just ... dead furniture or this ... super heavy history."[10]

Another important critical methodology that Youden used was to stitch surgical sutures into the leather surfaces of the objects, making them resemble real wounds, sores, and sites of pain, or a type of self-piercing. Here, Youden literally cut away the facade of masculine and ableist appearances, taking away the power of these objects. Alongside the stitching, piercing, and cutting, Youden decorated the furniture pieces with feminine, pink objects – trinkets, ribbons, and tassels that were more comforting and resonant with her own domestic design aesthetics, which she calls queer feminine. Just like that, Youden took away the sparkling clean luxury of these objects, ruining their so-called glamorization. The tassels could also be taken for talismans, warding off poisons. The humorous aspect of these objects is evident in some of the decorative choices that Youden incorporated into them, such as the brown and white cow rawhide rug on the reclining lounge. The title of this work, *Bitch, I'm a Cow*, is taken from a lyric of a popular Doja Cat song. Youden imagined that she was making the lounge into a cow with a sweetgrass tail, which smells good and has a cute little bow to alleviate the heaviness of the aforementioned topics. Youden also stitched different kinds of pills into the hung furniture objects, drawing from her own personal stock of medications, past and current, that help with pain management and with depression and anxiety. Within this medley of objects is also a sex toy, which the artist perceives to be an important tool of self-care and health practice, as well as some face masks and COVID-19 tests – a token of the pandemic.

An aspect of the work I haven't yet discussed is the title itself, *Venus in Scorpio*. This is another lighthearted touch that Youden brings to the work, suggesting that these new arrangements of forms and objects might share an affinity with the constellations of celestial bodies, such as planets and stars, within the sublunar world. An astrological reading of Venus in Scorpio spells out a romantic person who is prone to jealousy and who keeps their heart guarded. Their love is intense, dark, and mysterious, and is at once a confrontation with darkness and with overwhelming passion. Youden's installation is accompanied by poems that she has written, where the qualities of Venus in Scorpio are mentioned through reference to an astrologer. Youden was drawn to thinking through the work using astrology because of astrology's status as an "alt medicine" which scientists have never validated or supported in mainstream Western medicine. As Youden puts it, astrology is like an alternative way of looking at illness, not through a medical lens, but through a philosophical, magical lens instead. She also equates the dark, passionate love found in Venus in Scorpio to the feeling of being chronically ill itself, where there is strength and vulnerability in equal measure. There is also vulnerability in a hospital setting and in the medical system, of course, as a patient is vulnerable with doctors and care providers, and a codependency can arise that can be very intense. Astrology, mythology, and even snippets from popular culture have thus proven to be innovative and fun means for the artist to create interesting metaphors for chronic illness, moving beyond stereotypes of the weak, sickly victim. Instead, the person with the chronic illness becomes dynamic and amazing.

The overarching intention is to foster healing and catharsis. In Youden's act of confronting the violent history of these pieces of furniture – both medical and otherwise – she is literally and metaphorically healing those narratives by medicating them with literature, self-help books, pills, a vibrator, and other soothing queer feminine products. Youden particularly wanted to incorporate fiction and nonfiction books into her assembly of objects, as they have been important to her and friends within the chronically ill and disabled community in aiding with confrontation and survival in the face of unimaginable odds. Youden's *Venus in Scorpio* is about acceptance of oneself, an exercise in tapping into one's own knowledge and understanding of self, and how those qualities can be nurtured to support one's own mental health and navigating of the world. Youden says, "for me, yeah, astrology or tarot or poetry ... is all alternative healing practices, just as much as theory and literature ... I take those ... very seriously as healing forms."[11] Youden's general approach to alternative healing practices is also informed by the environment where she was raised on the West Coast of Canada, which has a large Indigenous population. Complex issues of sovereignty between colonial and Indigenous communities continue to play out, and healing takes on multifarious meanings within the political imperative to decolonize in Canada and beyond.

In the Introduction, I noted that hospital aesthetics is not concerned with the interior design of hospital spaces, nor is it concerned with calming imagery that offers soothing environments for patients. What distinguishes hospital aesthetics from these other practices is political intent and centering the disabled patient experience. What I find refreshing and exciting about Youden's work is how she reflects on her negative encounters with the medical industrial complex by drawing from the expanded field of architecture and design, pointing out that modernist design was actually informed by health, sickness, and wellness to begin with. So while designers may enter hospital interiors with the intent to fabricate environments of wellness, the reverse was historically the case: the state of sickness informed mainstream design, at least for some specific designers like Le Corbusier. This is a surprising discovery and suggests that health and sickness are made manifest all around us much more deeply than we may have previously thought. And yet disabled bodies and other marginalized bodies were ironically still left out of this equation. A further irony that Youden exposes through her work is that while mainstream society does its best to squash illness, or keep it contained, shunting it off to the hospital and other medical facilities and related industries, the mainstream world is in fact more filled with medical ephemera than we could have ever imagined. Thus none of us can entirely escape illness, in some shape or form. Youden forges a hospital aesthetics through modernist architecture and furniture design, unpacking the ableist beginnings, middle, and endings of these traditions.

An important German artist whose work can be seen as a precursor to Youden's work is Joseph Beuys. Beuys was interested in humanism, psychology, sociology, and politics. He was a key participant in the 1960s Fluxus movement, and he was known for incorporating materials such as fat and felt as recurring motifs into his works, which conveyed his political ideology and his personal outlook on everyday life. In one of his earlier works, entitled *Infiltration homogen für Konzertflügel (Homogenous Infiltration*

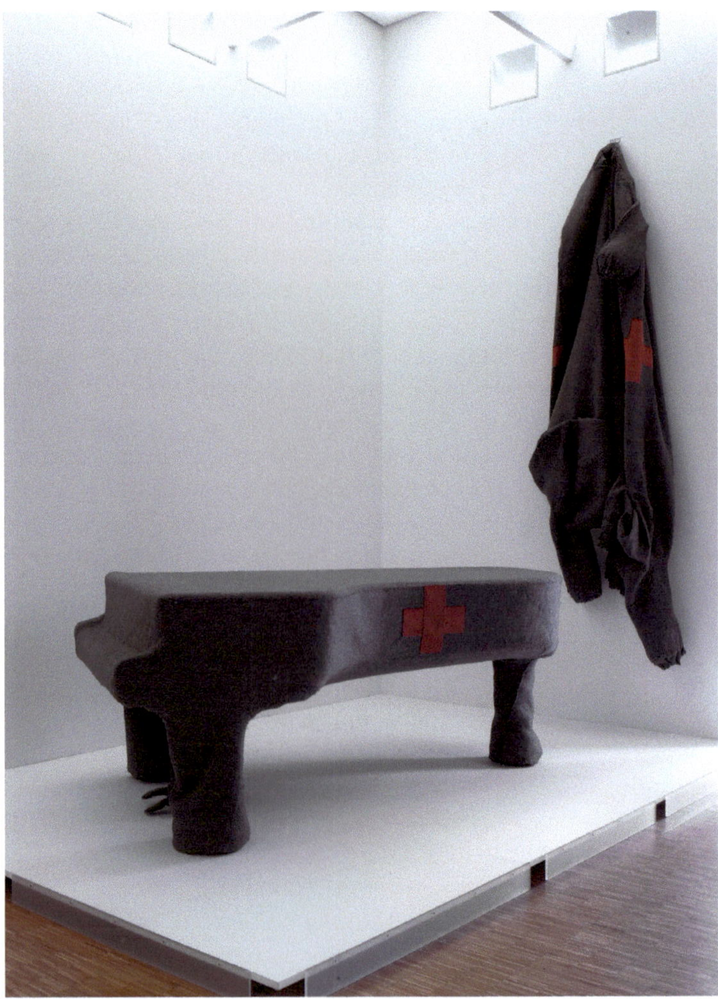

5.3 Joseph Beuys, *Homogenous Infiltration for Grand Piano (Infiltration homogen für Konzertflügel)*, 1966. Piano, felt, and febaric, 39.4 × 59.8 × 94.5in. (100 × 152 × 240 cm). Collection of Centre Georges Pompidou, Paris, Inv.: AM 1976-7. Photograph: Philippe Migeat. Art © 2024 Artists Rights Society (ARS), New York / VG Bild-Kunst, Bonn. Digital Image © CNAC/MNAM, Dist. RMN-Grand Palais / Art Resource, NY.

Image description 5.3: A sculpture in the shape of a dark gray baby grand piano with a small red cross painted on its side. Hanging on a wall next to the piano is a dark gray piano cover featuring the same red cross.

for Grand Piano) (1966), he used felt to cover up an entire grand piano (see Figure 5.3). A red cross was sewn onto each side of the felt cover, signaling emergency, as it still does today for organizations like the American Red Cross. By essentially 'silencing' the sounds that might be emitted from the piano keys, Beuys created a metaphor for the silencing of a medical scandal around thalidomide that was occurring in the late 1950s and 1960s. The drug was introduced in Germany and other parts of the world at that time and was used as a sedative and to treat pregnant women with nausea, vomiting, and other symptoms of morning sickness in the earlier stages of gestation. Unfortunately, little was known about the side effects of the drug, and it caused severe congenital birth defects and malformations. Both of these words are considered unsavory terms in disability studies, but are still associated with the outcomes of taking thalidomide today.

Beuys's work was originally conceived as a social action and performed on July 7, 1966 at the Staatliche Kunstakademie in Düsseldorf. Beuys interrupted a concert being given by Nam June Paik and Charlotte Moorman, and proceeded to cover the grand piano in felt, giving it both "thermal and acoustic insulation."[12] He then sewed red crosses on each side of the cover. Through this public action, Beuys was simultaneously showing how the medical scandal was being covered up (symbolized by the felt onesie) and that it must be made transparent (through the emergency crosses). Beuys aimed to provoke the audience to reflect on and debate a controversial topic. Indeed, many art historians have noted that Beuys perceived the function of art as both catharsis and therapy. Once Beuys's action was complete, the remaining part of the felt was hung on a wall near the piano, as can be seen in Figure 5.3. Other interpretations of Beuys's silencing of the piano with the felt equate it with the silencing of the impacted child who has become disempowered by the violence of medicine, underscoring that even we, as audience members, have a responsibility to give voice to minorities as a gesture of social justice.

Beuys's work is interesting to consider within a disability studies framework, given that many contemporary disabled artists have created work in response to being born with atypical bodily configurations as an outcome of their mother taking thalidomide, such as British actor and artist Mat Fraser. One might interpret Beuys's work to be inspired by similar questions to those driving disability justice practitioners in today's context, although it certainly was not disability justice informed, given the nascent nature of the disability rights movement at that time. The work falls squarely within Beuys's overall interest in humanism, sociology, and political subject matter, yet it is generative to consider alongside Youden's suspended furniture pieces. Both artists used found objects, ranging from the musical to the architectural, to manipulate and reinscribe their forms, crafting a broader political message that was tied to the misfortunes and misinformation surrounding medicine. While Beuys was pointing out how easily people would consume medicine despite little prior knowledge of it, Youden was showing the ways that people responded to illness without access to a cure. Beuys and Youden provide a clear alternative aesthetics to the historical ways that medicinal knowledge has been wielded.

Thinking about biocitizenship, intoxication, remedios, and alt medicine

The concept of biocitizenship is important to this chapter because it is endowed with a political apparatus that the artists and the artworks I discuss deeply contend with. Biocitizenship holds that beliefs about human biological existence are intertwined with conceptions of citizenship. Further, the health of our bodies, our society, and our environment affects the individual's ability to have agency.[13] In their introduction to the text *Biocitizenship: The Politics of Bodies, Governance, and Power*, editors Kelly E. Happe, Jenell Johnson, and Marina Levina state that it is important to consider who is fleshing out concepts of biocitizenship in the first place, because biocitizenship has neglected perspectives of race, class, and disability.[14] As an outcome of leaving certain voices out of the equation, notions of individual health become the narrow focal point and larger social inequities get ignored. Disabled artist Sharona Franklin helps us to better understand more complex conceptions of biocitizenship and activism through a disability perspective in the upcoming section.

In 2023, Mel Y. Chen published their highly anticipated second book entitled *Intoxicated: Race, Disability, and Chemical Intimacy Across Empire*.[15] The book also has great resonance with this chapter, given its focus on unpacking the word "intoxicated" in a generative discussion of the nexus of race and disability under imperialist and colonialist legacies. Chen uses "intoxication" in various ways in the book, but they mean for it to be capacious, incorporating intimacy, unlearning, slow constitution, and agitation. Overall, Chen suggests that "intoxication" rearranges the world much in the same way that disability does. They argue that when intoxication is positioned within a zone of exclusion, there may be generative knowledges that we miss out on. Chen suggests that medical practitioners in particular must be more open to different ways disabled patients are presenting and "thinking in difference."[16] Chen draws from disability theory to unravel ableist methodology, and embraces "intoxicated methodology" instead. They specifically apply this to the practice of allopathic medicine, writing that "a decolonial approach avoids the positing of hierarchies of medicating systems (for instance, the prioritizing of allopathy over other entrenched systems)."[17] A decolonial disability theory therefore shows how it might be possible for "dual modes of intoxication and intellectual difference" to coexist, free of the colonial hierarchization that still pervades Western medicine.[18] Chen is suggesting that the methods of surviving and thriving that may work for one person may not work for another, and it is important for medicine to be able to engage with alternative and multiple temporalities and states of being. As a discipline, the critical medical humanities were motivated at the outset by ethical considerations and calls for a more humanizing approach in the hospital room, the clinic, or the doctor's office.

If the discipline is seriously interested in these more humanizing approaches, then it must contend with the embodiment of disability, and, further, it must consider how disability may benefit from "alt medicine" intertwined with an "intoxicated method."

Chen's work provides a nice synergy with the work of Aurora Levins Morales, particularly the stories she weaves in her book *Medicine Stories: Essays for Radicals* (2019).[19] In one chapter of the book, Morales talks of the power of "remedios," which translates from Spanish to English as "cures." Like Chen, Morales adopts a word and reconstitutes how it is applied, setting it apart from more common or familiarized usages. Part of the work of remedios is to offer "medicinal" histories, where the history is retold in a new way, incorporating a subjugated perspective. Remedios are therefore different to conventional historical writing because within them, history is interrogated rather than being told. In this way, healing – or "medicinal" – stories can help to restore social justice to the oppressed and those who fall outside of mainstream and elitist narratives. Remedios are also a process of decolonization and making medicinal history most meaningful by centering minorities, telling untold stories, making absences visible, restoring global meaning (as opposed to a narrow imperialist focus on the West), and providing access and digestibility. The title of one of Morales's chapters is "The Historian as Curandera" – the meaning of the Spanish word "curandera" in English is "a healer who uses folk remedies." A curandero/a can also be compared to a shaman or a traditional native healer who is commonly found in Latin America; they are a specialist of medicine that can either be an alternative to or supplement Western medicine. Either way, a curandero/a has a different approach to the allopathic method of the West. By giving herself the title of curandera, Morales is suggesting that she is taking on the three-pronged role of historian-healer-activist. I appreciate Morales's approach as I have always called myself a curator-activist; I believe it is important to be outspoken about the new ways in which curatorship must be practiced, since it has long obscured and erased the needs of disabled artists and audiences. Morales uses medicine to rescript history so that alt medicine is effectively deployed through her storytelling, similar to the work by the contemporary disabled artists discussed in this chapter. The philosophical frameworks that biocitizenship, intoxication, and remedios provide all show how other scholars and thinkers turn to alt medicine in different ways for the same objectives – to think about new and better pathways that improve the situation for those that are typically forgotten, ignored, or oppressed. The work of this chapter is particularly potent because we are seeing problem-solving and solution-oriented artwork that builds on the work of the care collectives in Chapter 4.

There are numerous other contemporary artists who explore biocitizenship, rituals, and alt medicine. Carmen and Antonio Papalia's installation,

Tripping Hazard (Field Studio 1) (2023), was installed as part of curator Michael Birchall's *Interdependencies: Perspectives on Care and Resilience* exhibition at the Migros Museum in Zurich, Switzerland. The brothers set up a temporary housing structure in the middle of the gallery space where visitors could go inside to see their replication of cannabis cultivation, which included gardening tools, grow lights, running water, fans, a temperature control, and more. The work mimics efforts to grow weed within the context of a self-determined alt medicine. Antonio maintains the grow room for Carmen, who relies on marijuana as a nontraditional medicine to manage the pain he experiences as part of his chronic illness. In witnessing the work as a collaborative effort between two brothers, the visitor also sees how care work within alt medicine is about relational support. Alex Dolores Salerno's work *Offering* (2020) is also a meditation on cannabis as alt medicine that helps people to manage pain, and to nurture the body through relaxation and soothing pleasure. The work consists of a square-shaped pillow edged with used joint filters as a type of decorative frill. In this context, the frill suggests a medicinal support that literally frames the head of the pillow's user, offering a double or triple mode of relaxation and care. The head rests, ensconced within the soft stuffing of the pillow, compounding the relief that the marijuana brings.

In the same *Interdependencies* exhibition mentioned previously were two of Maryam Jafri's sculptures, entitled *Depression* (2017) (see Figure 5.4) and *Anxiety* (2017). These works were originally part of Jafri's solo exhibition, *War on Wellness*, held at the Kai Matsumiya gallery in New York in 2017, and were included in the series *Wellness-Postindustrial Complex*. The larger message Jafri wanted to convey was that Eastern self-care practices such as acupuncture or cupping to relieve pain and stress can help to optimize bodily functioning. These practices are becoming more aggressively sought after by many people as a result of the US government's indifference to the accessibility of healthcare, which in the gallery press release Jafri called a war on the wellness of "people's minds, bodies and spirits, waged by the current regime in Washington."[20]

From 2023 to 2024, the exhibition *Chronos: Health, Access, and Intimacy* was held at the Tensta Konsthall in Stockholm, Sweden, curated by artist Olivia Plender in collaboration with Cecilia Widenheim. The exhibition featured numerous artists and artworks that have resonance for the other work discussed in this chapter. Swedish-Canadian Black artist Cecilia Germain contributed several important works: *Grandmother as a Young Woman / The Okra Flower* (see Figure 5.5), *Grandmother as a Child / The Camphor Tree*, *Grandmother as a Mother / Papyrus*, and *Grandfather as a Young Man / Sassafras*, a series of four cyanotypes on paper from 2023. In these works, Germain created composites of black and white photographs of her grandmother or grandfather, layered with African diasporic plants that have alternative medicinal and ritual uses, including an okra flower

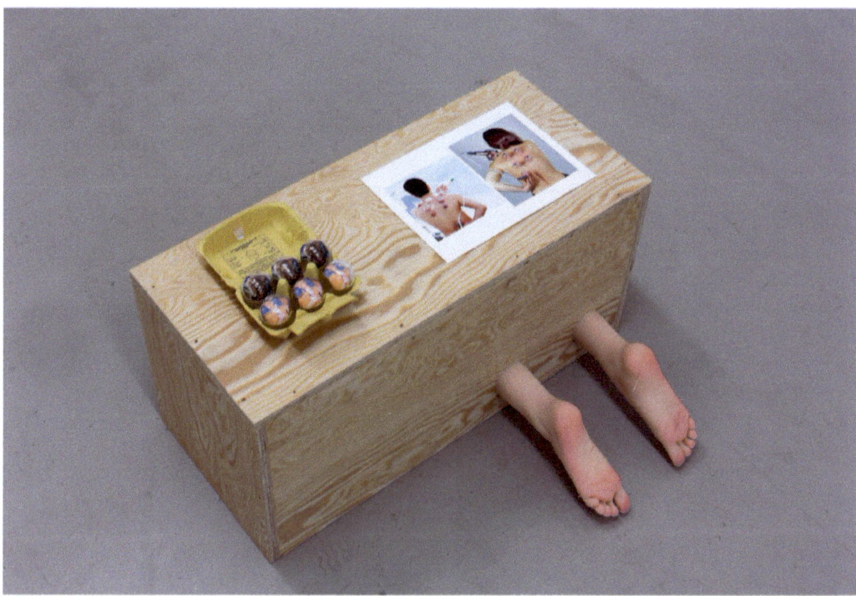

5.4 Maryam Jafri, *Depression*, from the series *Wellness-Postindustrial Complex*, 2017. Wood, silicone feet, acupuncture needles, glass cupping equipment, photograph, paper, and egg carton. 12 × 9 × 5in. (30.5 × 22.8 × 12.7cm). Courtesy of the artist.

Image description 5.4: A plywood box sitting on a cement floor. On top of the box is an egg carton full of glass cupping equipment and a color photograph of two people demonstrating how to use the equipment. On the floor, in front of the box, is a pair of sculpted human feet, laying with their heels facing upward and acupuncture needles delicately placed on the skin.

and the camphor tree. Germain has long been interested in the important role that plants play in spiritual traditions of the African diaspora, which she calls Black Flora or a Black Botany. In her research, she has uncovered numerous accounts where people of African origin who escaped slavery were able to survive thanks to the cultivation of medicinal plants. Germain's interdisciplinary practice is concerned with social justice in relation to public health, collective trauma and grief, alternative healing practices, colonial economies as they intersect with plants, and the historical role of botanicals and their impact on humans. Germain's work has explored local plant knowledge, herbalism, sleep as resistance, activism, and survival, as well as how ethnobotanical stories belong to a therapeutic landscape of radical knowledge.

Another important work from the *Chronos* exhibition was *Hospital for Selvmedicinering* (Hospital for Self-Medication) (2019), developed by Danish artist Jakob Jakobsen. The artist created this work in the attic of his own home, after a traumatic stay in the Gentofte Hospital in Copenhagen, Denmark. This work is a self-stylized imagining of what a better hospital

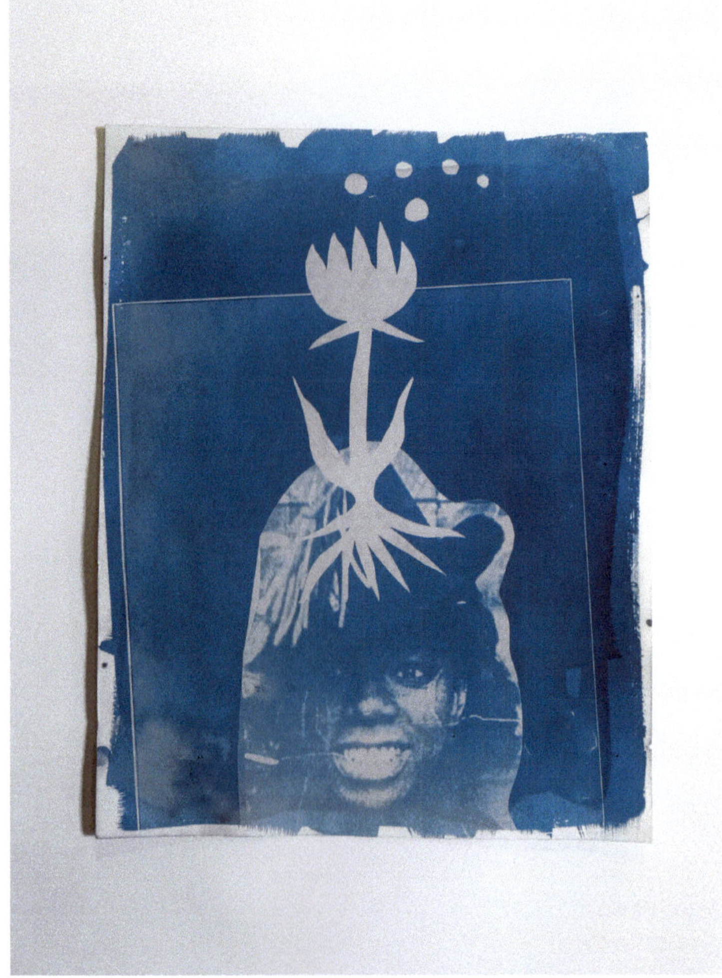

5.5 Cecilia Germain, *Grandmother as a Young Woman / The Okra Flower*, 2023. Cyanotype and watercolor on paper. Photograph: Wasim Harwill. Courtesy of the artist.

Image description 5.5: Blue and white mixed media work featuring a photograph of a smiling Black woman wearing a jaunty hat. A cyanotype (camera-less photographic print) has been made over the photograph using an okra flower, which produces a white silhouette emerging from the woman's hat.

could and should be, based on the artist's experience at the Gentofte. In an essay or manifesto entitled "We Are All Sick!," Jakobsen says,

> *Hospital for Self Medication* is a self-organized hospital. It is an experimental space for developing threads of health care with a communist texture; threads from which we can hopefully weave the fabric of a new community of the exhausted, the displaced, the ill, the disabled, the traumatized, the injured,

> the weathered, the suicidal. We need a new hospital built by the sick. *The Hospital for Self Medication* is an experimental institution that will work with critical forms of care and therapy. We want to lay bare and challenge the violent roots and practices of traditional health care. We will speculate, search for and try out new ways. Our bodies and minds have been dissected into increasingly smaller sections within the regime of present-day medical care. The specialization and separation of the capitalist system structuring our ideas of health care have to be countered by collective and everyday forms. We would like to put the mind-body back together and reclaim our own experience of the fuzzy contours of our physical selves.[21]

The remaining parts of Jakobsen's manifesto cover wide-ranging topics, including the urgency of addressing mental health issues, our social ills, how we must take more care of our carers, and how we must develop new language for madness and care. Jakobsen also challenges concepts of medication and recovery, and suggests that space itself can be designed as therapy if it is rid of furniture such as beds, chairs, and desks. Jakobsen designed his attic to feature a panoply of Persian rugs, with pillows and cushions scattered across the large area. In Jakobsen's vision, a space like this would be more conducive to conversation and collectivity, in contrast with how our bodies are typically segregated in hospital beds and rooms with a curtain to cut us off from neighboring patients. Also intriguing in Jakobsen's essay is how his work is a form of antitherapy, a layman's therapy, or even nontherapeutic therapy. His work questions the specialization of professional therapy practice, suggesting that we can all practice a form of therapy without needing to acquire specific qualifications. I also enjoy Jakobsen's remarks about how we need to abolish the word "patient."[22] He says, "to be a patient means suffering in silence. A lot of waiting rooms. The capitalist hospital wants you to become a patient, to accept the passivity of being a patient."[23] Jakobsen calls for deinstitutionalization of the hospital and the patient as part of the process of developing alternatives where communal life is embraced. Jakobsen's work evokes hospital aesthetics, creating a new aesthetics out of the relationship between hospitals and politics. And, importantly for this chapter, his work is an "alt medicine" or an "alt hospital" that achieves far greater comfort, care, and reclamation than that offered by the mainstream hospital.

All of these theoretical frameworks and additional artworks show how "alt-medicine" has been a wide-ranging concept for philosophers and artists. Imagining and building new worlds set apart from the repressed one we typically find ourselves in is a matter of survival and hope for a better place. This, too, is part of hospital aesthetics. I will now turn to the work of Sharona Franklin, who draws on the domestic aesthetics of wellness through quilting and baking to counteract the poisons of the medical industrial complex.

Domestic aesthetics of wellness: quilting and baking as antidote

Contemporary disabled artist, writer, and activist Sharona Franklin was born in Vernon, British Columbia, Canada, and has rare inflammatory, hematologic, and autoimmune diseases such as Still's disease, and endometriosis. Because of her illnesses and disabilities, she must sometimes use a wheelchair or other assistive devices, or undertake intensive treatments. Her lived experience with chronic illness and disabilities deeply informs her art practice. She states that "each of the modalities I work with speaks to the alienation and structural, societal, and interpersonal barriers that disabled people face in relation to able-centric norms."[24] Franklin is an interdisciplinary artist, and has explored many facets of her personal living space, where she administers her own medical care as a critical aspect of her domestic social practice. In her writing, she explores psychedelia and propaganda, and in her textile-based work she has created quilts, pillows, and tapestries. She has also produced videos and soundscapes, sculptures made from papier mâché, and sculptures that are edible. Franklin also uses social media to share her activism and her art, and maintains numerous Instagram accounts, including @paid.technologies, @star_seeded, and @ hot.crip, among other sites. Franklin grew up in several rural environments and in trailer homes, and as a consequence she was left to her own devices when it came to managing her disabilities and illnesses, an experience she describes as incredibly challenging. She graduated from high school in her twenties and eventually went to art school. She turned to skills that her grandmother taught her as primary mediums for her art-making practice, namely quilting and baking. In this section, I will examine two main forms of Franklin's work: her quilt-based work, and her jelly sculptures, which take baking to a new aesthetic and activist level.

Franklin has become most well known for her biodegradable botanical jelly sculptures. In these works the transparency, vulnerability, and fragility of the jelly acts as a metaphor for her lived experience, where disability and chronic illness are entwined with the ethical and environmental complexities of the pharmaceutical industrial complex. Within the jelly sculptures, Franklin incorporates flowers, herbs, syringes, hardware, nutritious foods, and expired pharmaceuticals. Franklin both injects and ingests pharmaceuticals on a daily basis to keep herself alive, and has a push–pull relationship with medication. The gelatinous composition of these sculptures requires much care, a necessity Franklin found to be equivalent to the care and accommodations required by disabled bodies. Franklin intimately understands the material of jelly because of her own jelly-like joints. Franklin acknowledges that she must be much more sensitive in handling jelly than during baking. Importantly, the process also involves working with temperature and alchemy. Franklin says, "temperature and alchemy are something that my life has been completely ruled by as a person with multiple inflammatory diseases. I have daily fevers and I have to navigate inflammation with ice and heat … ."[25] Franklin's ability to translate intangible, incommunicable sensorial experiences into chemical artistic materials is brilliant and revelatory.

In 2020, Franklin held her first US solo exhibition at the Kings Leap gallery in New York, entitled *New Psychedelia of Industrial Healing*. It's uncanny that Franklin's exhibition opened to the public shortly before the COVID-19 pandemic hit the world in March of 2020. The exhibition included several wall-mounted ceramic plates entitled *Hemichrome Plate* and *Amoebic Self Portrait of Pharmaceutical Preservation Methodologies*, which suggest how the domestic becomes tied up with the pharmaceutical industry; a large cone-shaped jelly sculpture on a pedestal in the center of the gallery space entitled *Mycoplasma Alter* (see Figure 5.6); and a large patchwork quilt entitled *Comfort Studies* (see Figure 5.7).

The gelatinous form of *Mycoplasma Alter* is filled with many items, including yellow daisies, kidney beans, methotrexate (an immunosuppressant), amoxicillin pills, tapioca pearls, and syringe vials filled with antibodies. During an interview with Franklin some years ago, I asked her how she kept the jelly structure from decomposing during the exhibition, and she explained that to prevent spoilage and fungus growth she had to inject it with a mold inhibitor, a substance that is commonly used in baked goods. While the work would thus be protected, it would still shrink and sink a little each day atop its ornate pedestal. In her review of the exhibition, Dana Kopel wrote that the work "resembles nothing so much as a 1950s dinner-party gelatin mould, the dusty yellow color of it like a sun-bleached page in a midcentury women's magazine. That visual association with the 1950s feels fitting, given the pharmaco-capitalist approach to the human body that began taking hold in that era."[26] The jelly sculpture oozes experimentation and openness; it provides an appropriate metaphor for Franklin's own illnesses, which have been difficult to diagnose, along with the kinds of medications she has been prescribed to treat them. Of this, Franklin says, "My work is about giving visibility to rare illnesses and the complicated treatments that are often undeveloped, and how we become used as test subjects."[27] Franklin and others have referred to her jelly sculptures as *bioshrines* that explore ongoing tensions in the biopharmaceutical industry. As a patient of biopharmaceutical and transgenic treatments for over twenty years, and through work such as this, Franklin hopes to reclaim the narratives of her disabilities. Her work helps us to question the power of medicine, whether its chemicals are hurting us or curing us, and what their true side effects are. Experiencing Franklin's work in the aftermath of the pandemic has raised our awareness of our own neuroplasticity, and how we must regard biocitizenship seriously and with self-care and resilience.

Comfort Studies, a large, colorful patchwork quilt hanging on a beam suspended from the ceiling, is a collage of images and texts on found

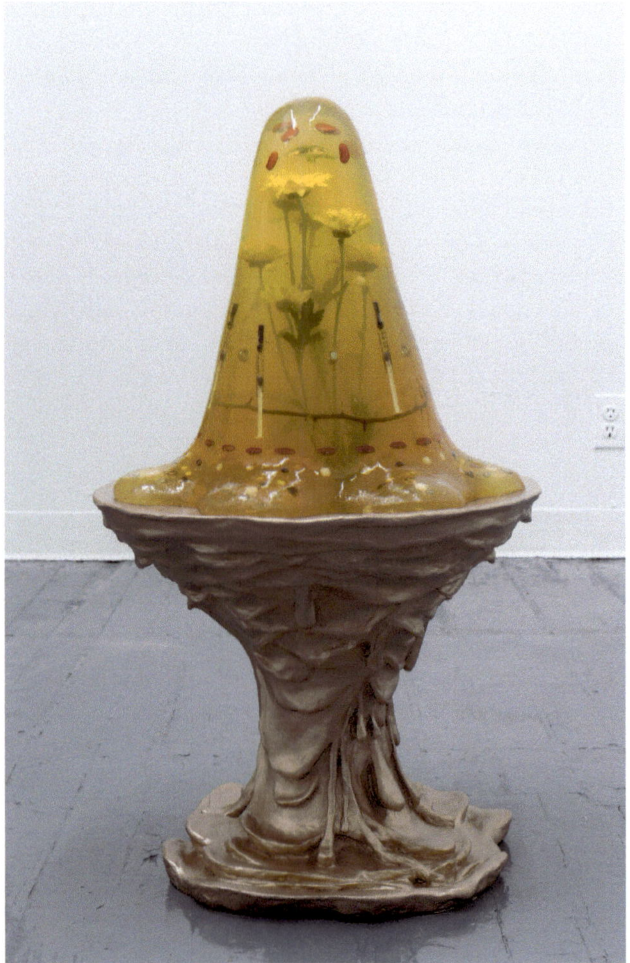

5.6 Sharona Franklin, *Mycoplasma Altar*, 2020. Gelatin powder, daisies, foraged rose thorns sourced by Wretched Flowers, baby's breath, juniper berry, metal nuts, kidney beans, amoxicillin pills, hydroxychloroquine pills, methotrexate pills, antibodies in glass syringe vials, tapioca pearls, sunflower seeds, metal button, almond extract, papier-mâché, wood, acrylic, plaster; Bone Dust Sculpture: 17 × 17 × 17 in. (43 × 43 × 43 cm); Plinth: 16 × 17 × 17 in. (41 × 43 × 43 cm); Overall: 33 × 17 × 17 in. (84 × 43 × 43 cm). Photograph: Stephen Faught. Images courtesy of the artist and King's Leap.

Image description 5.6: A phallic cone-shaped yellow gelatin mould filled with flowers, pills, syringes, and other objects. The sickly colored sculpture is perfectly perched on top of a short, beige-colored pedestal that has been carved to resemble organic rock formations.

fabrics (see Figure 5.7). Examples of the disability-justice-inspired aphorisms found across the quilt include, "who's anti-body is your body of?" and "pity is a sin greater than any sick-ness." The title of the piece speaks to the qualities often associated with the quilt, namely comfort and coziness

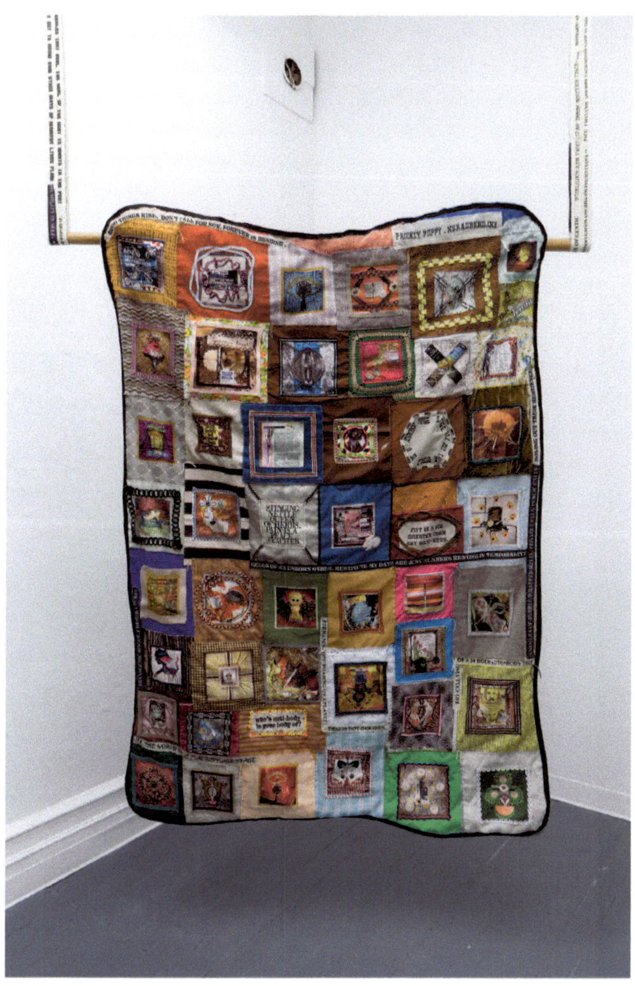

5.7 Sharona Franklin, *Comfort Studies*, 2020. Cotton, linen, velvet, silk, polyester, vinyl, wood, plastic, 72 × 55.5in. (183 × 141cm). Photograph: Stephen Faught. Images courtesy of the artist and King's Leap Fine Arts.

Image description 5.7: A multi-colored quilt made of mixed media.

within a domestic sphere. The quilt also evokes other dimensions of comfort because it has now become a fabric associated with social justice, empowerment, biocitizenship, and radical self-acceptance thanks to Franklin's intervention. The quilt is thus meant to bring comfort to Franklin herself and to us as the observers of the work, extending care within a larger medical system that can be cold, depersonalized, and harsh. The blanket as a protective cover and a pacifier during times of vulnerability is both antibody and antidote to the biorituals that have become incorporated into our lives to manage the smallest and the greatest personal and social ills.

Franklin's handmade quilt also points to how earlier generations of feminist artists have used domestic crafts to defy artistic categories and artistic mediums that are ostensibly masculine or feminine. These kinds of feminist labor practices open up possibilities for disabled and immunocompromised individuals to subvert the masculine and able-bodied perspective at the center of the biopharmaceutical industry. While it is true, then, that the quilt evinces feminine, nurturing qualities, Franklin's deployment of the domestic – both baking and quilting – is political in the same manner as works by feminist artists like Miriam Schapiro, Faith Ringgold, and Judy Chicago. Active in the 1960s and 1970s, these artists rejected the idea that specific mediums should be relegated to the category of "women's work"; they reclaimed these mediums in art galleries and museums, thus elevating them and cementing their status as art objects.

In 2022, Franklin's work was displayed in her first institution-based exhibition at the Massachusetts Institute of Technology List Visual Arts Center, which, coincidentally, is mere blocks away from the COVID-19 pharmaceutical heavyweights Moderna and Pfizer. The exhibition was entitled *List Projects 24: Sharona Franklin*, and the centerpiece was *Anti-Alpha Principles* (2022), a child-sized coffin made from wicker (see Figure 5.8). It is decorated with numerous materials such as syringes, seeds, pills, flowers, and grass, in the same manner as her jelly sculptures. The used and recycled medical waste is Franklin's, the product of the daily medical ritual through which she treats her various autoimmune diseases. Franklin layers flowers into the medical waste to counteract both the aesthetics and the origins of each symbol in the installation; the medical waste never disintegrates, while the flora decomposes over time, much like a body in a coffin buried beneath the ground. As Leah Triplett Harrington writes, "The constant evolution of form and aesthetic mimics how our bodies are in continual flux, strained with time and our physical environment."[28] Franklin's use of a child-size coffin conveys vulnerability and rawness, and strips her down to an essence that is painfully innocent, yet aware. On either side of the wicker coffin, Franklin placed two church pews, painted white to look less austere and graffitied with black handwritten ink scrawls proclaiming poetic and political inscriptions. The pews suggest that Franklin intends for us to sit and ponder the casket in the center in the context of a funeral, where we can pay homage to the fragility of life. Yet the seats are uncomfortable and hard, reminding us that this is a temporary pause only, where meditation is encouraged but kept to a minimum, just as in the timetable of our everyday existence. Franklin keeps reminding us of the push and pull tension inherent in the biopharmaceutical complex and in the healthcare industry at large, giving us an even wider lens through which to understand the complexity of hospital aesthetics.

Franklin's work is aesthetically and topically connected to that of collage and mixed-media New York City-based artist Thomas Lanigan-Schmidt,

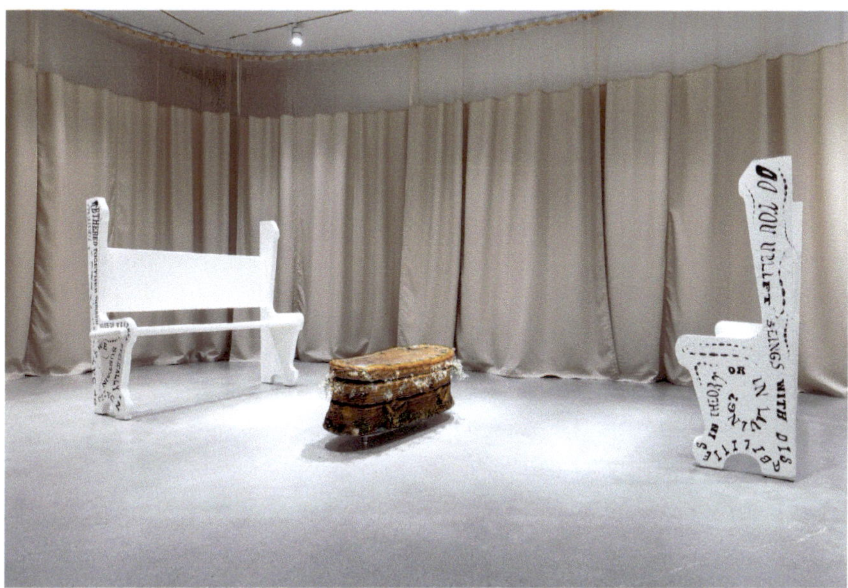

5.8 Exhibition view, *List Projects 24: Sharona Franklin*, MIT List Visual Arts Center, 2022. Photograph: Mel Taing. Image courtesy MIT List Visual Arts Center. Artworks courtesy of the artist and King's Leap.

Image description 5.8: A windowless gallery space with two white, high-back benches that resemble pews from a church. The benches are placed across from one another with a small sculpture resembling a child's casket in between.

who made tinfoil altars to memorialize the uncanny and the strange in the everyday in the 1960s and 1970s. Through his queer aesthetic, Lanigan-Schmidt explored themes of sex, religion, and class in his esoteric and idiosyncratic portraits and compositions. Like Franklin, Lanigan-Schmidt seamlessly blended a so-called high and low aesthetic, using materials some would describe as audacious, such as glitter, plastic, Mylar, colored foil, and staples. Franklin's work is akin as well to that of feminist and postminimalist artist Ree Morton, who also made work during the 1970s. Morton's collages, which incorporated text, autobiography, bold color, humor, and an obsession with the decorative, mirror Franklin's own aesthetic approach in their engagement with identity politics, specifically through questions of gender. The title of Morton's piece *The Plant That Heals May Also Poison* (1974) is an adage that can be applied to Franklin's work, alongside that of all the other artists described in this book. We are all implicated in a medical industrial system that is simultaneously keeping us alive and killing us.

Franklin's work is an important addition to the contemporary genre of pharma art, a body of work that is solely focused on pharmaceuticals in its themes and objects. Even though pharmacology itself is an ancient practice going back to the Greeks, pharmaceutical companies only started to emerge in the late nineteenth century. Developments in biochemistry, chemistry, and molecular biology drove the industry; the production of insulin and penicillin became the greatest achievements of the 1920s and 1930s, followed by the birth control pill, Valium, Prozac, and drugs to treat cancer and AIDS. Owing to the thalidomide controversy that occurred in the 1960s, as discussed previously, stricter regulations were put in place around the release and use of new medications, and today the pharmaceutical industry has a massive public profile, achieved through advertising, consumer culture, and social media campaigns. In the aftermath of the COVID-19 pandemic, when there was a race among large pharmaceutical companies all over the world to find a vaccine, the world is painfully aware of how we may all be at the mercy of pills and injections that can have a life-giving power. Yet the race to find the COVID-19 vaccine also made the world aware that access never was or will be equal, as the wealthier nations were able to treat their populations first, and within those nations the elite classes came first, while marginalized groups had higher rates of mortality. Pharma art touches on these themes, alongside the ever-present and urgent need to flee reality through drugs that help us cope by numbing us or, equally, that damage and tear up our lives. While other artists who contribute to the genre of pharma art are not at all removed from or oblivious to our culture of drug use and addiction, Franklin shares with us a vulnerability regarding her pain and her trauma that is honest and raw.

Well-known British artist Damian Hirst produced his large-scale *Pharmacy* installation at the Tate Modern in London in 2012 (see Figure 5.9). His installation imitated the look and feel of a pharmacy store, and worked so well that apparently some visitors didn't want to enter the installation, confusing it with a real-life pharmacy. The shelves are lined with a vast array of colorful prescription drugs, reminding us that we are living in an age of addiction and drug-dependence on a scale never experienced before. Included in the installation were four large apothecary bottles filled with green, yellow, red, and blue liquids, representing earth, air, fire, and water. An apothecary is another word for a pharmacist, someone who formulates and dispenses medicines. While the installation is familiar, even soothing perhaps, with its commonplace design and benign contents in a clean, unassuming environment, Hirst also skillfully shows us how easy it is for us to be swallowed by medicine, and that perhaps we have far less control over what we digest for our supposed wellness and betterment than we might imagine. Thus the pharmacy acts as a symbol of help and recovery, yet it is simultaneously ominous and threatening for its potential to incite addiction, dependence, and decay. Hirst's installation was inspired by a work by the same name by Marcel Duchamp, and by Joseph Cornell's *Pharmacies* series created in the 1940s and 1950s, which consisted of old

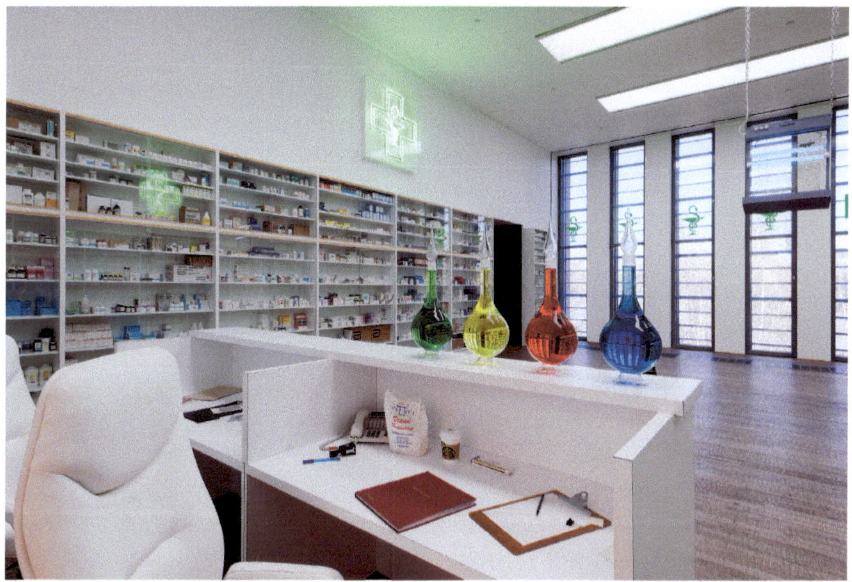

5.9 Damien Hirst, Installation of *Pharmacy*, Tate Modern, April 4–September 9, 2012. Photo © Tate (Andrew Dunkley). Art © Damien Hirst and Science Ltd. All rights reserved / DACS, London / ARS, NY 2024.

Image description 5.9: An installation that resembles a contemporary pharmacy: minimalist architecture, walls lined with shelves featuring products, and harsh fluorescent lighting.

wooden medicine chests stuffed with feathers, shells, colored powders and liquids, paper and leaves, all assembled in rows of glass bottles.

Another artist who preceded Youden in thinking about the biopharmaceutical industry through art praxis is Beverly Fishman, who has been interested in the aesthetics of medicine since the 1980s. Her work includes installations of larger-than-life medicine pills of all shapes and sizes, such as *In Sickness and In Health* (2015–16). The work is comprised of unique blown glass objects, carefully and carelessly scattered across a low-lying pedestal. The majority of works from Fishman's portfolio are convex and concave-shaped paintings inspired by the shapes of pills. Her paintings feature saturated fluorescent colors inspired by hard-edged geometric abstraction from the 1950s and 1960s, evoking both legal and illegal drugs. Her large-scale paintings that reference the palette and the shapes of medication shock us through their scale and theatricality. In making the ordinary extraordinary, Fishman forces us to reflect on the role that medication plays in our lives and in shaping culture at large.[29] For this reason, Fishman has much in common with Franklin and Hirst, as they each force the viewer to reckon with their participation in a society in which our dependency on drugs grows by the day.

Of course, before Hirst and Fishman, or Youden and Franklin, drugs and drug dependency had been prominent subjects in artists' autobiographies. The topics of addiction and substance use were taken up throughout the twentieth century by art historians and curators, who were most interested in categorical assessment and interpretation of how addictions might contribute to artistic madness and genius in equal measure. For example, the lives of Frida Kahlo and Vincent van Gogh have been discussed at great length alongside their talent for making some of the most evocative art of the modern period. In Kahlo's case, art historians and curators have drawn from significant events in her life, particularly the bus accident that caused numerous permanent injuries to the artist's body and the infidelity she bore while living in the shadow of her husband, Diego Riviera. The notorious episode in which Van Gogh cut off his ear in a fit of rage and mental anguish is seen as a preface for the final chapter of his story, in which the artist died by suicide. Van Gogh's art is consistently analyzed for the emotive and psychological qualities that are evidence of his so-called state of mind as a tortured artist, and thus his genius. Both artists relied heavily on a range of substances to cope with physical and mental ailments throughout their lifetimes (and it is said that Van Gogh was under the influence of drugs when he self-mutilated his ear).

In addition to these individual case studies where art and psychology come into conversation with medication, the entire field of outsider art is defined in terms of the self-taught artist on the margins of the art world, who might identify as Black, disabled, or female, and who may be addicted to prescription or illegal drugs in the context of their socioeconomic and medical circumstances. Art historians have written extensively on outsider art in the past few decades, pointing out how the connections between the Black folk art movement in America and Art Brut in France, which had both otherness and aesthetics in common, led to the founding of a genre. Outsider art has particular appeal in the commercial art industry, as it taps into people's inclination to marvel at the heroic and the rare talents of artists who are afflicted by incurable pathologies. In his text *Outsider Art: Spontaneous Alternatives*, Colin Rhodes says that the definition of artist outsiders suggests that they are "fundamentally different to their audience, often thought of as being dysfunctional in respect of the parameters for normality set by the dominant culture. What this means specifically is, of course, [that they are] subject to changes dictated by history and geographical location."[30] The artist outsider group is heterogeneous by virtue of the great assortment of people who might be assigned to this vast category, and so there is much slippage in this definition, as those deemed dysfunctional in society are often labeled due to social classifications like pathology, mental illness, criminality, or gender or sexuality. The list goes on. What Rhodes makes clear is that in the early days of Art Brut, the artists were mostly mentally ill patients and "self-taught visionaries," people working "outside" the art academy.[31] But I think it is fair to say that in the contemporary moment, agents who work with developmentally disabled artists have conveniently utilized the profitable "outsider art" label to promote their work within a recognizable, commercial, and "legitimate," if still contentious, category. In other words, developmentally disabled artists have been lumped into the "outsider art" category, wrongly or rightly, just as artists belonging to other minority positions have also been swept into the Otherness borderlands. While the word "outsider" may have historically had quite a different genealogy (as developmentally disabled artists had nothing to do with "outsider art"), it becomes tricky to disassociate the etymological and social implications of "outsider."

Beyond these facile efforts at categorization, problematic genres such as outsider art or the trope of the artist as tortured genius addicted to illicit drugs are related to art history's focus on biography (which might be compared to the medical and diagnostic chart of a patient). This narrow focus also severely limits the position that the art historian or critic can mediate from regarding the inclusion of minority and disabled subjects. Methodologies and categorizations such as this clearly need to be repudiated, but they also need to be reshaped and retooled by the contemporary disabled artists themselves. Art historians take for granted that, much like the clinician, the doctor, or the therapist, they wield disciplinary power through the interpretive act. Contemporary disabled artists show us how we can write about art history differently, producing histories where their voices are loudly and defiantly represented, but they also show us a hospital aesthetics that defies the supposedly correct and knowledgeable medical industry.

In the Introduction, I mentioned that there was a darker history of how disabled patients were "treated" by the medical industrial complex in the twentieth century. This was a period when disabled people were the subject of painful and inhumane medical experiments, and were considered utterly disposable under malevolent government regimes such as the Nazis. A recent book entitled *Disalienation: Politics, Philosophy, and Radical Psychiatry in Postwar France* by Camille Robcis provides revelatory new information about how one hospital broke with standardized approaches and understandings of madness during the early twentieth century, in a way that dovetails with the definition of hospital aesthetics I have crafted through these five chapters.[32] In the history of asylums and hospitals Robcis provides, she notes that there was a turn to more humane treatment of patients in one particular asylum in a rural village in France. In their act of rethinking both the practical and theoretical bases of psychiatric care, the Saint-Alban psychiatric hospital founded a new movement called institutional psychotherapy, which was characterized by a belief that theory and practice were inextricably linked. In other words, in order to treat a patient with a mental illness, they must take into account the patient's self-accounts and how social, familial, and cultural factors might impact the "genesis of mental processes" for the individual.[33] Robcis states that "the point of institutional psychotherapy was never to devise a fixed dogma or model that could be applied indiscriminately, but rather to offer an 'ethics' ... a practice of everyday life."[34] Institutional psychotherapy also emphasized that it was critical to account for the "political nature of all medical practice," given its "historical entanglement with structures of power, and its responsibility with the stigmatization of madness."[35] Robcis notes that many doctors were moved to come and spend time and work at Saint-Alban because they were tired of how other psychiatric hospitals were mired in biological essentialism, an exclusive "neurological approach to the brain," and a rigid approach of neutrality and objectivism.[36] Saint-Alban proved unique in its more compassionate and humanitarian approach to its patients, and its broad impact owed much to its efforts at not only curing patients but in curing humanity itself, as this hospital wished to disassociate itself from the eugenic and genocidal atrocities that were occurring during this period. Saint-Alban had many important admirers, including philosophers and psychoanalysts such as Frantz Fanon, Michel Foucault, and Félix Guattari, and given these great thinkers' contributions to poststructuralist thought, Saint-Alban has an obvious connection to their magnum opuses. Saint-Alban's refreshing and inspiring approach was clearly an anomaly among the more mainstream attitudes to madness, and today, while I perceive Saint-Alban's philosophy to be aligned with hospital aesthetics, it is still incongruous with most contemporary clinical methodologies.

I share this important account by Robcis because the theoretical and practical branches of hospital aesthetics have strong and clear historical precedents within the hospital setting itself, which I find exciting. This means that a desire for change and transformation was expressed in older forms of clinical practice itself, beyond aesthetics and the world of art. Specific case studies like Saint-Alban show that the institution of the hospital and its medical practitioners have recognized the limitations of neutrality and objectification in medical education, but that these limitations have yet to be fully and consistently absorbed into the hospital so that real transformation can take place.

Alongside institutional psychotherapy at Saint-Alban, Lauryn Youden and Sharona Franklin conclude the work of hospital aesthetics in this chapter with their myriad forms of "alt medicine," showing how alternative methodologies, processes, and experiences can be fruitful and generative. By combining histories of architecture with personal and domestic objects such as vibrators, quilts, books, and more, and engaging with biocitizenship and Western antibiotics, the artists offer us a chance to unravel all these complex ideological and political frameworks, demonstrating how they can cause pain and hardship on the one hand, while being reclaimed and used to empower on the other through artistic interventions. The artists also show us that alternative approaches to healthcare do not necessarily have to be the antithesis to allopathic medicine, and there are benefits to be gained by incorporating knowledge from both of these scripts to aid in an individual's healing and recovery from unwellness, both chronic and temporary. It is also fortuitous to include alt medicine in this last chapter because it is a powerful segue for the larger goals and arguments of this book: that alternatives must be deployed by the medical establishment at large. There are too many stories from disabled patients that recount how they are not being heard by the medical industrial complex. By offering literal alternatives through their transgressive artworks, the artists show us that there must also be alternatives to "business as usual" within the mainstream hospital world, where transformation is a critical necessity for improving the lives and the health of all of us.

Notes

1 Alice Hattrick, *Ill Feelings* (London: Fitzcarraldo Editions, 2021).
2 Brit Barton, "Interdependencies: Perspectives on Care and Resilience," *Mousse Magazine*, November 13, 2023, www.moussemagazine.it/magazine/interdependencies-brit-barton-migros-museum-zurich-2023 [accessed December 5, 2024].
3 Amanda Cachia interview with Lauryn Youden, Zoom, March 14, 2024.
4 Beatriz Colomina, *X-Ray Architecture* (Baden, Switzerland: Lars Müller Publishers, 2019).
5 Donna Schons, "Resting Place," *PW-Magazine*, March 19, 2023, https://pw-magazine.com/2023/resting-place [accessed December 5, 2024].
6 Schons, "Resting Place."
7 Schons, "Resting Place."
8 Margaret Campbell, "What Tuberculosis did for Modernism: The Influence of a Curative Environment on Modernist Design and Architecture," *Medical History: An International Journal for the History of Medicine and the Related Sciences* 49, no. 4 (2005): 463–88, https://doi.org/10.1017/s0025727300009169
9 Colomina, *X-Ray Architecture*.
10 Cachia interview with Youden, March 14, 2024.
11 Cachia interview with Youden, March 14, 2024.
12 Fanny Drugeon, *Collection art contemporain – La collection du Centre Pompidou, Musée national d'art moderne*, ed. Sophie Duplaix (Paris: Centre Pompidou, 2007).
13 Jenell Johnson, Kelly E. Happe, and Marina Levina, "Introduction," in *Biocitizenship: The Politics of Bodies, Governance, and Power*, ed. Kelly E. Happe, Jenell Johnson, and Marina Levina (New York: New York University Press, 2018), 1–18.
14 Johnson, Happe, and Levina, "Introduction," 1–18.
15 Mel Chen, *Intoxicated: Race, Disability, and Chemical Intimacy Across Empire* (Durham, NC: Duke University Press, 2023).
16 Chen, *Intoxicated*, 133.
17 Chen, *Intoxicated*, 134.
18 Chen, *Intoxicated*, 134.
19 Aurora Levins Morales, *Medicine Stories: Essays for Radicals* (Durham, NC: Duke University Press, 2019).
20 Kai Matsumiya gallery, "Maryam Jafri War on Wellness," press release, 2017, https://kaimatsumiya.com/maryam-jafri-war-on-wellness [accessed December 5, 2024].

21 Jakob Jakobsen, "We Are All Sick!," *Palette*, February 11, 2020, https://paletten.net/artiklar/we-are-all-sick [accessed December 5, 2024].
22 Jakobsen, "We Are All Sick!"
23 Jakobsen, "We Are All Sick!"
24 Robin Laurence, "How I Became an Artist: Sharona Franklin," ArtBasel, April 28, 2023, www.artbasel.com/stories/sharona-franklin-bioethics-disability-activism-statements-art-basel-2023?lang=en [accessed December 5, 2024].
25 Lutte Collective, "Sharona Franklin," February 2020, https://luttecollective.com/featured-artists/sharona-franklin [link no longer active].
26 Dana Kopel, "Sharona Franklin," Canadian Art, March 18, 2020, https://canadianart.ca/reviews/sharona-franklin/ [accessed December 5, 2024].
27 "Sharona Franklin's New Psychedelia of Industrial Healing," *Editorial Magazine*, March 19, 2020, https://the-editorialmagazine.com/sharona-franklin-kings-leap [accessed December 5, 2024].
28 Leah Triplett Harrington, "A Mediation on Biotech's Cycles of Healing and Harm," *Hyperallergic*, May 29, 2022, https://hyperallergic.com/736112/meditation-on-biotech-cycles-of-healing-harm [accessed December 5, 2024].
29 Bonnie Pitman, "Pharma Art – Abstract Medication in the Work of Beverly Fishman," *JAMA: Journal of the American Medical Association* 319, no. 4 (2018): 326–28. http://dx.doi.org/10.1001/jama.2017.18675
30 Colin Rhodes, *Outsider Art: Spontaneous Alternatives* (London: Thames & Hudson, 2000).
31 Rhodes, *Outsider Art*.
32 Camille Robcis, *Disalienation: Politics, Philosophy, and Radical Psychiatry in Postwar France* (Chicago, IL: University of Chicago Press, 2021).
33 Robcis, *Disalienation*, 3.
34 Robcis, *Disalienation*, 3.
35 Robcis, *Disalienation*, 3.
36 Robcis, *Disalienation*, 3.

Conclusion: moving the needle

In January 2024, Alice Wong (the subject of Riva Lehrer's portrait, which appears as the first image of discussion in the Introduction) posted on Instagram that she had just emerged from a serious medical situation that required a visit to the emergency room and a brief hospitalization in the intensive care unit. Wong was outraged by the fact that so many of the medical practitioners were not wearing N95 masks, particularly those attending to her. As a high-risk disabled patient, Wong is much more vulnerable and at risk of becoming infected by COVID-19. As Wong wrote in her Instagram post, "Disabled, immunocompromised, and chronically ill people know fully well that the world is not designed for us and how we are often dehumanized and considered burdens by the medical industrial complex. It is an exhausting struggle to be seen and heard while fighting to survive in the face of systemic oppression."[1] Wong's urgent call for more masking in hospitals, even when it is no longer mandated by the government in a post-pandemic world, has convinced me to end the book with a final installment of what hospital aesthetics should and can be. Hospital aesthetics must encompass the politics of masking, which is a visible manifestation of illness, safety, care, and compassion. During the height of COVID-19, when people were wearing masks the world over, the mask remained a controversial politic, and yet, because of its abundance, it remained prominent in mind and vision. Now, post-COVID, the mask has been tossed aside, and disabled bodies have also been left to fend for themselves. COVID-19 still causes deaths, and it remains a highly risky illness for disabled people and other minority communities, and it will continue to be for years to come.

Many artists, such as Ruth Cuthand and Pato Herbert, have in fact incorporated the mask into their art-making. The New York City-based artists Noah and Ezra Benus, who founded the Brothers Sick, a sibling artistic collaboration focusing on disability justice, illness, and care, offered potent statements about the nature of sickness and health in a society that disregards disabled bodies and does not acknowledge the merits of collective care. The brothers created a series of masks for an online exhibition at the nonprofit organization Visual AIDS in New York City in 2020. The masks bore statements typed in red text in a serif font, such as "networks of care CAN and SHOULD also be contagious," and "illness finds us all, but care unfortunately does not" (see Figures C.1 and C.2). They drew

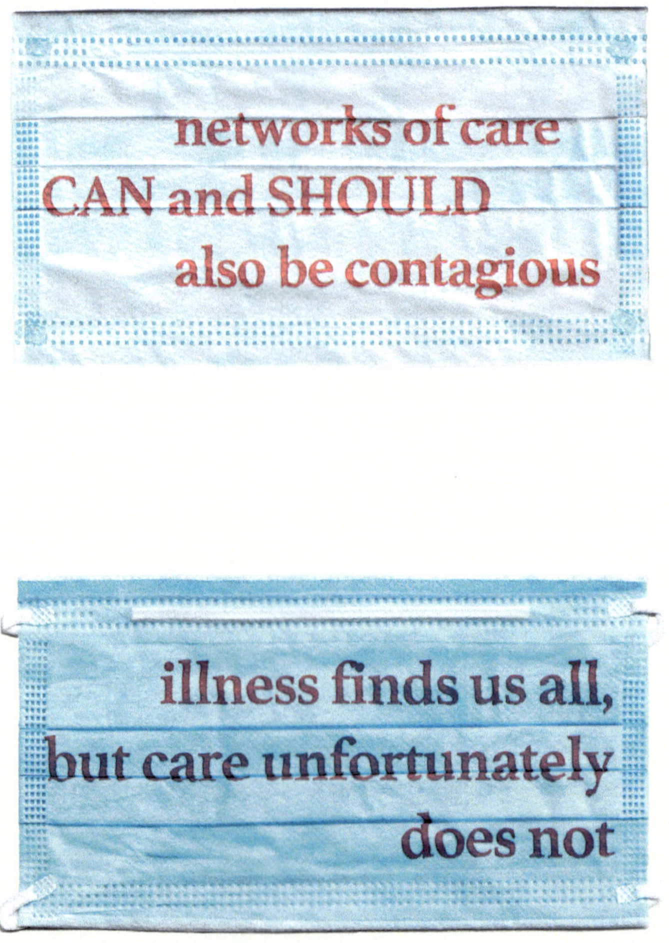

C.1, C.2 Brothers Sick (Ezra and Noah Benus), *Masks*, 2020. Digital prints, dimensions variable. Courtesy of Brothers Sick.

Image description C.1, C.2: Four blue surgical masks positioned one above the other, side by side, perfectly aligned. For the two masks on the left, the top mask has red text that reads "networks of care CAN and SHOULD also be contagious" and the bottom mask reads "illness finds us all, but care unfortunately does not." For the two masks on the right, the top mask has red text that reads "an army of the sick can't be defeated" and the bottom mask reads "to be scared of the sick is to be scared of [the] living."

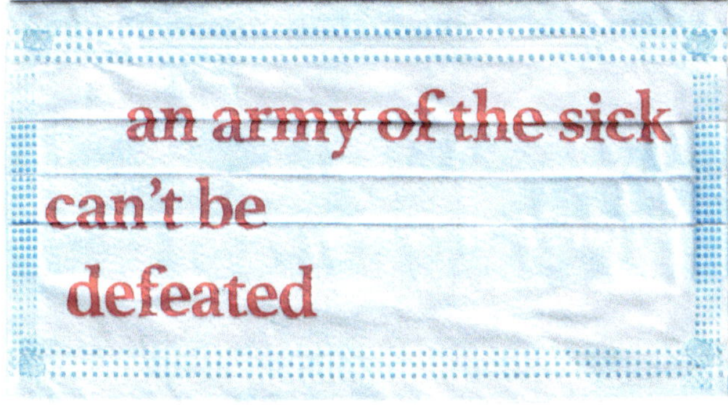

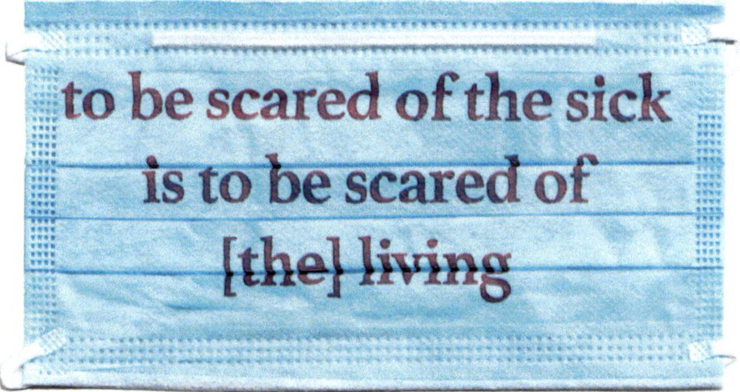

C.1, C.2 Continued

parallels between the AIDS epidemic and COVID-19, and considered questions such as who does get care, and who doesn't? Their reflections also remind us that as a society, in Ezra Benus's words, "we need to center and learn from sick and disabled communities not only during times of widespread illness but as an unwavering constant."[2] They essentially argue for a radical crip ecology, whereby disabled bodies are better protected, sustained, and nourished within interdependent networks of care. Hospital aesthetics thus embraces the mask for its political and aesthetic qualities: as a politic, it unmasks the bias and prejudice within the medical industrial complex, and as an aesthetic, it shows how yet another medical assistive device or prop can be reconstituted to give voice to disabled users and makers. Arguably, the mask has even more potency in promoting political change, given its immediate recognizability for disabled and nondisabled spectators alike.

The aesthetics and politics of the mask are the final step to fully defining hospital aesthetics. In this book, I have defined hospital aesthetics in both *aesthetic* and *political* terms, arguing that within this politics, contemporary disabled artists continue to reject the medical model of disability, as they did in the 1980s when the disabled art movement first emerged. The politics of hospital aesthetics is also deeply intersectional, responding to the medical industrial complex's oppression of minorities and disabled people. The themes I have developed across the chapters – charting immunocompromised bodies, making medical assistive devices and prosthetic devices strange, coupling disability with sexuality, feminist/queer collectives of care, and uncovering alternative medicines – have helped to enrich hospital aesthetics and endow it with a wealth of meaning and possibility, thanks to the work of Dominic Quagliozzi, Carolyn Lazard, Bhavna Mehta, Jesse Darling, Robert Andy Coombs, Panteha Abareshi, Black Womxn Flourish, the Feminist Health Care Research Group, Power Makes Us Sick, the Sick Affinity Group, Park McArthur, Constantina Zavitsanos, Lauryn Youden, Sharona Franklin, and many others. It is no coincidence that more and more artists have turned to this subject matter in the years following the pandemic, and that to be a disabled or immunocompromised artist today is not to be so unusual. Ten years ago when I curated the exhibition *What Can A Body Do?* at Haverford College in Pennsylvania, my show created what I perceive to be a small ripple of a materialist turn in disability art, or a turn away from representation. This interest in the aesthetics of access, or the materials of access, has been an incredibly important development in the history of disability art. This book argues that hospital aesthetics has been a critical development within this history as well, and will likely continue to have an impact in disabled artistic production and practice in the future.

Part of my method in this book has been to show how the work of contemporary disabled artists discussed here can be identified and compared with other art from the past fifty years, whose themes span intersectional identity, health, wellness, life and death, and more. Some of the artists I have mentioned include Bob Flanagan and Sheree Rose, Félix González-Torres, Robert Gober, Senga Nengudi, Katherine Sherwood, Donald Rodney, Matthew Barney, Joseph Beuys, Damian Hirst, and several others. I have employed this comparative methodology in my other writing projects because I have wanted to reinforce how important it is for contemporary disabled art to be perceived and understood as part of the canon of art history, and how it has historically been left out of the discourse. While my deployment of this methodology in this book is similarly motivated, rather than considering that the work in this book remains to be recognized, or has been left out owing to oppression and ableism in the art world, instead I am suggesting that contemporary disabled artists are filling a thematic void that only a few significant artists have addressed in the past fifty years. Artwork that addresses health, sickness, and disability has been scarce, and contemporary disabled artists are leading the way in powerfully engaging with a topic that is timely, and that impacts many more people in our world than previously acknowledged. These artists are also showing us that hospital aesthetics is a political approach to how disabled bodies are systemically ignored or repressed by the wellness industrial complex, and how important it has been and continues to be to vocalize this oppression and pain into a constructive work of art that speaks truth.

Hospital aesthetics: Disability, medicine, activism differs from my earlier monograph, *The Agency of Access: Contemporary Disability Art and Institutional Critique* (2024), in that it looks at how the medical model of disability is being rejected by contemporary disabled artists. This topic is particularly resonant for the post-pandemic climate in which we now all live. *The Agency of Access* traced how access aesthetics and sensory diversity were bringing more attention to the needs of both disabled artists and audiences in the museum, where less attention has been paid to empowering figurative representations of the disabled body by disabled artists in the past decade. The first book was interested in the social model of disability, but numerous other disability studies frameworks too, including crip theory, access intimacy, disability biopolitics, and the materiality of access. Finally, *The Agency of Access* makes a powerful case for the significance of this work in contemporary art worlds and as part of the legacy of art history. By contrast, *Hospital aesthetics* makes a strong case for the importance of recent work in which artists address the lived experiences of their health impairments. These range from chronic illness to life-changing significant injuries, and the artists incorporate the realities, temporalities, and materialities of long-term hospitalization and illness into their creative efforts. In the current moment, there is a wellspring of creativity and interest around this repudiation of the medical industrial complex. This is why I wanted to write *Hospital aesthetics*. I consider my two books to be companion volumes aiming to establish an authentic and critical disability art history that has yet to take hold in the art academy.

In February 2024, Julie McGarry, Professor of Nursing and Gender-Based Violence at the University of Sheffield in the United Kingdom, won an important award for her innovative arts-based healthcare research which she has used to empower domestic abuse survivors. I was particularly struck by how McGarry turned a simple question around to empower the survivor of domestic abuse: instead of the prevailing healthcare framing of "what is the matter with you?," McGarry reasoned that it was much more important to ask, "what matters to you?" This simple shift in the line of questioning – from one that proceeds from the curative imperative to one invested in what the patient actually needs – has the potential to truly change the way healthcare professionals respond to disabled patients. Indeed, all the contemporary art I have discussed in this book illustrates this desire to ask what matters and why. The medical industrial complex could certainly learn from this work and the artists behind it. While I'm pleased that medical scholars and practitioners like McGarry are taking the time to sit down and actually listen to their patients, this type of reflective thinking is sorely overdue.

When I first started working on disability arts curating and activism in 2010, I thought work that addressed representations of the sick body was less common than works that deal with challenging the senses, which is the subject of my first book, *The Agency of Access*. In fact, I thought that straightforward, even mechanical, representations of the disabled body as refutations of the medical model of disability were outdated and no longer a useful or relevant topic. But COVID-19 in 2020 changed all that, and I was forced to step back and examine all the work exploding around me that was dealing with artists' misgivings about the medical system. While it is still true that some contemporary disabled artists have stepped away from representation and instead offer more abstract and material explorations of the disabled body in their practices, critiques of the medical industrial complex are stronger than ever before. While this is, in part, due to COVID-19 putting health, access, and wellness at the forefront of all our minds, particularly in the art world, this book has shone a light on the many artistic predecessors who paved the way for younger generations of disabled artists to advance their medical critiques, their activism, and their politics. In a way, it is almost disappointing that there needs to be so much work that explores these grievances with the health industrial complex, because it means our heath and wellness system is unhealthy and unwell, particularly in its ongoing systemic violence and mistreatment of disabled patients.

At the same time as this work was unfolding during a worldwide pandemic, the art world was also being shaken up by the urgent call to decolonize the museum in the context of the recent Black Lives Matter movement. Given the parallel emergence of Black Lives Matter and the pandemic, it made sense that the hospital and the art gallery should be in a productive dialogue about how their spaces can help one another to support the most vulnerable people in our population. Simply put, galleries should and must show more work by disabled, BIPOC, and intersectionally identifying artists. As I mentioned in the Introduction, hospital aesthetics can help to challenge and transform both the hospital and the art gallery into more welcoming sites, where the two venues can share critical dialogue and resources regarding the treatment of disabled bodies. Both the art gallery and the hospital can benefit from *talking with* disabled users (visitors and patients if you will) instead of *talking to* them. In lieu of a depersonalized, top–down approach, these institutions can invite disability in and have a productive conversation. Hospitals and art galleries play an important role in our society; we need them, but they also need us. Hospitals would not exist if there wasn't a need from patients, and art galleries would not thrive if they did not have audiences. Both of these institutions should pay heed to the people who use them, and shed the obsolete policies and practices passed down from their historical origins in colonialism and capitalism.

The revolt against hierarchy in the hospital is mirrored in the art museum, because artists are annoyed with how they are being treated when they go to the hospital *and* when they go to the art gallery. I've been annoyed too, so I get it. It is up to us to change it. The rationale for the hospital and the gallery to be in communication is simply that they can help one another, and learn new things and gain new perspectives. This idea is not exactly new, as I outlined in the Introduction. There is a massive industry dedicated to how the arts can help the hospital and its patients, encompassing professional and academic organizations such as the National Organization for Arts in Health (NOAH), conferences, and working groups. But the industry I'm talking about here is not the wellness industry (which is also a capitalist marketing scheme that many of the artists in this book detest). It is a hospital aesthetics rendered and enacted by contemporary disabled and sick artists, providing unique insights that can be incorporated by both the hospital and the art gallery in powerful, game-changing ways. Similarly, the hospital – and certainly the desire for healing – is being brought more frequently and with more urgency into the gallery by many artists, including Grace Ndiritu as discussed in the Introduction, and others like Simone Leigh and Guadalupe Maravilla. But the contemporary disabled artists discussed in this book are set apart from these artists because they are offering a uniquely disabled perspective that insists on a wider scope of consideration and reflection by those in power. So the hospital and the art museum could serve to become more *hospitable* as an outcome of studying and implementing hospital aesthetics.

While I have attempted to cover some of the major trajectories and missions of contemporary disabled artists working today, it is also impossible to cover everyone, and I hope that other scholars and art critics will bring more attention to these vital practices in the near future. One major area that needs more attention is the critique of the medical industrial complex by patients with mental health issues including depression and anxiety, and from the perspective of artists with intellectual disabilities. I sincerely hope these topics can be covered in more depth by other art historians committed to topics of disability, and by scholars in the critical medical humanities committed to arts-based issues. While it is true that an aesthetics of health is more popular and relevant than ever before, we must remind ourselves that disabled individuals and other minorities need to be centered in these conversations and dialogues.

Now that we have reached the end of the book, what can be done about the treatment of disabled patients in the medical industrial complex? What is an ideal, or above average, scenario? What if there was no need for hospital aesthetics anymore, and instead I could change the title of the book to hospitable aesthetics after all? Not too long ago, I gave a brief presentation of hospital aesthetics for some colleagues in the arts and medical humanities field. I told these colleagues the story of how my genetics and maternity care providers wanted to give me the option of terminating my pregnancy once we all learned that my daughter had achondroplasia after some testing. There was a silence on the Zoom call, which I took to signal a collective reaction of shock, but also perhaps an indication that others in the virtual room were unable to relate to this experience of ableism that had transpired in a medical setting. Indeed, they seemed lost for words. It left me with the impression that many folks still don't really understand or are not even aware of the kinds of problematic exchanges that take place between disabled patients and doctors, hence the importance of hospital aesthetics. The work of this book is raising awareness; it is helping to show how the hospital and the art gallery have a lot in common because both spaces must decolonize to become more inclusive, and that both spaces could really learn to proactively listen and empathize. While there are increasing partnerships and collaborations between galleries and hospitals as they recognize that they each have resources that could benefit the pedagogical development of professionals across both sectors, I hope that disability frameworks can enter into these conversations with more frequency.

I wish I could say that hospital aesthetics is a term that will be short-lived. But it is more likely that it will become a tool that will be further sharpened by contemporary disabled artists to incise an industry in dire need of radical crip care and critique.

Notes

1 Wong, Alice (@disability_visibility), "Help me urge @ucsfhealth to require all staff, patients, and visitors to wear N95 masks. My recent column in Teen Vogue about the surge and its impact on me as a high risk disabled person became a terrifying reality when I had a medical emergency that required a visit to the ER and brief hospitalization in the ICU. Disabled, immunocompromised, and chronically ill people know fully well that the world is not designed for us and how we are often dehumanized and considered burdens by the medical industrial complex. It is an exhausting struggle to be seen and heard while fighting to survive in the face of systemic oppression. While I was in the hospital I tweeted some of my experiences because I needed to document what was happening and do something while filled with fear. Writing and organizing is a way to channel my rage and process my medical trauma. I call upon you all to help me push for a N95 mask mandate at UCSF Health. No one should

have to delay care or risk infection from COVID when receiving necessary medical care. Image description: A picture of me, an Asian American disabled woman. There is a tracheostomy at my throat connected to a ventilator tube. A white gauze dressing is tucked around the tracheostomy. I am wearing a camouflage jacket. My eyes are swollen after crying uncontrollably for hours and barely able to open. I look miserable." Instagram post, January 25, 2024, www.instagram.com/p/C2iRdEIPz7L/?hl=en [accessed December 5, 2024].

2 Visual AIDS, "April Web Gallery Curator Talk: Ezra and Noah Benus," https://visualaids.org/events/detail/benus-curator-talk [accessed January 19, 2025].

Bibliography

Primary sources

"Art, Health, and Accessibility: A Conversation with Laura Lulika of the Sickness Affinity Group." Podcast, 44:59, October 26, 2021. *Critical Diversity Podcast*, produced by Critical Diversity AG, Berlin University of the Arts. https://anchor.fm/critical-diversity/episodes/Art—Health—and-Accessibility-A-Conversation-With-Laura-Lulika-of-the-Sickness-Affinity-Group-e19a8p6 [accessed December 5, 2024].

Benevedes, Jeffrey Mouton. "Shifting Identity, Emerging Self: An Interview with Robert Andy Coombs, aka CripFag." *JungJournal: Culture & Psyche* 14, no. 1 (2020): 103–23. https://doi.org/10.1080/19342039.2020.1706393

Black Women's Health Imperative. https://bwhi.org [accessed April 10, 2024].

Black Womxn Flourish. "Our Collective Update: We're Entering an Extended Period of Trans Formation." Instagram post (@blackwomxnflourish), March 15, 2023. www.instagram.com/p/Cp0gSPbuLq9 [accessed December 5, 2024].

——. www.blackwomxnflourish.co [accessed April 10, 2024].

Damman, Catherine. "Carolyn Lazard by Catherine Damman [Interview]." *BOMB*, September 10, 2020. https://bombmagazine.org/articles/2020/09/10/carolyn-lazard [accessed December 5, 2024].

Grigely, Joseph. "Cripping the World." Email to his SAIC students, shared by Corbett O'Toole with permission. Facebook post, April 24, 2020.

Jakobsen, Jakob. "We Are All Sick!" *Palette*, February 11, 2020. https://paletten.net/artiklar/we-are-all-sick [accessed December 5, 2024].

Laurence, Robin. "How I Became an Artist: Sharona Franklin." ArtBasel, April 28, 2023. www.artbasel.com/stories/sharona-franklin-bioethics-disability-activism-statements-art-basel-2023?lang=en [accessed December 5, 2024].

Lazard, Carolyn. "How to Be a Person in the Age of Autoimmunity." *Cluster Magazine*, January, 2013.

——. "The World is Unknown" [digital project]. *Triple Canopy*, April 19, 2019. https://tc3.canopycanopycanopy.com/issues/24/contents/the-world-is-unknown [accessed December 5, 2024].

Mitchell, David T., and Sharon L. Snyder, dirs. *Vital Signs: Crip Culture Talks Back*. Brooklyn, NY: Icarus Films, 1995. VHS, 48 minutes.

Plender, Olivia. *Our Bodies Are Not the Problem, the Problem is Power* [installation, Glasgow Women's Library]. https://oliviaplender.org/many-maids-make-much-noise/installation-life-support–forms-of-care-in-art [accessed April 10, 2024].

Power Makes Us Sick. https://powermakesussick.noblogs.org/about-us/ [accessed January 19, 2025].

——. "Most of us are not doctors and some of us can't go to the doctor, but everything that is living will at some point fall ill. Although we prefer to thrive amongst the well, illness rests like the other side of the coin. And in another way, we are all sick under late capitalism or, we are all sick when alienated from our activity, from the places where we rest, from one another. We are all crazy when someone or something else has the ability to diagnose us against our will. When the air we breathe is toxic, we all suffer indeterminately. As we learn to take care of one another's health the state can't but fail, or at least we would no longer be bothered if it did. In May PMS led a workshop called How Are You Feeling Today? We facilitated a playful discussion to dissect the vocabulary of sickness and illness. We closed with a visualization exercise towards an aspirational idea of 'health'." Tumblr post, 2018. https://powermakesussick.tumblr.com/post/175046750302/workshop-in-the-st%C3%A4ndige-vertretung-we-call-it [accessed December 1, 2021].

Saltz, Jerry. "Yes, This is Me: Robert Andy Coombs Shows Us a Gorgeous Orchidology of Sexual Desire." *New York Magazine*, February 3, 2020.

Schons, Donna. "Resting Place." *PW-Magazine*, March 19, 2023. https://pw-magazine.com/2023/resting-place [accessed December 5, 2024].

Smith, Roberta. "Bob Flanagan, 43, Performer Who Fashioned Art From His Pain." *New York Times*, January 6, 1996.

Taylor, Sunaura. "Artist Statement." Wynn Newhouse Awards. www.wnewhouseawards.com/sunaurataylor2.html [accessed December 9, 2023].

——. "What Would Health Security Look Like?" *Boston Review*, May 28, 2020. www.bostonreview.net/articles/sunaura-taylor-title-forthcoming [accessed December 5, 2024].

Visual AIDS. "April Web Gallery Curator Talk: Ezra and Noah Benus." https://visualaids.org/events/detail/benus-curator-talk [accessed January 19, 2025].

Watlington, Emily. "Chronicling Illness." *Art in America*, September 2, 2021. www.artnews.com/art-in-america/features/chronicling-illness-guadalupe-maravilla-carolyn-lazard-1234602858 [accessed December 5, 2024].

——. "'Golem Girl': An Interview with Riva Lehrer." *Art Papers*, Winter 2018/19. www.artpapers.org/golem-girl-an-interview-with-riva-lehrer [accessed June 30, 2023].

—— and Panteha Abareshi. "Between Bondage and Bandage." Podcast, 67:00, May, 2023. *Kunsthall Trondheim Podcast*, produced by Kunsthall Trondheim. https://soundcloud.com/kunsthalltrondheim/18-panteha-abareshi [accessed December 5, 2024].

Wong, Alice. "Alice Wong on Hospitalization, Crowdfunding Medical Care, and Finding Love in Community." *Teen Vogue*, February 14, 2023. www.teenvogue.com/story/alice-wong-hospitalization-crowdfunding-community [accessed December 5, 2024].

——. "Help me urge @ucsfhealth to require all staff, patients, and visitors to wear N95 masks. My recent column in Teen Vogue about the surge and its impact on me as a high risk disabled person became a terrifying reality when I had a medical emergency that required a visit to the ER and brief hospitalization in the ICU. Disabled, immunocompromised, and chronically ill people know fully well that the world is not designed for us and how we are often dehumanized and considered burdens by the medical industrial complex. It is an exhausting struggle to be seen and heard while fighting to survive in the face of systemic oppression. While I was in the hospital I tweeted some of my experiences because I needed to document what was happening and do something while filled with fear. Writing and organizing is a way to channel my rage and process my medical trauma. I call upon you all to help me push for a N95 mask mandate at UCSF Health. No one should have to delay care or risk infection from COVID when receiving necessary medical care. Image description: A picture of me, an Asian American disabled woman. There is a tracheostomy at my throat connected to a ventilator tube. A white gauze dressing is tucked around the tracheostomy. I am wearing a camouflage jacket. My eyes are swollen after crying uncontrollably for hours and barely able to open. I look miserable." Instagram post (@disability_visibility), January 25, 2024. www.instagram.com/p/C2iRdEIPz7L/?hl=en [accessed December 5, 2024].

Secondary sources

Abareshi, Panteha. "Disabled, Chronically Ill, Severe Artist." *Massachusetts Review* 63, no. 4 (Winter 2022): 681–92. https://dx.doi.org/10.1353/mar.2022.0100

Aristarkhova, Irina. *Arrested Welcome: Hospitality in Contemporary Art*. Minneapolis, MN: University of Minnesota Press, 2020.

Barton, Brit. "Interdependencies: Perspectives on Care and Resilience." *Mousse Magazine*, November 13, 2023. www.moussemagazine.it/magazine/interdependencies-brit-barton-migros-museum-zurich-2023 [accessed December 5, 2024].

Beilin, Caren and Feminist Health Care Research Group. "Medicine & Misogyny." *Art in America*, October 8, 2021. www.artnews.com/art-in-america/interviews/feminist-health-care-research-group-caren-beilin-1234606473 [accessed December 5, 2024].

Bellamy, Dodie. *When the Sick Rule the World*. Cambridge, MA: MIT Press, 2015.

Berne, Patty. "Disability Justice – A Working Draft." Sins Invalid (blog), June 10, 2015. For more information, see https://sinsinvalid.org/10-principles-of-disability-justice/ [accessed January 19, 2025].

Billimore, Yvonne. "Introduction: Matter(s) of Security." In *Rehearsing Hospitalities Companion 3*, edited by Yvonne Billimore and Jussi Koitela, 13–29. Berlin: Archive Books, 2022.

Birkett, Richard. "A Promise and a Practice: Carolyn Lazard." *Mousse Magazine*, October 13, 2020. www.moussemagazine.it/magazine/carolyn-lazard-richard-birkett-2020 [accessed December 5, 2024].

Bishop, Claire. *Artificial Hells: Participatory Art and the Politics of Spectatorship*. London: Verso, 2012.

Bonn, Julia, Inga Zimprich, and Chloe Stead. "The Feminist Health Care Research Group Fights Art-World Exploitation." *Frieze*, April 19, 2021. www.frieze.com/article/feminist-health-care-research-group-fights-art-world-exploitation [accessed December 5, 2024].

Bourriaud, Nicolas. *Relational Aesthetics*. Dijon: Les presses du reel, 1998.

Bradley, Rizvana. "Transferred Flesh: Reflections on Senga Nengudi's 'R.S.V.P.'" *Drama Review* 59, no. 1 (Spring 2015): 161–66.

Cachia, Amanda. "Disability, Curating, and the Educational Turn: The Contemporary Condition of Access in the Museum." *OnCurating* 24 (December 2014). www.on-curating.org/issue-24-reader/disability-curating-and-the-educational-turn-the-contemporary-condition-of-access-in-the-museum.html [accessed December 5, 2024].

——. "Disabling Surrealism: Reconstituting Surrealist Tropes in Contemporary Art." In *Disability and History*, edited by Ann Millett-Gallant and Elizabeth Howie, 132–54. New York: Routledge, 2017.

Campbell, Margaret. "What Tuberculosis did for Modernism: The Influence of a Curative Environment on Modernist Design and Architecture." *Medical History: An International Journal for the History of Medicine and the Related Sciences* 49, no. 4 (2005): 463–88. https://doi.org/10.1017/s0025727300009169

Cartwright, Lisa. *Screening the Body: Tracing Medicine's Visual Culture*. Minneapolis, MN: University of Minnesota Press, 1995.

Chen, Mel. *Intoxicated*. Durham, NC: Duke University Press, 2023.

Colomina, Beatriz. *X-Ray Architecture*. Baden, Switzerland: Lars Müller Publishers, 2019.

Das, Jareh. "Illness as Metaphor: Donald Rodney's X-ray Photographs." *Nka: Journal of Contemporary African Art* 45 (November 2019): 88–98. https://muse.jhu.edu/article/738989 [accessed December 5, 2024].

Derrida, Jacques. *Hospitality*, Vol. 1, translated by E. S. Burt, edited by Pascale-Anne Brault and Peggy Kamuf. Chicago, IL: University of Chicago Press, 2023.

Dokumaci, Arseli. *Activist Affordances: How Disabled People Improvise More Habitable Worlds*. Durham, NC: Duke University Press, 2023.

Drugeon, Fanny. *Collection art contemporain – La collection du Centre Pompidou, Musée national d'art modern*. Paris: Centre Pompidou, 2007.

Eschner, Kat. "In 1913, Henry Ford Introduced the Assembly Line: His Workers Hated it." *Smithsonian Magazine*, December 1, 2016. www.smithsonianmag.com/smart-news/one-hundred-and-three-years-ago-today-henry-ford-introduced-assembly-line-his-workers-hated-it-180961267 [accessed December 5, 2024].

Feldman, Julia Pelta. *Carolyn Lazard, Support System (for Tina, Park, Bob): Sunday, October 30, 2016*. Brooklyn, NY: Room & Board, 2016. https://roomandboard.nyc/wp-content/uploads/2018/04/support-system-book-with-cover.pdf [accessed January 22, 2024].

Feminist Health Care Research Group. *Being in Crises Together*. www.think-tank.nl/health/zines.html [accessed December 1, 2021].

Fink, Marty. *Forget Burial: HIV Kinship, Disability, and Queer/Trans Narratives of Care*. New Brunswick, NJ: Rutgers University Press, 2020.

Folland, Thomas. "Felix Gonzalez-Torres, 'Untitled' *(Billboard of an Empty Bed)*." Smarthistory. https://smarthistory.org/felix-gonzalez-torres-untitled-billboard-of-an-empty-bed [accessed January 22, 2024].

Funk, Tiffany. "The Prosthetic Aesthetic: An Art of Anxious Extensions." https://digitalcommons.wayne.edu/macaa2012scholarship/1/ [accessed January 20, 2025].

Garland-Thomson, Rosemarie. "Dares to Stares: Disabled Women Performance Artists & the Dynamics of Staring." In *Bodies in Commotion: Disability & Performance*, edited by Carrie Sandahl and Philip Auslander, 30–41. Ann Arbor, MI: University of Michigan Press, 2005.

——. "Feminist Disability Studies." *Signs: Journal of Women in Culture and Society* 30, no. 2 (Winter 2005): 1557–87. https://doi.org/10.1086/423352

——. *Staring: How We Look*. Oxford: Oxford University Press, 2009.

Getsy, David J. "How to Teach Manet's Olympia after Transgender Studies." *Art History* 45, no. 2 (2022): 342–69. https://doi.org/10.1111/1467-8365.12647

Gillberg, Claudia. "Disability Experiences, Memoirs, Autobiographies, and Other Personal Narratives." *Disability & Society* 35, no. 9 (2020): 1527–29. https://doi.org/10.1080/09687599.2020.1744253

Gleeson, Sinéad. "A Different Kind of Healing." *Frieze*, September 7, 2020. www.frieze.com/article/different-kind-healing [accessed December 5, 2024].

Gruwell, Leigh. *Making Matters: Craft, Ethics, and New Materialist Rhetorics*. Denver, CO: University Press of Colorado, 2022.

Gupta, Kristina. *Medical Entanglements: Rethinking Feminist Debates About Healthcare*. New Brunswick, NJ: Rutgers University Press, 2020.

Hadley, Bree. *Disability, Public Space, Performance and Spectatorship*. New York: Palgrave Macmillan, 2014.

Happe, Kelly E., Jenell Johnson, and Marina Levina, eds. *Biocitizenship: The Politics of Bodies, Governance, and Power*. New York: New York University Press, 2018.

Harrington, Leah Triplett. "A Mediation on Biotech's Cycles of Healing and Harm." *Hyperallergic*, May 29, 2022. https://hyperallergic.com/736112/meditation-on-biotech-cycles-of-healing-harm [accessed December 5, 2024].

Hattrick, Alice. *Ill Feelings*. London: Fitzcarraldo Editions, 2021.

Hawkins, Anne Hunsaker. *Reconstructing Illness: Studies in Pathology*. West Lafayette, IN: Purdue University Press, 1998.

Hedva, Johanna. "Sick Woman Theory + Get Well Soon (both 2020)." Kunstverein Hildesheim. www.kunstverein-hildesheim.de/caring-structures-ausstellung-digital/johanna-hedva/ [accessed December 5, 2024].

——. "Sick Woman Theory," edited by Hanna Hurr and Isabelle Nastasia. *Mask Magazine*, January, 2016.

Hickman, Louise, and David Serlin. "Towards a Crip Methodology for Critical Disability Studies." In *Interdisciplinary Approaches to Disability: Looking Towards the Future*, edited by Katie Ellis, Rosemarie Garland-Thomson, Mike Kent, and Rachel Robertson, 131–41. New York: Routledge, 2019.

Holmes, Heather. "On Jesse Darling." *Journal of Visual Culture* 19, no. 2 (2020): 272–76. https://doi.org/10.1177/1470412920944482

Jackson, Shannon. *Social Works: Performing Art, Supporting Publics*. New York: Routledge, 2011.

Jacobs, Keisha. "Motifs of Social Maladies Abide: Remembering the Artistic Legacy of Donald Rodney." Arts Help website, 2021. www.artshelp.com/donald-rodney [accessed February 10, 2024].

Jain, Sarah S. "The Prosthetic Imagination: Enabling and Disabling the Prosthesis Trope." *Science, Technology & Human Values* 24, no. 1 (Winter 1999): 31–54. www.jstor.org/stable/690238 [accessed December 5, 2024].

Kafai, Shayda. *Crip Kinship: The Disability Justice and Arts Activism of Sins Invalid*. Vancouver: Arsenal Pulp Press, 2021.

Kai Matsumiya gallery. "Maryam Jafri *War on Wellness*." Press release, 2017. https://kaimatsumiya.com/maryam-jafri-war-on-wellness [accessed December 5, 2024].

Kaino, Lorna. *The Necessity of Craft: Development and Women's Craft Practices in the Asian-Pacific Region*. Perth: UWA Publishing, 1995.

Kester, Grant. *Conversation Pieces: Community and Communication in Modern Art*. Berkeley, CA: University of California Berkeley Press, 2004.

——. *The One and the Many: Contemporary Collaborative Art in a Global Context*. Durham, NC: Duke University Press, 2011.

Kittay, Eva Feder. *Learning from My Daughter: The Value and Care of Disabled Minds*. Oxford: Oxford University Press, 2019.

——. *Love's Labor: Essays on Women, Equality, and Dependency*. New York: Routledge, 1999.

——. *Love's Labor: Essays on Women, Equality and Dependency*, 2nd ed. New York: Routledge, 2020.

——. "The Ethics of Care, Dependency, and Disability." *Ratio Juris* 24, no. 1 (February 2011): 49–58. https://doi.org/10.1111/j.1467-9337.2010.00473.x

Knadler, Stephen. *Vitality Politics: Health, Debility, and the Limits of Black Emancipation*. Ann Arbor, MI: University of Michigan Press, 2019. Kindle.

Kopel, Dana. "Sharona Franklin." Canadian Art, March 18, 2020. https://canadianart.ca/reviews/sharona-franklin [accessed December 5, 2024].

Kudlick, Catherine. "Comment: On the Borderland of Medical and Disability History." *Bulletin of the History of Medicine* 87, no. 4 (Winter 2013): 540–59. https://doi.org/10.1353/bhm.2013.0086

Kuppers, Petra. *The Scar of Visibility: Medical Performances and Contemporary Art*. Minneapolis, MN: University of Minnesota Press, 2007.

Kurzman, Steven L. "Presence and Prosthesis: A Response to Nelson and Wright." *Cultural Anthropology* 16, no. 3 (August 2001): 374–87. www.jstor.org/stable/656681 [accessed December 5, 2024].

Lee, James Kyung-Jin. *Pedagogies of Woundedness: Illness, Memoir, and the Ends of the Model Minority*. Philadelphia, PA: Temple University Press, 2021.

Lehrer, Riva. *Golem Girl*. New York: Penguin Random House, 2020.

Lerner, Rosalia. "'Get Well Soon!' Sick Bodied Performance of Chronic Conditions." PhD dissertation, University of California, Riverside, 2022. https://escholarship.org/uc/item/90q3435t [accessed December 5, 2024].

Loviglio, Joann. "Albert M. Kligman, Dermatologist Who Patented Retin-A, Dies at 93." *Washington Post*, February 21, 2010. www.washingtonpost.com/wp-dyn/content/article/2010/02/21/AR2010022104116.html [accessed December 5, 2024].

Lutte Collective. "Sharona Franklin." February 2020. https://luttecollective.com/featured-artists/sharona-franklin [link no longer active].

MacPhee-Pitcher, Sam. "Undeliverable and What it is to Care." Akimblog (blog). Akimbo, October 29, 2021. https://akimbo.ca/akimblog/undeliverable-what-it-is-to-care-by-sam-macphee-pitcher.

McArthur, Park and Constantina Zavitsanos. "Ode to 1 & Under." *Arika*. https://arika.org.uk/ode-1-under/ [accessed January 19, 2025].

——, and Other Forms of Conviviality: The Best and Least of Which is Our Daily Care and the Host of Which is Our Collaborative Work." *Women & Performance: A Journal of Feminist Theory* 23, no. 1 (2013): 126–32. https://doi.org/10.1080/0740770X.2013.827376

McMillan, Uri. *Embodied Avatars: Genealogies of Black Feminist Art and Performance*. New York: New York University Press, 2015. Kindle.

Meldon, Perri. "Disability History: Early and Shifting Attitudes of Treatment." National Park Service. www.nps.gov/articles/disabilityhistoryearlytreatment.htm [accessed December 9, 2023].

Mercer, Kobena, ed., *Pop Art and Vernacular Cultures*. Cambridge, MA: MIT Press, 2007.

Millett-Gallant, Ann. *The Disabled Body in Contemporary Art*. New York: Palgrave Macmillan, 2010.

Minich, Julie Avril. *Radical Health: Unwellness, Care, and LatinX Expressive Culture*. Durham, NC: Duke University Press, 2023.

Mitchell, David T., and Sharon L. Snyder. "Talking About Talking Back: Afterthoughts on the Making of the Disability Documentary *Vital Signs: Crip Culture Talks Back*." *Michigan Quarterly Review* 37, no. 2 (Spring 1998). http://hdl.handle.net/2027/spo.act2080.0037.216 [accessed December 5, 2024].

Molesworth, Helen. "Art is Medicine: Helen Molesworth on the Work of Simone Leigh." *Artforum* 56, no. 7 (March 2018).

Morales, Aurora Levins. *Medicine Stories: Essays for Radicals*. Durham, NC: Duke University Press, 2019.

Mulvey, Laura. "Visual Pleasure and Narrative Cinema." *Screen* 16, no. 3 (Autumn 1975): 6–18. https://doi.org/10.1093/screen/16.3.6

Musser, Amber Jamilla. "From Our Body to Yourselves: The Boston Women's Health Book Collective and Changing Notions of Subjectivity, 1969–1973." *Women's Studies Quarterly* 25, no. 1/2 (Spring/Summer 2007): 93–109. www.jstor.org/stable/27649656 [accessed December 5, 2024].

Nishida, Akemi. *Just Care: Messy Entanglements of Disability, Dependency, and Desire*. Philadelphia, PA: Temple University Press, 2022.

Nochlin, Linda. *The Body in Pieces: The Fragment as a Metaphor of Modernity*. London: Thames and Hudson, 1994.

O'Brien, Martin. "Lie Back and Take It: BDSM, Biomedicine and the Hospital Bed in the Work of Bob Flanagan and Sheree Rose." *Body, Space & Technology* 15 (2016). http://doi.org/10.16995/bst.18

Ott, Katherine. "The Sum of its Parts: An Introduction to Modern Histories of Prosthetics." In *Artificial Parts, Practical Lives: Modern Histories of Prosthetics*, edited by Katherine Ott, David Serlin, and Stephen Mihm, 1–43. New York: New York University Press, 2002.

Ozga, Kasia. "The Internal Frontier: How Art at Once Problematizes Borders and Draws Us Closer to Them." *Contemporaneity: Historical Presence in Visual Culture* 6, no. 1 (2017): 1–18. https://doi.org/10.5195/contemp.2017.186

Palmer, Abi. *Sanatorium*. London: Penned in the Margins, 2020.

Papalia, Carmen. "A New Model for Access in the Museum." *Disability Studies Quarterly* 33, no. 3 (2013). http://dsq-sds.org/article/view/3757/3280 [accessed December 5, 2024].

——. "Bodies of Knowledge: Open Sourcing Disability Experience." *Journal of Cultural and Literary Disability Studies* 9, no. 3 (2015): 357–64. https://muse.jhu.edu/article/596373 [accessed December 5, 2024].

Piepzna-Samarasinha, Leah Lakshmi. *Care Work: Dreaming Disability Justice*. Vancouver: Arsenal Pulp Press, 2018.

Pitman, Bonnie. "Pharma Art – Abstract Medication in the Work of Beverly Fishman." *JAMA: Journal of the American Medical Association* 319, no. 4 (2018): 326–28. http://dx.doi.org/10.1001/jama.2017.18675

Puar, Jasbir. *The Right to Maim: Debility, Capacity, Disability*. Durham, NC: Duke University Press, 2017.

Quaintance, Don. "Modern Art in a Modern Setting: Frederick Kiesler's Design of Art of This Century." In *Peggy Guggenheim and Frederick Kiesler: The Story of Art of This Century*, edited by Susan Davidson and Philip Rylands, 207–73. New York: Guggenheim Museum Publications, 2004.

"Refuge in the Means." Recess Art website. www.recessart.org/projects/50-refuge-in-the-means [accessed April 11, 2024].

Reznick, Jordan. "Through the Guillotine Mirror: Claude Cahun's Theory of Trans Against the Void." *Art Journal* 81, no. 3 (Fall 2022): 53–69. https://doi.org/10.1080/00043249.2022.2110440

Rhodes, Colin. *Outsider Art: Spontaneous Alternatives*. London: Thames & Hudson, 2000.

Riva, Anna. *Secrets of Magical Seals: A Modern Grimoire of Amulets, Charms, Symbols and Talismans*. New York: International Imports, 1975.

Robcis, Camille. *Disalienation: Politics, Philosophy, and Radical Psychiatry in Postwar France*. Chicago, IL: University of Chicago Press, 2021.

Rose, Sarah F. *No Right to be Idle*. Chapel Hill, NC: University of North Carolina Press, 2017. Kindle.

Schalk, Sami. *Black Disability Politics*. Durham, NC: Duke University Press, 2022.

"Sharona Franklin's New Psychedelia of Industrial Healing." *Editorial Magazine*, March 19, 2020. https://the-editorialmagazine.com/sharona-franklin-kings-leap [accessed December 5, 2024].

Sherwood, Katherine. "How a Cerebral Hemorrhage Altered My Art." *Frontiers in Human Neuroscience* 6 (April 2012): 1–5. https://doi.org/10.3389/fnhum.2012.00055

Shildrick, Margrit. "Contested Pleasures: The Sociopolitical Economy of Disability and Sexuality." *Sexuality Research and Social Policy: Journal of NSRC* 4, no. 1 (March 2007): 53–66. https://doi.org/10.1525/srsp.2007.4.1.53

Shuttleworth, Russell, and Linda R. Mona, eds. *The Routledge Handbook of Disability and Sexuality*. New York: Routledge, 2021.

Siebers, Tobin. *Disability Aesthetics*. Ann Arbor, MI: University of Michigan Press, 2010.

Slater, Ella. "Grace Ndiritu Heals the Museum." *Frieze*, April 24, 2023. www.frieze.com/article/grace-ndiritu-heals-museum-review-2023 [accessed December 5, 2024].

Slavin, Ruth, Ray Williams, and Corinne Zimmermann, eds. *Activating the Art Museum: Designing Experiences for the Health Professions*. New York: Rowman & Littlefield, 2023.

Small, Zachary. "For Chronically Ill Artists, Coronavirus is the Worst-Case Scenario." *ARTnews*, March 13, 2020. www.artnews.com/art-news/artists/coronavirus-artists-chronic-illnesses-resources-1202681100 [accessed December 5, 2024].

Smith, Giulia. "Chronic Illness as Critique: Crip Aesthetics Across the Atlantic." *Art History* 44, no. 2 (April 2021): 286–310. https://doi.org/10.1111/1467-8365.12559

——. "Health v Wealth." *Art Monthly*, July–August 2018. www.artmonthly.co.uk/magazine/site/article/health-v-wealth-by-giulia-smith-jul-aug-2018 [accessed December 5, 2024].

Smith, Marquard, and Joanne Morra, eds. *The Prosthetic Impulse: From a Posthuman Present to a Biocultural Future*. Cambridge, MA: MIT Press, 2005.

Sobchack, Vivian. *Carnal Thoughts: Embodiment and Moving Image Culture*. Berkeley, CA: University of California Press, 2004.

Stiker, Henri-Jacques. *A History of Disability*. Ann Arbor, MI: University of Michigan Press, 1999.

Stramondo, Joseph A. "A Critique of the Curative Imperative." *Surgery* 171, no. 4 (2020): 1121–22. www.surgjournal.com/article/S0039-6060(21)00966-1/abstract [accessed December 5, 2024].

Tagg, John. *The Burden of Representation: Essays on Photographies and Histories*. Minneapolis, MN: University of Minnesota Press, 1993.

"What Would an HIV Doula Do?" *HIV Doula Work*. https://hivdoula.work [accessed April 15, 2024].

Willems, Laureanne. "On Caring Through Sharing and Reading When Seeing: Attending to Formal Potentialities of Illness Narratives." *Literature and Medicine* 40, no. 1 (Spring 2022): 38–54. https://doi.org/10.1353/lm.2022.0008

Wong, Alice. *Year of the Tiger: An Activist's Life*. New York: Vintage, 2022.

Yi, Chun-Shan (Sandie). "Res(crip)ting Art Therapy: Disability Culture as a Social Justice Intervention." In *Art Therapy for Social Justice: Radical Intersections*, edited by Savneet K. Talwar, 161–77. New York: Routledge, 2019.

——. "From Imperfect to I am Perfect: Reclaiming the Disabled Body Through Making Body Adornments in Art Therapy." In *Materials and Media in Art Therapy: Critical Understanding of Diverse Artistic Vocabularies*, edited by Catherine Hyland Moon, 103–17. New York: Routledge, 2010.

Zimprich, Inga, and Julia Bonn. *Practices of Radical Health Care: Materials of the Health Movement of the Seventies and Eighties*. Berlin: Self-published by Feminist Health Care Research Group, 2019.

Index

An 'n' after a page reference indicates the number of a note on that page.